STEROIDS AND NEURONAL ACTIVITY

The Ciba Foundation is an international scientific and educational charity. It was established in 1947 by the Swiss chemical and pharmaceutical company of CIBA Limited—now CIBA-GEIGY Limited. The Foundation operates independently in London under English trust law.

The Ciba Foundation exists to promote international cooperation in biological, medical and chemical research. It organizes about eight international multidisciplinary symposia each year on topics that seem ready for discussion by a small group of research workers. The papers and discussions are published in the Ciba Foundation symposium series. The Foundation also holds many shorter meetings (not published), organized by the Foundation itself or by outside scientific organizations. The staff always welcome suggestions for future meetings.

The Foundation's house at 41 Portland Place, London W1N 4BN, provides facilities for meetings of all kinds. Its Media Resource Service supplies information to journalists on all scientific and technological topics. The library, open five days a week to any graduate in science or medicine, also provides information on scientific meetings throughout the world and answers general enquiries on biomedical and chemical subjects. Scientists from any part of the world may stay in the house during working visits to London.

STEROIDS AND NEURONAL ACTIVITY

A Wiley-Interscience Publication

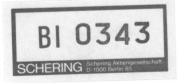

1990

JOHN WILEY & SONS

Chichester · New York · Brisbane · Toronto · Singapore

Published in 1990 by John Wiley & Sons Ltd.
Baffins Lane, Chichester
West Sussex PO19 1UD, England

Other Wiley Editorial Offices

John Wiley & Sons, Inc., 605 Third Avenue,
New York, NY 10158-0012, USA

Jacaranda Wiley Ltd, G.P.O. Box 859, Brisbane,
Queensland 4001, Australia

John Wiley & Sons (Canada) Ltd, 22 Worcester Road,
Rexdale, Ontario M9W 1L1, Canada

John Wiley & Sons (SEA) Pte Ltd, 37 Jalan Pemimpin 05-04,
Block B, Union Industrial Building, Singapore 2057

Suggested series entry for library catalogues:
Ciba Foundation Symposia

Ciba Foundation Symposium 153
x + 284 pages, 56 figures, 10 tables

Library of Congress Cataloging-in-Publication Data
Steroids and neuronal activity.
       p.   cm.—(Ciba Foundation symposium : 153)
    'Symposium on steroids and neuronal activity, held at the Ciba
Foundation, London, 23–25 January 1990'—Contents p.
    Editors: Derek Chadwick, organizer, and Kate Widdows.
    'A Wiley–Interscience publication.'
    Includes bibliographical references. Includes indexes.
    ISBN 0 471 92689 2
    1. Neuroendocrinology—Congresses.   2. Steroid hormones—
Physiological effect—Congresses.   3. Neurons—Congresses.
I. Chadwick, Derek.   II. Widdows, Kate.   III. Symposium on Steroids
and Neuronal Activity (1990: Ciba Foundation)   IV. Series.
[DNLM: 1. Brain—physiology—congresses.   2. Neuroendocrinology—
congresses.   3. Neurons—drug effects—congresses.   4. Neurons—
physiology—congresses.   5. Steroids—pharmacology—congresses.
W3 C161F v. 153 / WL 102.5 S839 1990]
QP356.S85   1990
612.8′14—dc20
DNLM/DLC
for Library of Congress   90-12763
                                                                                    CIP

British Library Cataloguing in Publication Data
Steroids and neuronal activity.
    1. Man. Nervous system. Effects of Steroids
    I. Ciba Foundation   II. Series
    612.8
    ISBN 0 471 92689 2

Phototypeset by Dobbie Typesetting Service, Tavistock, Devon.
Printed and bound in Great Britain by Biddles Ltd., Guildford.

Contents

Participants

T. Bäckström Department of Obstetrics & Gynaecology, Academic Hospital, S-751 85 Uppsala and Department of Obstetrics & Gynaecology, University Hospital, S-90185 Umeå, Sweden

E. E. Baulieu INSERM U 33, Département de Chimie Biologique, Faculté de Médecine de Bicêtre, Université de Paris Sud, 78 Avenue de General Leclerc, F-94275 Bicêtre Cedex, France

E. R. de Kloet Faculty of Medicine, Magnus Institute for Pharmacology, Vondellaan 6, 3521 GD Utrecht, The Netherlands

G. Deliconstantinos Department of Experimental Physiology, University of Athens Medical School, Goudi, GR-115 27 Athens, Greece

B. Dubrovsky Department of Psychiatry, Neurophysiology Laboratory, McGill University, 1033 Pine Avenue West, Montreal, Quebec, Canada H3A 1A1

S. Feldman Department of Neurology, Hadassah University Hospital, PO Box 12000, IL-91120 Jerusalem, Israel

K. W. Gee School of Pharmacy, University of Southern California, University Park, Los Angeles, CA 90089, USA

J. Glowinski GRP NB, INSERM U 114, Collège de France, 11 Place Marcelin Berthelot, F-75231 Paris Cedex 05, France

E. D. Hall CNS Diseases Research, 7251-209-4, The Upjohn Company, 301 Henrietta Street, Kalamazoo, MI 49001, USA

G. A. R. Johnston Department of Pharmacology, University of Sydney, Sydney, New South Wales 2006, Australia

D. Joubert-Bression INSERM U 223, Faculté de Médecine, Pitié-Salpêtrière, 105 Boulevard de l'Hôpital, F-75634 Paris Cedex 13, France

H. J. Karavolas   Department of Physiological Chemistry, University of Wisconsin, 587 Medical Sciences Building, 1300 University Avenue, Madison, WI 53706, USA

C. Kordon   Neuroendocrinology Unit, INSERM U 159, Centre Paul Broca, 2ter rue d'Alésia, F-75014 Paris, France

C. Kubli-Garfias   Instituto Mexicano del Seguro Social, Unidad Investigacion Biomedica, Apartado Postal 73032, Mexico City 03020 DF, Mexico

J. J. Lambert   Department of Pharmacology & Clinical Pharmacology, University of Dundee, Ninewells Hospital, PO Box 120, Dundee, DD1 9SY, UK

M. D. Majewska   Addiction Research Center, National Institute on Drug Abuse, Building C, PO Box 5180, Baltimore, MD 21224, USA

A. Makriyannis   Medicinal Chemistry U-92, University of Connecticut, Storrs, CT 06268, USA

L. Martini   Department of Endocrinology, University of Milan, Via G Balzaretti 9, I-20133 Milan, Italy

B. S. McEwen   Neuroendocrinology Laboratory, Rockefeller University, 1230 York Avenue, New York, NY 10021-6399, USA

R. W. Olsen   Department of Pharmacology, UCLA School of Medicine, Los Angeles, CA 90024, USA

M. Perusquia (*Ciba Foundation Bursar*)   Instituto Politecnico Nacional, Escuela Superior de Medicina, Seccion de Graduados, Prof Diaz Miron y Plan de San Luis, Mexico City 17 DF, Mexico

V. D. Ramirez   Department of Physiology & Biophysics, College of Liberal Arts & Sciences, University of Illinois, 524 Burrill Hall, 407 South Goodwin Avenue, Urbana, IL 61801, USA

M. A. Simmonds (*Chairman*)   Department of Pharmacology, School of Pharmacy, University of London, 29/39 Brunswick Square, London WC1N 1AX, UK

S. S. Smith   Department of Anatomy, Mail Stop 408, Hahnemann University, Broad & Vine, Philadelphia, PA 19102-1192, USA

T.-P. Su   Neurochemistry Unit, Neuropharmacology Laboratory, Addiction Research Center, National Institute on Drug Abuse, PO Box 5180, Baltimore, MD 21224, USA

A. J. Turner   Department of Biochemistry, Leeds University, Leeds LS2 9JT, UK

Introduction

Michael A. Simmonds

Department of Pharmacology, School of Pharmacy, University of London, 29/39 Brunswick Square, London WC1N 1AX, UK

We have brought together for this symposium scientists with diverse expertise, ranging through endocrinology, neurochemistry, electrophysiology and physical chemistry. About half of the participants would not claim to be endocrinologists but they have all worked with steroids because these substances have interesting effects in the neuronal systems they are studying. Some steroidal interactions with the nervous system are genomic but there is particular interest in the non-genomic effects that are elicited most potently by reduced metabolites of progestagens, androgens and corticosteroids.

The idea of holding this symposium originated from the discoveries that, in electrophysiological experiments on slice preparations of rat brain, the steroid anaesthetic alphaxalone potentiated both stimulus-evoked inhibition (Scholfield 1980) and the actions of the inhibitory amino acid γ-aminobutyric acid (GABA) at $GABA_A$ receptors (Harrison & Simmonds 1984). Subsequent work had shown that closely related steroids, some of which are produced endogenously, could also potentiate GABA and its analogue muscimol (Callachan et al 1987, Harrison et al 1987, Turner & Simmonds 1989). These observations raised the question of whether the long-known central depressant properties of cholesterol (Cashin & Moravek 1927) and a wide range of pregnane derivatives (Selye 1942, Atkinson et al 1965, Holzbauer 1976) might be attributed to potentiation of GABA.

This and other aspects of the non-genomic steroidal modulation of neurotransmitter systems will be explored during the symposium and attempts will be made to relate such effects to the actions of steroids on the functioning of the nervous system. The issues and problems that I hope we shall be able to address include the following:

1. To what extent have structure–activity relationships been determined for various non-genomic effects of steroids? Is there a common structure–activity relationship for some of the effects or are they all distinct? Where there is a clear relationship between structure and activity, what does it imply?

2. To what extent may perturbations of the lipid structure of cell membranes by steroids underlie some or all of their effects on receptor proteins and non-genomic effects in general?

3. Are there existing classes of drug that mimic or antagonize particular non-genomic effects of steroids by acting at a common site with the steroids?

4. Is there any evidence that modulation of specific transmitter/receptor systems by steroids may be physiologically relevant?

5. Can 'genomic' and 'non-genomic' effects of steroids be clearly distinguished? Do some steroids, perhaps together with their metabolic products, cause both types of effect to operate in concert or opposition?

If the formal presentations do not give answers to these questions, I hope that they will be addressed in the discussion periods.

References

Atkinson RM, Davis B, Pratt MA, Sharpe HM, Tomich EG 1965 Action of some steroids on the central nervous system of the mouse. II. Pharmacology. J Med Chem 8:426–432

Callachan H, Cottrell GA, Hather NY, Lambert JJ, Nooney JM, Peters JA 1987 Modulation of the GABA$_A$ receptor by progesterone metabolites. Proc R Soc Lond B Biol Sci 231:359–369

Cashin MF, Moravek V 1927 The physiological action of cholesterol. Am J Physiol 82:294–298

Harrison NL, Simmonds MA 1984 Modulation of the GABA receptor complex by a steroid anaesthetic. Brain Res 323:287–292

Harrison NL, Majewska MD, Harrington JW, Barker JL 1987 Structure–activity relationships for steroid interaction with the γ-aminobutyric acid$_A$ receptor complex. J Pharmacol Exp Ther 241:346–353

Holzbauer M 1976 Physiological aspects of steroids with anaesthetic properties. Med Biol 54:227–242

Scholfield CN 1980 Potentiation of inhibition by general anaesthetics in neurones of the olfactory cortex in vitro. Pflügers Arch Eur J Physiol 383:249–255

Selye H 1942 Correlations between chemical structure and the pharmacological actions of the steroids. Endocrinology 30:437–453

Turner JP, Simmonds MA 1989 Modulation of the GABA$_A$ receptor complex by steroids in slices of rat cuneate nucleus. Br J Pharmacol 96:409–417

Steroid effects on neuronal activity: when is the genome involved?

Bruce S. McEwen, Hector Coirini and Michael Schumacher

Laboratory of Neuroendocrinology, Rockefeller University, 1230 York Avenue, New York, NY 10021, USA

Abstract. For over four decades steroids have been regarded first as facilitators of enzymic reactions and subsequently as activators of genomic activity. The brain, long studied in terms of its bioelectric properties and anatomical connectivity, has now been recognized as a complex target tissue for genomic effects of steroid hormones, which bring about long-lasting alterations in brain structure and neurochemistry as well as changes in behaviour and neuroendocrine function. Studies of steroid effects on brain bioelectric activity have also shown rapid effects which are difficult to explain by a strictly genomic mechanism. One way to distinguish between genomic and non-genomic effects is by the time course, with extremely rapid effects being non-genomic and delayed effects being genomic. Effects with onset latencies of minutes to an hour may be due to either mechanism. Examples illustrating genomic actions include delayed effects of oestrogen which alter oxytocin and $GABA_A$ receptors and induce spines on dendrites and delayed glucocorticoid effects on neuronal survival. There are also examples of apparent genomic effects of oestradiol which interact with rapid and apparently non-genomic effects of progesterone: progesterone rapidly promotes spread of oestrogen-induced oxytocin receptors in ventromedial hypothalamus and rapidly modifies oestrogen-regulated $GABA_A$ receptor density in hypothalamus. The former effect is one produced by progesterone itself whereas the latter effect may be related to the ability of progesterone metabolites to interact with the chloride channel of the $GABA_A$–benzodiazepine receptor complex.

1990 Steroids and neuronal activity. Wiley, Chichester (Ciba Foundation Symposium 153) p 3–21

Since the purpose of this Ciba Foundation Symposium is to examine the membrane actions of steroids, it is essential at the outset to put into perspective the various cellular mechanisms of action of steroid hormones that have been considered over the last four decades. However, because the focus of this symposium is upon the neural actions of steroids, we shall pay particular attention to the relationship between excitable membranes and the genome. The thesis of this paper is twofold: first, that steroids can act on the genome to affect neuronal activity via changes in neurochemistry and morphology; and, second,

3

that genomic and membrane actions are undoubtedly interdependent and interactive with each other. This dualistic but interactive view of steroid action is schematically represented in Fig. 1.

Historical perspective

We now recognize that intracellular receptors for steroid and thyroid hormones are members of a family of DNA-binding proteins, so-called *trans*-acting factors, which enhance gene expression by binding to specific DNA sequences that are usually located up-stream of the promotor region of regulated genes (Evans 1988). This realization is the culmination of 30 years of investigation which began at a time when steroid hormones were thought to act as cofactors in enzymic reactions and/or as allosteric modulators (Williams-Ashman 1965). During the past 30 years, investigations of steroid actions on the nervous system have focused on identifying and mapping the intracellular receptors (McEwen et al 1979) that had been first identified and studied elsewhere in the body. However, one could never lose sight of the fact that steroids have rapid effects on neuronal electrical activity which cannot be explained by a genomic activation (Kelly et al 1977). We also know that some genomic effects of steroids can be very rapid,

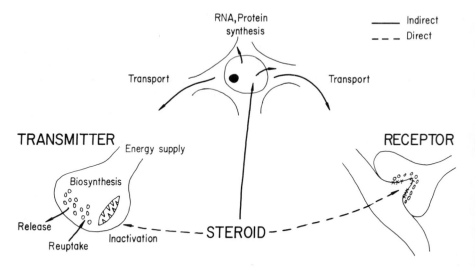

FIG. 1.   Genomic and non-genomic effects of steroid hormones on pre- and postsynaptic events. Non-genomic (direct) effects (dashed line) may involve the action of hormones on the pre- or postsynaptic membrane to alter the permeability of neurotransmitters or their precursors and/or the functioning of neurotransmitter receptors. Genomic (indirect) action of the steroid (unbroken line) leads to altered synthesis of proteins, which, after axonal or dendritic transport, may participate in pre- or postsynaptic events. (Reproduced from McEwen et al 1978 by permission of Raven Press.)

but still taking not less than 10 or 20 minutes (Mosher et al 1971). A time scale such as is shown in Fig. 2 serves to distinguish the most rapid, non-genomic effects from the slower, genomically mediated ones, with an intermediate zone of ambiguity in the range of minutes to an hour. One should bear in mind the caveat that steroids acting at the membrane to activate or modulate second messenger systems such as cyclic AMP generation (Finidori-Lepicard et al 1981) may exert delayed and prolonged effects on gene expression via those second messengers.

In one way the pursuit of genomic mechanisms in the case of the nervous system has been counter-intuitive, because the nervous system works by electrical signals transmitted by chemical neurotransmitters within a short time frame. However, the brain has gradually become recognized as a living, changing organ in which the synaptic structure and neurochemical apparatus are subject to continual modification and reshaping over long time periods (Fig. 2). Let us now examine some of these events and consider their possible relationship to the membrane actions of steroids, which will be the major focus of this volume.

Steroid hormone actions on neuronal morphology which appear to be genomically mediated

Changes in neuronal, especially synaptic, structure and number can have a profound effect on the operation of neural circuits that incorporate the changing structures. Receptors of the steroid/thyroid hormone gene family mediate effects on the nervous system that have been divided into two broad categories: organizational effects, which refer to developmental effects that are largely permanent; and activational effects, which refer to effects that can occur at

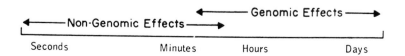

Non-Genomic Effects
    RAPID IN ONSET - Seconds, Minutes
    SHORT IN DURATION - following disappearance of steroid from tissue

Genomic Effects
    SLOWER IN ONSET - Minutes, Hours
    LONGER IN DURATION - persist after steroid disappears from tissue

FIG. 2.   Time scale of genomic and non-genomic effects of steroids. (Reproduced from McEwen et al 1978 by permission of Raven Press.)

any time during the lifespan and are largely reversible. Previously, organizational effects were thought to be largely structural, whereas activational effects were regarded as not at all structural but rather neurochemical and metabolic. These distinctions are breaking down somewhat (Arnold & Breedlove 1985), in the sense that reversible morphological changes do occur in conjunction with activational effects. For example, the number of dendritic spines increased and decreased during the oestrous cycle in the female rat in both the ventromedial nuclei (VMN) and the apical dendrites of CA1 neurons in the hippocampus (Frankfurt et al 1990, Gould et al 1990a). Ovariectomy caused spine density to decrease, whereas oestrogen replacement enhanced spine formation in both structures (Frankfurt et al 1990, Gould et al 1990a). These effects of oestradiol may be contrasted with those of increased levels of the thyroid hormone, triiodothyronine (T3), which permanently enhanced dendritic branching and spine density in CA3 hippocampal neurons during neonatal development in the rat but did not produce the same effect when given during adult life (Gould et al 1990b,c). A change in the number of dendritic spines may mean several things: first, it may indicate changes in synapse formation, and indeed there is evidence that oestradiol induces an increase in synaptic density in the VMN (Carrer & Aoki 1982) together with the increased spine density (Frankfurt et al 1990); second, the appearance of new spines may indicate a change of existing synapses to a new postsynaptic configuration with different electrical properties from those of synapses on dendritic shafts (Harris & Stevens 1989). Further research is necessary to elucidate these possibilities.

Another aspect of neuronal morphology which is susceptible to the actions of steroid hormones is seen in the hippocampal formation in relation to glucocorticoids. The absence of glucocorticoids after adrenalectomy caused granule cell neurons of the dentate gyrus to become smaller and less branched (Gould et al 1990d). In addition, there was increased neuronal death (Gould et al 1990d). Glucocorticoid replacement restored neuronal size and shape and prevented neuronal death (Gould et al 1990d). We are now exploring the significance of these changes in relation to the variation in circulating glucocorticoids which accompanies the diurnal rhythm and the response to stress.

In contrast to the dentate gyrus, which is positively dependent on glucocorticoids, excess glucocorticoids caused CA3 neurons in the hippocampus to become less branched (Gould et al 1990d). When this treatment was prolonged for 12 weeks, large CA3 neurons disappeared and presumably died (Sapolsky et al 1986). This mimicked an effect seen in the ageing hippocampus (Sapolsky et al 1986). Moreover, glucocorticoids potentiated neuronal death resulting from hypoxia or the actions of exogenous excitotoxins (Sapolsky et al 1986). Neither the trophic nor the neuronal loss-promoting effects of glucocorticoids have been studied in enough detail to reveal the cellular or molecular mechanisms. However, preliminary evidence would suggest that intracellular adrenal steroid receptors, which are found in large numbers in hippocampus (McEwen et al

1990), are involved. Nevertheless, the specific relationship of these receptors to genomic and non-genomic processes remains to be elucidated.

Examples of interacting genomic and non-genomic effects

Activational effects of steroids also include changes in neurochemistry, and some of these effects illustrate the duality of steroid actions shown in Fig. 1. Two further examples from our own work will serve to illustrate this point.

The first example deals with the neuropeptide, oxytocin, which is associated with reproduction, lactation and maternal behaviour. Oestrogen treatment induced oxytocin receptors in the female reproductive tract and also in the VMN (Johnson et al 1989). This induction took at least 24 hours and involved a 4–5-fold increase in receptor density in VMN (Johnson et al 1989). Because it is delayed and prolonged and occurs in the part of the VMN which contains intracellular oestrogen receptors, where oestrogen also induces large increases in genomic activity and protein synthesis (McEwen et al 1987), oxytocin receptor induction in the VMN is most probably a genomic event. On the other hand, progesterone, the second of the important female reproductive steroid hormones, produced a further and very rapid modification of the oxytocin receptors induced by oestradiol (Schumacher et al 1989a). As shown in Fig. 3, this modification involved a spread of the oxytocin receptor field into an area lateral and dorsal to the VMN. The spread occurred within 30 minutes and was produced *in vitro* by progesterone applied to unfixed brain sections (Schumacher et al 1990). We do not know if the spread of oxytocin receptors represents a movement of receptors along dendrites or the activation of receptors already there. What is becoming evident, however, is that this activation or movement is a correlate of the ability of oxytocin to elicit female reproductive behaviour; that is, low amounts of oxytocin will only activate reproductive behaviour when infused into the VMN if progesterone is given after oestrogen priming (Schumacher et al 1989a). It therefore appears that the combination of a genomic effect of oestradiol and a non-genomic effect of progesterone, which requires the prior oestrogen priming, produces the changes in oxytocin receptor level and location that are needed for reproductive behaviour to occur.

The second example of possibly interacting genomic and membrane effects of steroids concerns the $GABA_A$ receptor system. In the VMN, arcuate nucleus and midbrain central grey, oestrogen priming induced a decrease in $GABA_A$ receptor binding (Schumacher et al 1989b), as is shown in Fig. 4 (left). In contrast, in the CA1 subfield of the hippocampus, oestrogen priming induced an increase in $GABA_A$ receptor binding (Schumacher et al 1989b), as is shown in Fig. 4 (right). None of these effects was produced by *in vitro* exposure to oestradiol. Progesterone administration *in vivo* had no effects on $GABA_A$ receptor binding in the areas of the brain where oestradiol effects were found, unless the rats had been primed with oestrogen. Then, progesterone reversed

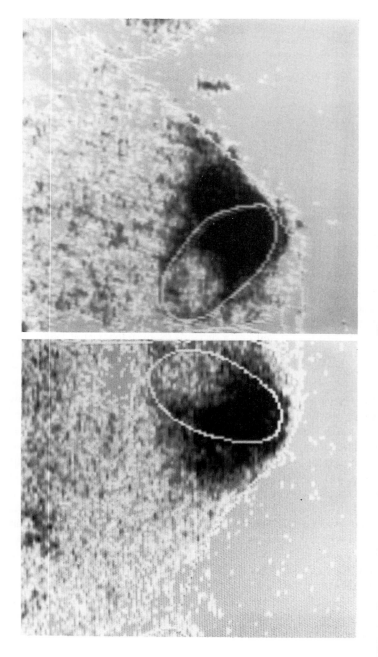

FIG. 3.   Representative autoradiograms showing the binding of ^{125}I-labelled ornithine vasotocin analogue ([d(CH$_2$)$_5$], Tyr (Me)^2, Thr^4, Tyr-NH$_2$^{9}]-ornithine vasotocin) to oxytocin receptors in the ventromedial hypothalamus. Female rats were ovariectomized and adrenalectomized and were injected with oestradiol benzoate ($2 \times 10\,\mu g$) (left) or successively with oestradiol benzoate and progesterone (0.5 mg) (right). The ventromedial nuclei of the hypothalamus (VMN) have been drawn on each side of the third ventricle by apposing stained sections to the autoradiograms. The results show that progesterone causes the oestrogen-induced oxytocin receptors to spread laterally.

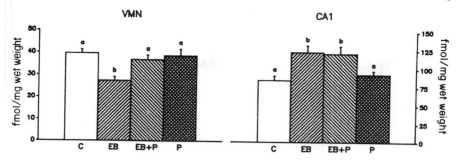

FIG. 4. High affinity GABA$_A$ receptor binding in the ventromedial nuclei of the hypothalamus (VMN) (*left*) and the CA1 region of the dorsal hippocampus (*right*). Female rats were ovariectomized and adrenalectomized and were injected with vehicle (C), with oestradiol benzoate (EB, $2 \times 10\mu g$), progesterone (P, 0.5 mg) or successively with EB and P (EB + P). The binding of [^{3}H] muscimol was quantified by the method of *in vitro* receptor autoradiography. Letters (a,b) above columns denote statistical differences within each area at least at the $P < 0.05$ level by Duncan multiple range tests. (Modified from Schumacher et al 1989a,b.)

the effects of oestradiol in the VMN and midbrain central grey, but not in the arcuate nucleus or hippocampal CA1, and it did so rapidly, within four hours (Schumacher et al 1989b,c). This is shown in Fig. 4. The direction of these progesterone effects (namely, to increase GABA$_A$ receptor binding) is consistent with either an *in vivo* genomic action or an *in vitro* effect produced by progesterone itself or by a metabolite such as 5α-pregnan-3α-ol-20-one (3α-OH-dihydroprogesterone, 3α-OH-DHP). The generation of such metabolites from progesterone by enzymes present in neural tissue is well documented (see Karavolas & Hodges 1990). The direct membrane actions of steroids like 3α-OH-DHP enhance binding of ligands to both the benzodiazepine and GABA$_A$ sites (Harrison et al 1987). If this mechanism is involved in the *in vivo* effects of progesterone already described, what is particularly surprising is the selectivity of the action of progesterone on the oestrogen sensitive structures, as noted above. This might be explained by the heterogeneity of GABA$_A$ receptor subtypes, expression of which might be differentially regulated by oestrogens and result in receptor complexes that are differentially sensitive to the effects of steroids (for review see Schumacher & McEwen 1989). Such speculations must, however, be replaced by experimental data.

In contrast to the specific effects of progesterone metabolites on the GABA$_A$–benzodiazepine–chloride channel complex (Gee et al 1988), progesterone itself appears to be more effective in producing the spread of oxytocin receptors (Schumacher et al 1990). Moreover, progesterone is also effective, even when conjugated to bovine serum albumin, in modulating the release of luteinizing hormone releasing hormone (LHRH) and dopamine from neural tissue (Ramirez et al 1990). Thus, both progesterone and its metabolites

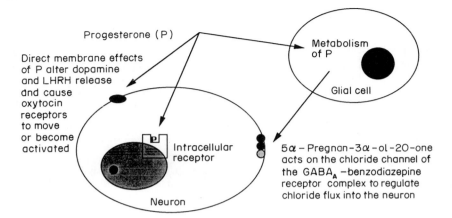

FIG. 5. Schematic diagram of various ways in which progesterone (P) affects neuronal properties, as discussed in this article.

exert membrane effects in neural tissue which complement the genomic actions of progesterone that are mediated by intracellular receptors (Fig. 5).

Conclusions

Steroid hormones have many and diverse effects on neural structure, neurochemistry and activity which cannot be explained by a single mechanism involving only the genome or only effects on excitable cell membranes. In fact, both types of actions are undoubtedly involved. We have illustrated the interaction between these two modes of action wth several examples from our laboratory, but other illustrations could be given. For example, the iontophoretic application of oestradiol-17β hemisuccinate to preoptic-septal neurons in the female rat results in single unit electrical responses which vary from excitation to inhibition during various stages of the oestrous cycle (Kelly et al 1977). It would appear likely that some type of priming via the genomic mechanism may alter the sensitivity of the membrane response mechanisms for the same steroid. Other examples will undoubtedly be presented in the course of the symposium.

One of the lessons to be learned from the multitude of effects of steroids on brain cells is that these molecules do too many things to be easily adapted as therapeutic agents. This knowledge has led in at least one instance to attempts to create molecules with only one of the multiple effects of a particular steroid hormone. The development of a non-glucocorticoid steroid analogue of methylprednisolone which shows protective effects against lipid peroxidation-induced membrane damage is one example of this strategy (Hall et al 1987). Future developments of this type offer considerable hope for new classes of therapeutic agents.

Acknowledgements

Research on this topic in the authors' laboratory is supported by USPHS grants NS07080 and MH41256. H.C. and M.S. are both Fogarty Fellows of the National Institutes of Health. H.C. was also supported by CONICET (Argentina) and M.S. by fellowships from NATO and EMBO.

References

Arnold A, Breedlove S 1985 Organizational and activational effects of sex steroids on brain and behavior: a reanalysis. Horm Behav 19:469–498

Carrer H, Aoki A 1982 Ultrastructural changes in the hypothalamic ventromedial nucleus of ovariectomized rats after estrogen treatment. Brain Res 240:221–223

Evans R 1988 The steroid and thyroid hormone receptor superfamily. Science (Wash DC) 240:889–895

Finidori-Lepicard J, Schorderet-Slatkine S, Hanoune J, Baulieu E 1981 Progesterone inhibits membrane bound adenylate cyclase in *Xenopus laevis* oocytes. Nature (Lond) 292:255–257

Frankfurt M, Gould E, Woolley C, McEwen BS 1990 Gonadal steroids modify dendritic spine density in ventromedial hypothalamic neurons: a golgi study in the adult rat. Neuroendocrinology, in press

Gee K, Bolger M, Brinton R, Coirini H, McEwen BS 1988 Steroid modulation of the chloride ionophore in rat brain: structure–activity requirements, regional dependence and mechanism of action. J Pharmacol Exp Ther 246:803–812

Gould E, Woolley C, Frankfurt M, McEwen BS 1990a Gonadal steroids regulate dendritic spine density in hippocampal pyramidal cells in adulthood. J Neurosci 10:1286–1291

Gould E, Westlind-Danielsson A, Frankfurt M, McEwen BS 1990b Sex differences and thyroid hormone sensitivity of hippocampal pyramidal cells. J. Neurosci 10:996–1003

Gould E, Woolley C, McEwen BS 1990c The hippocampal formation: morphological changes induced by thyroid, gonadal and adrenal hormones. Psychoneuroendocrinology, in press

Gould E, Woolley C, McEwen BS 1990d Short term glucocorticoid manipulations affect neuronal morphology and survival in the adult hippocampal formation. Neuroscience, in press

Hall ED, McCall JM, Chase RL, Yonkers PA, Braughler JM 1987 A nonglucocorticoid steroid analog of methylprednisolone duplicates its high-dose pharmacology in models of central nervous system trauma and neuronal membrane damage. J Pharmacol Exp Ther 242:137–142

Harris KM, Stevens JK 1989 Dendritic spines of CA1 pyramidal cells in the rat hippocampus: serial electron microscopy with reference to their biophysical characteristics. J Neurosci 9:2982–2997

Harrison NL, Majewska MD, Harrington JW, Barker JL 1987 Structure–activity relationships for steroid interaction with the γ-aminobutyric acid$_A$ receptor complex. J Pharmacol Exp Ther 241:346–353

Johnson A, Coirini H, Ball G, McEwen BS 1989 Anatomical localization of the effects of 17β-estradiol on oxytocin receptor binding in the ventromedial hypothalamic nucleus. Endocrinology 124:207–211

Karavolas HJ, Hodges DR 1990 Neuroendocrine metabolism of progesterone and related progestins. In: Steroids and neuronal activity. Wiley, Chichester (Ciba Found Symp 153) p 22–55

Kelly M, Moss R, Dudley C 1977 The effects of microelectrophoretically applied estrogen, cortisol and acetylcholine on medial preoptic-septal unit activity throughout the estrous cycle of the female rat. Exp Brain Res 30:53–64

McEwen BS, Krey L, Luine V 1978 Steroid hormone action in the neuroendocrine system: when is the genome involved? In: Reichlin R et al (eds) The hypothalamus. Raven Press, New York, p 255–268

McEwen BS, Davis P, Parsons B, Pfaff D 1979 The brain as target for steroid hormone action. Annu Rev Neurosci 2:65–112

McEwen BS, Jones K, Pfaff D 1987 Hormonal control of sexual behaviour in the female rat: molecular, cellular and neurochemical studies. Biol Reprod 36:37–45

McEwen BS, Brinton R, Chao H et al 1990 The hippocampus: a site for modulatory interactions between steroid hormones, neurotransmitters and neuropeptides. In: Muller E et al (eds) Neuroendocrine perspectives. Springer-Verlag, New York, in press

Mosher K, Young D, Munck A 1971 Evidence for irreversible, actinomycin D-sensitive, and temperature-sensitive steps following the binding of cortisol to glucocorticoid receptors and preceding effects on glucose metabolism in rat thymus cells. J Biol Chem 246:654–659

Ramirez VD, Dluzen DE, Ke FC 1990 Actions of progesterone metabolites on neuronal membranes. In: Steroids and neuronal activity. Wiley, Chichester (Ciba Found Symp 153) p 125–144

Sapolsky R, Krey L, McEwen BS 1986 The neuroendocrinology of stress and aging: the glucocorticoid cascade hypothesis. Endocr Rev 7:284–301

Schumacher M, McEwen BS 1989 Steroid and barbiturate modulation of the $GABA_A$ receptor: possible mechanisms. Mol Neurobiol 3:275–304

Schumacher M, Coirini H, Frankfurt M, McEwen BS 1989a Localized actions of progesterone in hypothalamus involve oxytocin. Proc Natl Acad Sci USA 86:6798–6801

Schumacher M, Coirini H McEwen BS 1989b Regulation of high-affinity $GABA_A$ receptors in the dorsal hippocampus by estradiol and progesterone. Brain Res 487:178–183

Schumacher M, Coirini H, McEwen BS 1989c Regulation of high-affinity $GABA_A$ receptors in specific brain regions by ovarian hormones. Neuroendocrinology 50:315–320

Schumacher M, Coirini H, Pfaff DW, McEwen BS 1990 Behavioural effects of progesterone associated with rapid modulation of oxytocin receptors. Science (Wash DC), in press

Williams-Ashman H 1965 New facets of the biochemistry of steroid hormone action. Cancer Res 25:1096–1120

DISCUSSION

Baulieu: I would like to comment first of all on the general problem of genomic versus non-genomic effects of steroids in terms of what we know in a system other than the CNS. Steroid hormones essentially work through intracellular mechanisms, via nuclear receptors which operate at the gene level, as described by Bruce McEwen. However, non-genomic mechanisms are also very important to consider for the entire field of steroid action. (Incidentally, I am unaware of any informational ligands that are thought to work at both levels in the same cell, namely the genomic level and the membrane level.)

We worked formerly in the *Xenopus laevis* oocyte system, where we showed that a steroid hormone (progesterone) can act at the cell membrane level, promoting the reinitiation of meiosis (Baulieu & Schorderet-Slatkine 1983). I was interested by the fact that there was no way of demonstrating an intracellular progesterone receptor in that oocyte system, but that we could initiate the resumption of meiosis with a 'macromolecular steroid' (a progesterone analogue chemically linked to polyethylene oxide) which could not enter the cell (Godeau et al 1978). We did show that progesterone could decrease adenylate cyclase activity in an oocyte membrane preparation (Finidori-Lepicard et al 1981), reproducing our observations in the intact oocyte. This result is still unexplained mechanistically, because this inhibitory action of the steroid on adenylate cyclase activity is not inhibited by pertussis toxin, unlike what is observed on G protein-associated receptors.

Steroid specificity similar to that observed for the activity of progesterone in the brain, to which Dr McEwen referred (Kelly et al 1977), was not observed in the oocyte membrane system, where testosterone or deoxycorticosterone worked as well as progesterone, although oestrogens did not. We concluded at that time that there was different steroid specificity for binding to a putative membrane receptor and to the intracellular progesterone receptor which is found in conventional target organs in all species. This was one criterion for saying that we have a signalling system at the surface level distinct from the intracellular system.

This leads to the question to which Dr Simmonds referred in his Introduction, of whether we have a steroid receptor molecule in the cell membrane. Is it a receptor protein, or are we just observing an effect on the lipid component of the membrane which may, in turn, change adenylate cyclase activity? The problem is a difficult one because steroids are lipids and cell membranes are also mainly lipid. When a membrane is exposed to lipidic ligands, there is a problem in terms of the ordinary methods used in binding studies. It took some time to characterize a binding activity in the oocyte membrane which was associated with a 30 000 M_r protein that could be affinity labelled (Blondeau & Baulieu 1984). This receptor system is, in molecular and also functional terms, totally different from the intracellular receptor for progesterone (Evans 1988, Savouret et al 1989).

In the brain (Baulieu 1981), are we dealing with proteins at the membrane level which are similar or identical to nuclear receptors, or are there different kinds of receptor proteins specifying activities at the nuclear and membrane levels, respectively?

Simmonds: The membrane protein that you describe is not involved in the internalization of the steroid, as far as you know?

Baulieu: We have no evidence for protein-mediated internalization of the steroid in the oocyte system. We only have evidence for a mechanism which involves adenylate cyclase, and also for the involvement of receptors for IGF (insulin-like growth factor) and insulin (El Etr et al 1979, Wallace et al 1980). The two receptors do cooperate.

Kordon: We have previously described a membrane effect of oestrogens on the hypothalamus. We think it is a direct one, because it works in rat brain slices as well as in synaptosomes (Drouva et al 1984, 1985). It concerns a selective capacity of 17β-oestradiol to enhance depolarization-induced release of GnRH from the hypothalamus. There are several indications that this is a non-genomic effect. It works in the absence of cell nuclei; it takes about one minute after addition of the steroid to develop *in vitro*. It is probably specific, since it is highly peptide selective; other hypothalamic neuropeptides, such as somatostatin or GHRH, are not affected. The pharmacology of this membrane effect looks rather like that of nuclear receptors; progesterone (in the absence of oestrogens), testosterone and 17α-oestradiol are inactive and oestrogen antagonists block the effect.

The paradox here is that the effect is fast (about 1 min), but it is not terminated very readily. You can even treat the rat with oestrogen before sampling the brain slices and still see the oestrogen effect on GnRH release, which persists for two hours in the perfusion system. So there seems to be no symmetry between the onset and the termination of the effect.

Although that membrane effect on GnRH release was not completely characterized from a pharmacological point of view, we can say that the pharmacology is quite similar to that of nuclear oestrogen receptors. Could you comment on the possibility that a molecule sharing large homologies with the nuclear receptor, at least in the recognition domain, could be combined by alternative splicing with sequences providing membrane attachment domains? Such a receptor could thus become inserted into plasma membranes, but still share pharmacological properties with the nuclear oestrogen receptor.

McEwen: This emphasizes an important point about the time considerations, that the onset may be rapid with a membrane effect of a steroid but if a second messenger system or some secondary or tertiary consequence is involved, the response to a steroid may not 'turn off' as rapidly as the steroid disappears from the tissue.

Baulieu: It seems plausible that the membrane receptor could be composed of a ligand-binding domain and a 'response domain'; the size we have measured for the receptor in the oocyte, namely M_r of about 30 000, makes this possible (Blondeau & Baulieu 1984). However, from specificity studies, the oocyte receptor does not look similar to the ligand-binding domain (C-terminal) of intracellular receptors (Evans 1988), as would be expected to explain some of Dr Kordon's results.

In fact, as far as I know, the $GABA_A$ receptor is the only brain membrane receptor that has as yet been described in terms of reactivity to certain steroids. This receptor is completely different from the classical intracellular steroid receptors, but is also different from the receptor for steroids found in *Xenopus laevis* oocytes.

Karavolas: Many have seen lag periods in the induction of certain progesterone effects, but when particular metabolites are used instead of the parent compound, shorter induction times are observed. Bruce McEwen is correct to identify a time between minutes and hours where the mechanism may be either genomic or non-genomic. During this interval a number of metabolic changes and steroid conversions can occur. In a sense, the steroid is not available to exert its effect when it is attached to the metabolizing enzyme; then, when the metabolic product is released, it produces its biological effect. This processing of the steroid hormone can occur in this period when the mechanism can be either genomic or non-genomic. Additionally, much like many growth factors, there can be a self-priming effect by the hormone whereby it generates some enabling protein, which has a permissive effect, and then the hormone can act very quickly. So the effect takes minutes, but you may be seeing a slightly delayed non-genomic effect. We therefore need to be careful when we distinguish genomic and non-genomic effects just by the time they take.

On another point of timeliness, I would add that Hans Selye back in 1942 provided many of the observations on steroid structures and anaesthetic effects that we shall be discussing with more specificity in this meeting.

Baulieu: Bruce McEwen said that there is a problem with describing a brief action of a steroid as a non-genomic action. There is no reason to believe that there is not a desensitization mechanism for the membrane effects of steroids. It may be recalled that at the same time as insulin receptor down-regulation was observed, independently we showed down-regulation of the intracellular progesterone receptor (Milgrom et al 1973), which becomes evident in a few hours and is possibly due to negative feedback activity on receptor synthesis.

Karavolas: On another point, I wonder if Dr Simmonds can tell us whether the effects of phenobarbitone on the $GABA_A$ receptor have been observed in ovariectomized and adrenalectomized animal models? The absence of endogenous steroids in such animals would remove lower threshold operating effects of some of these steroids.

Simmonds: I am not aware of anyone having done that experiment. The nearest we can get to it is in culture, where the cultured neuron has been deprived of the normal exposure to steroidal hormones. The barbiturates still work perfectly well as GABA potentiators in cultured neurons, so I can't see that there is any major steroid dependence there, although that's not to say that there may not be some influence of changing levels of steroids on responses to barbiturates. Indeed, as Jeremy Lambert will no doubt show us (see Lambert et al 1990), 5β-pregnan-3α-ol-20-one can increase the potency of phenobarbitone as a potentiator of GABA on both chromaffin cells and spinal cord neurons in culture.

Feldman: We showed in adrenalectomized cats a greater sensitivity of the reticular formation and the hypothalamus, electrophysiologically, to barbiturates than in intact animals (Feldman 1962). The cats were supported with low levels of steroids after the operation and we studied evoked potentials in these brain areas. Our experiments showed that the multisynaptic system in the reticular formation and hypothalamus is much more sensitive to pentobarbitone anaesthesia than the medial lemniscus in the adrenalectomized cats. We therefore used this system and showed a suppression of evoked potentials in the hypothalamus and the reticular formation with much smaller amounts of barbiturates than in control animals.

We also showed that what is called the long-latency, 'secondary response' can be recorded in the cortex and the hypothalamus under high levels of pentobarbitone anaesthesia. This response appeared in the hypothalamus, after sciatic nerve stimulation, with much smaller amounts of this agent in adrenalectomized cats than in controls. We also found delayed synaptic transmission using recovery cycles in these adrenalectomized animals. We concluded that a synaptic disturbance in the adrenalectomized cats was probably responsible for the greater sensitivity to barbiturates.

de Kloet: As Bruce McEwen has pointed out, the various signalling pathways activated by the hormone can be distinguished on the basis of onset and duration of the hormone action. On the basis of this time factor one can, therefore, design the appropriate experiments for demonstrating either a direct membrane effect or a genomic effect of the steroid. An experimental design that we both like involves removing an endocrine gland and then giving the particular hormone either *in vivo*, or *in vitro* to tissue slices. If one waits until the hormone is eliminated from the circulation, and after a couple of hours the effects appear, this is suggestive evidence for a genomic effect. This is, for instance, what we saw when we examined *in vitro* adrenal steroid effects on hippocampal neurons of adrenalectomized rats. We exposed the tissue to glucocorticoid for 20 min, then washed away the steroid and waited 60 min. At that time neuronal excitability was suppressed in response to the glucocorticoid (Joëls & de Kloet 1989). The question I would like to raise is whether one can extrapolate from the effects observed after acute administration of the steroids to the physiological role these hormones have during the slow changes in circulating level in the oestrous cycle.

McEwen: With the oestrous cycle you are looking over a period of several days and are seeing events that are mimicked by a schedule of hormone injections that also extends over days, in the case of oestrogens. Given that we are talking about apparently major structural changes in the cell (the formation of new dendritic spines and new synapses), I think it likely that a genomic mechanism is operating. When you consider the additional effects of progesterone, which in the hippocampus within four hours further enhanced the number of spines, or if you are considering the rather rapid disappearance of the spines over pro-oestrus and oestrus, again it is still in the order of hours, and I suspect genomic mechanisms are operating. But I wouldn't rule out, in the case of the rapid effects of progesterone, some local actions on the membrane to a system that has already been revved up, where the materials for new spines are at hand and the effects of progesterone are helping to put them in their place. As far as your general comment goes, I think that further detailed studies of time course in the oestrous cycle, and after exogenous treatment with oestradiol and progesterone, will clarify the relationship between the natural cycle and the hormone replacement.

Kubli-Garfias: Some steroid hormones have both genomic and non-genomic effects. Szego (1971) showed that the effect of oestrogens on the uterus is characterized initially by histamine release a few seconds after the addition of 17β-oestradiol. On the other hand, this steroid also has a remarkable effect on the genome, whereby it induces protein synthesis (among other effects) in the endometrium. It is clear that oestrogens have a short latency, with almost immediate action via non-genomic effects, whereas the genomic ones take place later with a long latency. Progesterone and some adrenocortical steroids also have both kinds of effects, genomic and non-genomic. Moreover, most of these compounds induce brain electrical changes a few seconds after their administration.

Besides the latencies, it is important to consider the chemical structure of the steroids. For instance, 17β-oestradiol, with the aromatized A ring, seems to persist in its biological action more than the Δ^4 compounds or C-5-reduced forms. Thus, oestrogens in many cases have a more lasting action than progesterone. Likewise, C-5-reduced progestins and androgens are to some extent less persistent than progesterone or testosterone. In fact, C-5-reduced compounds have a very short latency and also a short half-life in both *in vitro* and *in vivo* conditions.

Therefore, if we know the compound's chemical structure, the latency, what kind of biological action it has, its half-life and the nature of the target organ, we can deduce what kind of phenomena we are observing—genomic or non-genomic. As examples we have oestrogens, progesterone and testosterone with both kind of effects, whereas the C-5-reduced steroids, which are more vulnerable to chemical inactivation *in vivo*, show only non-genomic effects.

Feldman: I would like to describe some of our results on the non-genomic and genomic effects of glucocorticoids in the hypothalamus of adult male rats of the Hebrew University strain. We have recorded electrophysiological responses, to iontophoretically applied neurotransmitters and glucocorticoids, from neurosecretory cells in the paraventricular nucleus (PVN), which project to the median eminence. Glutamate increases the rate of firing. Hydrocortisone and corticosterone have a profound inhibitory effect on the spontaneous electrical activity. The spontaneous electrical activity of the majority of these neurosecretory cells in the dorsal medial area of the PVN, which is the main site of the corticotropin-releasing factor (CRF)-containing cells, is inhibited by these steroids. This inhibition may represent an electrophysiological correlate of the negative feedback exerted by glucocorticoids at the level of the cell membrane; the inhibition occurs within seconds, so it involves a non-genomic mechanism (Saphier & Feldman 1988).

A variety of neural stimuli, such as acoustic, photic and sciatic nerve stimulation, cause an increase in ACTH and corticosterone secretion by way of a mechanism which is mediated by CRF-41 (Weidenfeld et al 1989). We examined the effect of sciatic nerve stimulation on single paraventricular neurons, antidromically identified as projecting to the median eminence, in the area of the CRF-producing cells. Electrical stimulation of the sciatic nerve increases the rate of firing of such PVN neurons. After iontophoretic application of hydrocortisone there is a depression of the spontaneous activity of the neurons and a significant depression of the activity evoked by sciatic nerve stimulation (Fig. 1). The iontophoretic application of hydrocortisone to the membrane of such PVN cells, which have glucocorticoid receptors, most probably inhibits the response of CRF-secreting cells to sensory stimuli (D. Saphier & S. Feldman, unpublished work).

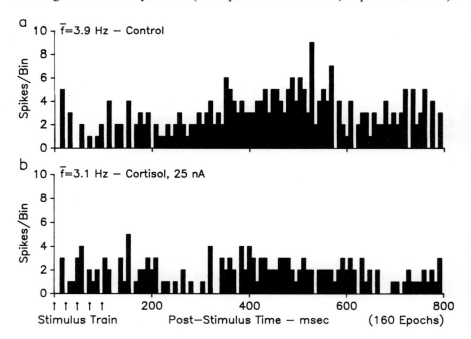

FIG. 1 (*Feldman*). Post-stimulus histogram showing the response of a single para-ventricular nucleus neuron identified as projecting to the rat median eminence, following a train of sciatic nerve stimulation (arrows). (a) Control trace, with the cell showing an increase in firing in response to the stimulation; (b) during iontophoretic application of hydrocortisone (25 nA), when an overall decrease in spontaneous activity was recorded and there is no response to sciatic nerve stimulation.

Similar results are seen in freely moving rats with electrodes implanted in the paraventricular nucleus. Intraperitoneal injection of 0.5 mg of corticosterone, which gives a plasma concentration of about 20 µg/100 ml, inhibits the increase in electrical activity induced by acoustic stimulation. This effect is seen after about 30 minutes, so it might be a non-genomic or a genomic effect (Mor et al 1986).

We have implanted cholesterol, corticosterone and dexamethasone in the area above the paraventricular nucleus and looked at the effect on responses to photic and acoustic stimulation. Four hours after implantation of cholesterol, photic stimulation resulted in a significant increase in plasma corticosterone levels. However, in rats with corticosterone or dexamethasone PVN implants, this response was greatly inhibited, and even more so after 24 hours (Fig. 2). This inhibitory effect is partially mediated by CRF, because six days after implantation of corticosterone there is a significant depletion of CRF in the median eminence.

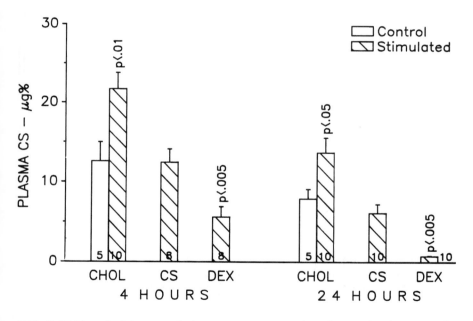

FIG. 2 (*Feldman*). Adrenocortical responses, expressed as changes in plasma corticosterone (CS) levels (mean ±SEM), after photic stimulation, in rats in which cholesterol (CHOL), corticosterone (CS) or dexamethasone (DEX) had been implanted above the paraventricular nucleus four or 24 hours before stimulation. Control animals were subjected to the same surgical procedure and a cholesterol implant but were not exposed to the photic stimulation. The number at the base of each column represents the number of experimental animals. *P* values calculated using Student's *t*-test.

Thus, it appears that the response of CRF-secreting cells to various neural stimuli can be blocked by the action of glucocorticoids at the level of the membrane or at the genomic level.

McEwen: Have you measured activity during sustained infusion of glucocorticoid, rather than using pulses of glucocorticoid? Domingo Ramirez showed that pulsatile application of progesterone facilitates release of LHRH or amphetamine-evoked dopamine release, whereas sustained application is inhibitory or ineffective. In your experiments, pulsatile application of glucocorticoid causes an inhibition of activity. Does a sustained application also have this effect?

Feldman: The rats that had electrodes chronically implanted in the PVN were given an intraperitoneal injection of 0.5–5.0 mg corticosterone. Recording commenced half an hour after injection, when there was a sustained plasma level of corticosterone.

McEwen: Steroid levels are still declining, though. Rate-sensitive feedback occurs only when levels are increasing or decreasing: I'm wondering about what would happen if levels were constantly high. We don't know what would happen to your observed membrane effects under a condition of truly sustained application.

Feldman: During iontophoresis there was a sustained application of glucocorticoid and, with the intraperitoneal injection, 5 mg of corticosterone should have resulted in sustained levels.

Ramirez: How long was the iontophoretic application?

Feldman: It was for up to 100 seconds.

References

Baulieu EE 1981 Steroid hormones in the brain: several mechanisms? In: Fuxe K et al (eds) Steroid hormone regulation of the brain. Pergamon Press, Oxford, p 3–14

Baulieu EE, Schorderet-Slatkine S 1983 Steroid and peptide control mechanisms in membrane of *Xenopus laevis* oocytes resuming meiotic division. In: Molecular biology of egg maturation. Pitman, London (Ciba Found Symp 98) p 137–158

Blondeau JP, Baulieu EE 1984 Progesterone receptor characterized by photoaffinity labelling in the plasma membrane of *Xenopus laevis* oocytes. Biochem J 20:301–306

Drouva SV, Epelbaum J, Laplante E, Kordon C 1984 Calmodulin involvement on the Ca^{2+}-dependent release of LHRH and SRIF in vitro. Neuroendocrinology 38:189–192

Drouva SV, Laplante E, Kordon C 1985 Progesterone induced LHRH release in vitro is an estrogen as well as Ca^{2+} and calmodulin dependent secretory process. Neuroendocrinology 40:325–331

El Etr M, Schorderet-Slatkine S, Baulieu EE 1979 Meiotic maturation in *Xenopus laevis* oocytes initiated by insulin. Science (Wash DC) 205:1397–1399

Evans RM 1988 The steroid and thyroid hormone receptor family. Science (Wash DC) 240:889–895

Feldman S 1962 Electrophysiological alterations in adrenalectomy. Arch Neurol 7:106–116

Finidori-Lepicard J, Schorderet-Slatkine S, Hanoune J, Baulieu EE 1981 Steroid hormone as regulatory agent of adenylate cyclase. Inhibition by progesterone of the membrane bound enzyme in *Xenopus laevis* oocytes. Nature (Lond) 292:255–256

Godeau JF, Schorderet-Slatkine S, Hubert P, Baulieu EE 1978 Induction of maturation in *Xenopus laevis* oocytes by a steroid linked to a polymer. Proc Natl Acad Sci USA 75:2353–2357

Joëls M, de Kloet ER 1989 Effects of glucocorticoids and norepinephrine on the excitability in the hippocampus. Science (Wash DC) 245:1502–1505

Kelly M, Moss R, Dudley C 1977 The effects of microelectrophoretically applied estrogen, cortisol and acetylcholine on medial preoptic-septal unit activity throughout the estrous cycle of the female rat. Exp Brain Res 30:53–64

Lambert JJ, Peters JA, Sturgess NC, Hales TG 1990 Steroid modulation of the GABA$_A$ receptor complex: electrophysiological studies. Wiley, Chichester (Ciba Foundation Symposium 153) p 56–82

Milgrom E, Luu Thi M, Atger M, Baulieu EE 1973 Mechanisms regulating the concentration and the conformation of progesterone *receptor*(s) in the uterus. J Biol Chem 248:6366–6374

Mor G, Saphier D, Feldman S 1986 Inhibition by corticosterone of paraventricular nucleus multiple unit activity responses in freely moving rats. Exp Neurol 94:391–399

Saphier D, Feldman S 1988 Iontophoretic application of glucocorticoids inhibits identified neurones in the rat paraventricular nucleus. Brain Res 453:183–190

Savouret JF, Misrahi M, Loosfelt H et al 1989 Molecular and cellular biology of mammalian progesterone receptor. Recent Prog Horm Res 45:65–120

Selye H 1942 Correlations between the chemical structure and pharmacological actions of the steroids. Endocrinology 30:437–453

Szego MC 1971 The lysosomal membrane complex as a proximate target for steroid hormone. In: McKerns KW (ed) The sex steroids. Appleton-Century-Crofts, New York, p 1–51

Wallace RA, Misulovin Z, El Etr M, Schorderet-Slatkine S, Baulieu EE 1980 The role of zinc and follicle cells in insulin-initiated meiotic maturation of *Xenopus laevis* oocytes. Science (Wash DC) 210:928–930

Weidenfeld J, Rougeot C, Dray F, Feldman S 1989 Adrenocortical response following acute neurogenic stimuli is mediated by CRF-41. Neurosci Lett 107:189–194

Neuroendocrine metabolism of progesterone and related progestins

Harry J. Karavolas and Donald R. Hodges

Department of Physiological Chemistry, The University of Wisconsin, Madison, WI 53706, USA

Abstract. In mammalian neuroendocrine structures the metabolic processing of progesterone and related natural progestins is primarily a reductive process involving the C-4,5 double bond and the C-3 and C-20 ketones. The principal products of the neuroendocrine metabolism of progesterone in female rats are the two 5α- and 3α-reduced metabolites, 5α-dihydroprogesterone and 3α,5α-tetrahydroprogesterone, with lesser amounts of the corresponding 20α-reduced products. Certain of these metabolites produce some, but not all, of progesterone's biological effects. 5α-Dihydroprogesterone and 3α,5α-tetrahydroprogesterone, in particular, have potent progesterone-like effects on neuroendocrine functions, such as gonadotropin regulation. The two other principal ovarian progestins, 20α-dihydroprogesterone and 17α-hydroxyprogesterone, are metabolized in an analogous manner. The major neuroendocrine progestin conversions therefore appear to be 5α-reduction and 3α-hydroxysteroid oxidoreduction. In the hypothalamus and anterior pituitary, the enzymic activities that catalyse these conversions appear to be under ovarian control and appear to vary with changing reproductive states. These quantitative changes in processing, together with the potent progesterone-like effects of certain metabolites, suggest that these neuroendocrine conversions may provide an important mechanism for mediating some of the effects of progesterone. Alternatively, some metabolites, by duplicating selected effects of progesterone, may provide a means of prolonging certain of its effects while others are terminated.

1990 Steroids and neuronal activity. Wiley, Chichester (Ciba Foundation Symposium 153) p 22–55

Progesterone has significant neuroendocrine effects. Either alone or in combination with other hormones it affects gonadotropin regulation, ovulation, sexual behaviour, body temperature, brain excitability and sleep behaviour. The metabolic processing of progesterone and related natural progestins by neuroendocrine tissues in female rats is primarily a reductive process involving the C-4,5 double bond and the C-3 and C-20 ketones (Karavolas & Nuti 1976,

Karavolas et al 1979, 1984, Celotti et al 1979). The formation of these metabolites in anterior pituitary and neural tissues may provide a means whereby the parent steroid (progesterone or related progestin) is converted to inactive, more active, less active or equipotent forms (Karavolas et al 1984). The diverse effects of progesterone could theoretically result from the actions of progesterone itself or from one or more specific metabolites.

Since some of the metabolites that are formed share neuroendocrine effects in common with progesterone and some do not, the consequences of this metabolic processing provide a means of ending progesterone's effects by converting it to inactive metabolites. On the other hand, this processing could generate active metabolites which, among other possibilities, could (a) produce some or all of progesterone's effects in certain tissues, (b) exhibit variable progesterone-like biopotencies, (c) be duplicative of some or all of progesterone's effects, such that both progesterone and the metabolite are active on some or all functions, or (d) be requisite for some or all of progesterone's effects, the conversion being necessary to generate mediators for some or all of progesterone's effects (Karavolas et al 1984). To understand the mechanisms by which progestins exert their neuroendocrine effects, one must understand, among other things, the characteristics of their metabolism in neuroendocrine target tissues and the nature of the active steroidal compounds.

In this chapter we report our findings on characteristics of the neuroendocrine metabolism of progesterone and the other principal ovarian progestins, 20α-dihydroprogesterone (20α-DHP) and 17α-hydroxyprogesterone (17α-OH-P), especially in the hypothalamus and anterior pituitary of female rats. We discuss the nature of the steroidal products, their progesterone-like neuroendocrine effects, tissue differences in metabolic processing, changes in metabolism during altered physiological states, and the characteristics of the principal progestin-metabolizing enzymes. Finally, we shall discuss how these ubiquitous progesterone-metabolizing steps can generate progesterone-specific target tissue responses.

Nature of the steroidal products and metabolic pathways

Progesterone metabolism

We used both *in vitro* and *in vivo* studies, with reverse isotopic dilution analyses, to determine which metabolites were formed, and in what relative amounts, in several rat neuroendocrine structures. These structures included the anterior pituitary, hypothalamus,* midbrain-tectum, pineal and cerebellum (Karavolas

---

*The term 'hypothalamus' will be used interchangeably with 'medial basal hypothalamus' unless otherwise indicated.

& Nuti 1976, Karavolas et al 1984). In all these tissues, and especially so in the anterior pituitary and the hypothalamus, the principal metabolites of progesterone were usually 5α-dihydroprogesterone (5α-DHP) and 3α,5α-tetra-hydroprogesterone (3α,5α-THP) (Fig. 1, top half); this indicates the presence of substantial progesterone 5α-reductase and 5α-DHP-3α-hydroxysteroid oxidoreductase enzymic activity. We found generally minor amounts of the corresponding 20α-reduced metabolites, 20α-DHP, 5α,20α-tetrahydro-progesterone (5α,20α-THP) and 3α,5α,20α-hexahydroprogesterone (3α,5α,20α-HHP), indicating some 20α-hydroxysteroid oxidoreductase activity (Fig. 1, bottom half). There were quantitative, but no qualitative, differences in the metabolism of progesterone among the tissues examined. Others have also reported similar conversions of progesterone to 5α-, 3α- and 20α-reduced products in brain and anterior pituitary tissues of female and male rats and other species, such as chickens, guinea pigs, dogs, subhuman primates and humans; some workers have reported 5β- and 3β-reduced products in chickens and dogs (Rommerts & Van der Molen 1971; for review see Celotti et al 1979).

Formation of 5β- and 3β-isomers and other metabolites

In our studies there was no definitive evidence for the production of 5β-, 3β- or 20β-reduced isomers. Using reverse isotopic dilution analyses and separation systems that distinguish α and β isomers, we found significant amounts of radioactivity to be associated only with 5α-, 3α- and 20α-reduced products. However, because the radioactivity that was occasionally associated with carrier 5β, 3β or 20β compounds was too low for meaningful analysis, their existence remains a possibility. If these derivatives were present, they could not have formed more than a trace of the metabolized radio-activity ($<0.05\%$). Other metabolites may have been present, because in some tissue incubations small amounts of unidentified radioactivity (usually 1–5% of the total) were associated with TLC zones corresponding to compounds, probably hydroxylated derivatives, more polar than the metabolites mentioned above.

Metabolism of 20α-DHP by anterior pituitary and hypothalamus

When 20α-DHP was used as substrate in female rat hypothalamus and anterior pituitary we observed conversions analogous to those seen when progesterone was the substrate (Karavolas et al 1984). The metabolic pathway is essentially that shown in the lower half of Fig. 1. We detected no appreciable conversion to progesterone ($<1\%$). The principal metabolites were the corresponding 5α- and 3α-reduced derivatives, 5α,20α-THP and 3α,5α,20α-HHP.

25

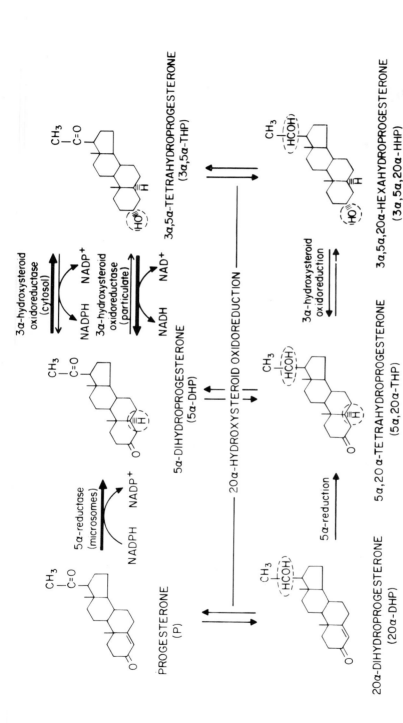

FIG. 1. Major and minor metabolic pathways for the processing of progesterone by female rat neuroendocrine structures. The major pathway, denoted by bold arrows (top half), is through 5α-dihydroprogesterone (5α-DHP) and 3α,5α-tetrahydroprogesterone (3α,5α-THP). Details are in the original publications referenced in the text.

Metabolism of [³H]17α-OH-P by anterior pituitary and hypothalamus

This was the last of our studies on the metabolism of the major ovarian progestins by the anterior pituitary and the hypothalamus (Karavolas et al 1988). The presence of the 17α-hydroxyl moiety offered the exciting possibility that we might observe side-chain cleavage to C_{19} products. Because certain brain structures, including the hypothalamus, can convert certain C_{19} androgens to oestrogens, there was also the possibility that *in situ* aromatization might be seen (Martini 1982). We found conversions analogous to those obtained with [³H]progesterone or [³H]20α-DHP as substrates (Fig. 2). The major products in both tissues were 17α-hydroxy-5α-pregnane-3,20-dione and 3α,17α-dihydroxy-5α-pregnan-20-one, with small amounts of the corresponding 20α-reduced products. There was no evidence for the formation of C_{19} metabolites. Thus, with the three major ovarian progestins (progesterone, 20α-DHP and 17α-OH-P) as substrates, the principal anterior pituitary and hypothalamic progestin-metabolizing activities are 5α-reduction and 3α-hydroxysteroid oxidoreduction, with minor amounts of 20α-hydroxysteroid oxidoreduction. The resulting metabolites accounted for nearly all of the metabolized radioactivity in the two tissues. We know little about the effects in the anterior pituitary and the hypothalamus of 20α-DHP and 17α-OH-P (see below) but their availability as alternative substrates may be important for the regulation of progesterone processing in these regions.

Biological effects of progesterone metabolites

Several of the progesterone metabolites described above, especially 5α-DHP and 3α,5α-THP, share some, but not all, of the biological endpoint effects traditionally associated with progesterone, neuroendocrine ones in particular (Table 1). Neither 5α-DHP nor 3α,5α-THP have progesterone-like effects on uterine progestational parameters (such as those tested in Table 1). Some early studies, which revealed the absence of any effects of 5α-DHP and 3α,5α-THP on the uterus, led to the false supposition that these metabolites would also have no effects on other processes mediated by progesterone, such as gonadotropin regulation, ovulation and sexual behaviour.

With respect to gonadotropin regulation (Table 1), 5α-DHP, 3α,5α-THP, 20α-DHP and 3α,5α,20α-HHP exhibit progesterone-like facilitatory and inhibitory effects on luteinizing hormone (LH) and follicle stimulating hormone (FSH) in rats (Nuti & Karavolas 1977, Karavolas et al 1984, Zanisi et al 1984). 5α-DHP and 3α,5α-THP also modulate the hypothalamic content and release of luteinizing hormone releasing hormone (LHRH) (Zanisi et al 1984). 5α-DHP and 20α-DHP, but not 3α,5α-THP, facilitate ovulation, although both are less potent than progesterone (Karavolas et al 1984). Neither of the 20α-DHP metabolites (5α,20α-THP or 3α,5α,20α-HHP)

27

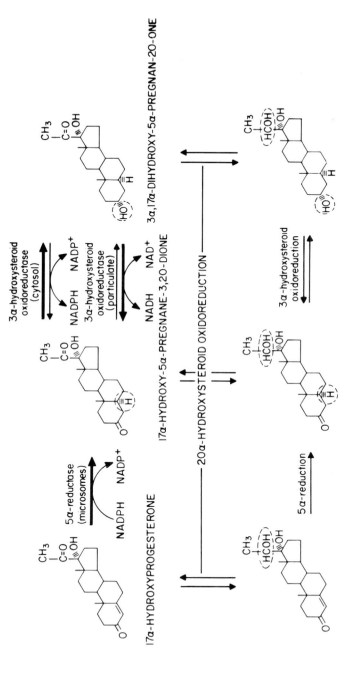

FIG. 2. Metabolic pathway for the processing of 17α-hydroxyprogesterone by female rat anterior pituitary and hypothalamus. The major pathway is denoted by bold arrows. Details are in the original publication cited in the text.

TABLE 1 Progesterone-like effects of some 3α-, 5α- and 20α-reduced metabolites[a] of progesterone

Effect	5α-DHP	3α,5α-THP	20α-DHP	5α,20α-THP	3α,5α,20α-HHP
Facilitation and inhibition of LH and FSH release (in vivo)	≤P	≤P	≤P	No	≤P
Facilitation and inhibition of LHRH-induced LH release (in vitro)	≥P	<P	<P	—	—
LHRH content and release	<P	<P	No	No	No
Facilitation of ovulation	<P	No	<P	No	No
Facilitation of inhibition of lordosis	≥P	<P	≤P	—	No
Uterine effects (decidual reaction, parturition, pregnancy maintenance)	No	No	—	—	—
Modulation of GABA receptor	>P	>P	—	—	≥P
Anaesthetic effect	>P	≥P	—	—	>P

[a]The ovarian progestin 17α-hydroxyprogesterone, also has progesterone-like effects on the facilitation and inhibition of LH release. We have no information on its 5α,20α-reduced and 3α,5α,20α-reduced metabolites. Details can be found in the original publications referenced in the text or in a previous review (Karavolas et al 1984).

P, progesterone; DHP, dihydroprogesterone; THP, tetrahydroprogesterone; HHP, hexahydroprogesterone; LH, luteinizing hormone; LHRH, luteinizing hormone releasing hormone; FSH, follicle stimulating hormone; —, no report.

facilitates ovulation. 5α-DHP exerts potent progesterone-like effects in facilitation of lordosis behaviour in rats, guinea pigs and hamsters (Karavolas et al 1984). When bioavailability problems are eliminated, 5α-DHP appears to be as potent as, or more potent than, progesterone is in facilitating lordosis (Celotti et al 1979, Gorzalka & Whalen 1977). 3α,5α-THP also exerts behavioural effects, but its bioactivity is less than that of progesterone (Kubli-Garfias 1984). 3α,5α-THP may act as a barbiturate-like modulator of the GABA receptor complex (Majewska 1987). This may explain how 3α,5α-THP, which is a more potent anaesthetic than progesterone (Holzbauer 1976), modulates neuronal excitability.

Little is known about the effects of 17α-OH-P and its metabolites. 20α-DHP does exhibit some progesterone-like effects, but with lower potency (Gilles & Karavolas 1981); but because 20α-DHP (unlike 5α-DHP) can be converted back to progesterone, it is unclear whether the active compound is 20α-DHP itself, or progesterone or its 5α- and 3α-reduced metabolites.

Tissue differences in the metabolic processing of progesterone

The production of metabolites that are more or less active than progesterone or that retain only certain biological effects could be important in regulating progesterone's neuroendocrine effects on reproduction. Thus, there could be differences in the metabolic processing of progesterone between different tissues (e.g. target vs non-target) and between different reproductive states (e.g. oestrous cycle, pregnancy and reproductive senescence).

Tissue differences: in vitro studies

We examined the anterior pituitary, the hypothalamus and the major brain areas of the rat shown in Table 2 and found all of them to be capable of converting progesterone to all the metabolites shown in Fig. 1 (Hanukoglu et al 1977, Karavolas et al 1984). There were quantitative, but no apparent qualitative, differences among the tissues. Although 5α- and 3α-reduction and some 20α-reduction of progesterone are common properties of these neural tissues, the relative levels of 3α-, 5α- and 20α-reduced metabolites formed by these tissues vary (Table 2). The highest levels of 5α-DHP and 3α,5α-THP occurred in the anterior pituitary and the hypothalamus, followed by the medulla (5α-DHP) or the cerebellum (3α,5α-THP) and the other brain regions shown; the pineal had the lowest levels. The formation of 20α-reduced metabolites was highest in the pineal and the cerebellum and lowest in the anterior pituitary and the hypothalamus. With respect to the localization of these metabolic activities within the anterior pituitary and the hypothalamus, we and others have found higher progesterone 5α- and 3α-

TABLE 2   **Relative levels of progesterone metabolites in various brain areas and anterior pituitary**

Metabolite(s)	Relative levels
5α-DHP	Anterior pituitary (30–35%) > hypothalamus, medulla (18–22%) > thalamus, midbrain-tectum, tegmentum, cerebellum (10–12%) > pineal (<1%)
3α,5α-THP	Anterior pituitary, hypothalamus (11–15%) > cerebellum (4%) > thalamus, midbrain-tectum, tegmentum, medulla (1–2%) > pineal (<1%)
20α-Reduced metabolites	Cerebellum, pineal (0.1%) > thalamus, midbrain-tectum, tegmentum, medulla (0.05–0.08%) > anterior pituitary, hypothalamus (≤0.05%)

reduction in progesterone target areas such as gonadotropes and the median eminence (Lloyd & Karavolas 1975, Bertics et al 1987, Melcangi et al 1985, Martini 1982, Rommerts & Van der Molen 1971). Studies of anterior pituitary and hypothalamic levels of progesterone metabolizing enzymes are discussed later.

Tissue differences: in vivo *studies*

We examined the *in vivo* metabolism and selective retention (accumulation) of [^{3}H]progesterone and [^{3}H]5α-DHP and their metabolites by female rat anterior pituitary, hypothalamus and some other neural tissues relevant to progesterone's effects on gonadotropin regulation and sexual behaviour. We found large, selective accumulations of 5α-DHP by the anterior pituitary and the hypothalamus after injections of either [^{3}H]progesterone or [^{3}H]5α-DHP (as compared to non-target tissues). In those studies (Karavolas et al 1979) we collected tissue and plasma samples from ovariectomized (OVX) and oestrogen-treated ovariectomized (E-OVX) rats injected for 10 minutes with either radiolabelled progesterone or radiolabelled 5α-DHP, and analysed the samples for the identity and concentration of accumulated ^{3}H-labelled steroids. In addition to the hypothalamus, the anterior pituitary and some extra-hypothalamic target sites for progesterone (namely midbrain-tectum, pineal and cerebellum), we also examined the uterus (as a well-established progesterone target tissue), muscle (as a non-target tissue), and the cerebral cortex (as a putative non-target neural tissue). Most radioactivity in the tissue and plasma samples was *not* the original ^{3}H-labelled steroid (i.e. [^{3}H]progesterone or [^{3}H]5α-DHP), except after injection of [^{3}H]5α-DHP in the anterior pituitary, hypothalamus, and pineal. The accumulated

TABLE 3 Selective tissue accumulation of progesterone and its metabolites after injection of [^{3}H] progesterone into ovariectomized rats

Progesterone metabolite accumulated	Tissue examined	Relative levels versus non-target tissues and plasma[a]	
		Without oestrogen priming	With oestrogen priming
Progesterone	Anterior pituitary	No significant accumulation above non-target tissues	No differences except for:
	Hypothalamus	1.3-fold > c. cortex; 2-fold > plasma	Pineal 5-fold > c. cortex; 6-fold > plasma
	Cerebellum	No selective accumulation	Uterus 20-fold > muscle; 6-fold > plasma
	Midbrain-tectum	No selective accumulation	
	Pineal	2.5-fold > c. cortex; 4-fold > plasma	
	Uterus	No selective accumulation	
5α-DHP	Anterior pituitary	20-fold > muscle and plasma	No differences
	Hypothalamus	2-fold > c. cortex; 13-fold > plasma	
	Cerebellum	2-fold > c. cortex; 11-fold > plasma	
	Midbrain-tectum	3-fold > c. cortex; 17-fold > plasma	
	Pineal	No selective accumulation	
	Uterus	No selective accumulation	
3α,5α-THP	Anterior pituitary	5-fold > muscle; 4-fold > plasma	No differences except for:
	Pineal	2.5-fold > c. cortex; 4-fold > plasma	Uterus 9-fold > muscle; 6-fold > plasma
	Uterus	4-fold > muscle; 3.5-fold > plasma	Midbrain 1.4-fold > c. cortex;
	Other tissues	No selective accumulation	2-fold > plasma
20α-Reduced steroids[a]	Anterior pituitary	5α,20α-THP: 13-fold > muscle; 5-fold > plasma; 3α,5α,20α-HHP: 9-fold > muscle; 2.5-fold > plasma	No differences except for:
	Pineal	20α-DHP: 4-fold > c. cortex and plasma; 5α,20α-THP: 4-fold > c. cortex and plasma	Pineal 20α-DHP: 30-fold > c. cortex; 8-fold > plasma
	Other tissues	No selective accumulation	

[a]Only those metabolite levels that are significantly different from levels in non-target tissues (muscle, cerebral cortex) are listed. Details and statistical comparisons are in the original publication referenced in the text.

TABLE 4 Selective tissue accumulation of 5α-DHP and metabolites after injection of [³H] 5α-DHP into ovariectomized rats

5α-DHP/ metabolite accumulated	Tissue examined	Relative levels versus non-target tissues and plasma[a]	
		Without oestrogen priming	With oestrogen priming
5α-DHP	Anterior pituitary	50-fold>muscle; 18-fold>plasma	No differences except for:
	Hypothalamus	3-fold>c. cortex; 25-fold>plasma	Pineal 2-fold>c. cortex; 13-fold>plasma
	Cerebellum	No selective accumulation	
	Midbrain-tectum	1.3-fold>c. cortex; 11-fold>plasma	
	Pineal	No selective accumulation	
	Uterus	No selective accumulation	
3α,5α-THP	Midbrain-tectum	1.4-fold>c. cortex; 2-fold>plasma	No differences except for:
	Other tissues	No selective accumulation	Anterior pituitary 1.4-fold>muscle; 2-fold>plasma
			Uterus 1.4-fold>muscle; 2-fold>plasma
20α-Reduced steroids[a]	Pineal	5α,20α-THP: 3-fold>c. cortex and plasma	Pineal No selective accumulation
	Other tissues	No selective accumulation	
Progesterone	All tissues	No conversion to progesterone from [³H] 5α-DHP was detected in either group	

[a]Only those metabolite levels that are significantly different from levels in non-target tissues (muscle, cerebral cortex) are listed. Details and statistical comparisons can be found in the original publication referenced in the text.

tissue and plasma radioactivity was mostly associated with the metabolites of progesterone and 5α-DHP that are shown in Fig. 1. To make meaningful comparisons between tissue and plasma, we determined the concentrations of these [3H]-labelled steroids. Reverse isotopic dilution analyses of the radioactivity accumulated by plasma and selected tissues were made for progesterone, 5α-DHP, 3α,5α-THP, 20α-DHP, 5α,20α-THP and 3α,5α,20α-HHP. As summarized in Tables 3 and 4, we observed significant differences between tissues in the steroidal compounds that they accumulated to levels above those accumulated by plasma and non-target tissue.

[3H]Progesterone injections (Table 3). Tissue levels of [3H]progesterone were not significantly greater than plasma and non-target tissue levels except in the hypothalamus and the pineal. [3H]5α-DHP was the predominant metabolite in the anterior pituitary and was the major [3H]-labelled steroid besides [3H]progesterone in neural tissues other than the pineal. Concentrations of [3H]5α-DHP in the anterior pituitary, hypothalamus, midbrain-tectum and cerebellum were greater than those in plasma, muscle and cerebral cortex. Muscle and uterine concentrations of [3H]progesterone and [3H]5α-DHP were equivalent to plasma levels. In most of the tissues, lesser amounts of [3H]3α,5α-THP were found and only anterior pituitary and pineal concentrations of this metabolite were greater than plasma and non-target tissue levels. Tissue concentrations of 20α-DHP and its metabolites were generally low and comparable to plasma levels, except in the case of [3H]20α-DHP and [3H]5α,20α-THP in the pineal, and [3H]5α,20α-THP and [3H]3α,5α,20α-HHP in the anterior pituitary. Treatment with oestrogen before injection of the radiolabelled steroid enhanced tissue accumulations of progesterone and its metabolites only in the pineal, midbrain-tectum and uterus.

[3H]5α-DHP injections (Table 4). 5α-DHP and 3α,5α-THP accounted for most radioactivity in all tissues tested. Small amounts of tritium were associated with 5α,20α-THP and 3α,5α,20α-HHP, but tritium associated with progesterone or 20α-DHP was equivalent to background levels. Most tissue tritium (80–90%) was associated with these four carrier steroids. 5α-DHP was the major [3H]-labelled steroid in the anterior pituitary, hypothalamus and pineal, whereas 3α,5α-THP predominated in plasma, tectum, muscle and uterus. Although anterior pituitary and neural levels of 5α-DHP were greater than those of plasma, only in the anterior pituitary, the hypothalamus and the midbrain-tectum were they also greater than levels in the putative non-target neural tissue, namely cerebral cortex. Tissue levels of 3α,5α-THP, 5α,20α-THP and 3α,5α,20α-HHP generally did not differ from levels in plasma and non-target tissues, except in the accumulation of 3α,5α-THP by the mid-brain and 5α,20α-THP by the pineal. There were few differences after pretreatment with oestrogen; the only differences evident were the

accumulation of 5α-DHP in the pineal and that of 3α,5α-THP in anterior pituitary and uterus.

In summary, the anterior pituitary accumulated large amounts of radiolabelled 5α-DHP after injection of *either* steroid, but progesterone levels did not differ from levels in plasma and non-target tissues. The hypothalamus accumulated significant amounts of *both* 5α-DHP *and* progesterone. The midbrain accumulated 5α-DHP to levels comparable to those seen in the hypothalamus and anterior pituitary in both groups (i.e. OVX controls and oestrogenized OVX rats) after injection of *either* steroid. The pineal showed the greatest accumulation of progesterone in both groups, but it did not accumulate 5α-DHP above non-target tissue levels after [^{3}H]progesterone injection. The pineal also accumulated significant amounts of the 20α-reduced metabolites. In the uterus, there was little accumulation of 5α-DHP; significant accumulation of progesterone was seen only after oestrogen priming.

These results clearly indicate that significant differences exist between tissues in their accumulation of [^{3}H]progesterone, [^{3}H]5α-DHP and their metabolites. The formation and accumulation of a particular metabolite may provide an active intermediary or an inactive metabolite which represents a means of inactivating the parent compound. It is important to correlate selective tissue accumulations with the progesterone-like effects of the metabolites on these tissues. We noted that large amounts of 5α-DHP were selectively accumulated in the hypothalamus and the anterior pituitary, but not in the uterus, after injections of either [^{3}H]progesterone or [^{3}H]5α-DHP. 5α-DHP has progesterone-like effects on gonadotropin regulation, ovulation, and lordosis, which are ostensibly functions of the hypothalamus and anterior pituitary. Also, the absence of a selective accumulation of 5α-DHP in the uterus is consistent with the reported inability of 5α-DHP to elicit a uterine progestational response and the notion that it is progesterone *per se* that is the active hormone form in this tissue. Thus, these and other results suggest that the diverse effects of progesterone may result from actions of progesterone itself, or its metabolites, or from the effects of combinations (Fig. 3).

Anterior pituitary and hypothalamic metabolism of progesterone during changed physiological states

If the processing of progesterone by the anterior pituitary and the hypothalamus were important in the regulation of reproduction, there might be differences in metabolite formation during altered reproductive states. In a series of *in vitro* studies we determined the levels of progesterone metabolites formed by the rat anterior pituitary and hypothalamus during pregnancy, reproductive senescence and various stages of the oestrous cycle. We saw changes in progesterone 5α-reduction in the anterior pituitary (but not in the hypothalamus) at different stages of pregnancy (Marrone & Karavolas 1981). The formation of 5α-DHP

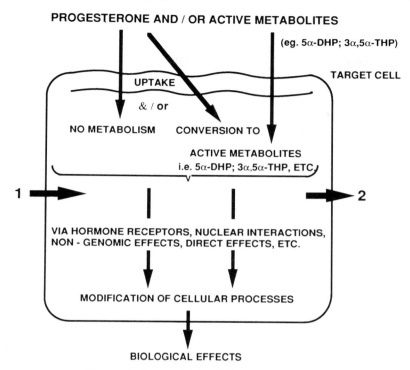

PROGESTERONE AND / OR ACTIVE METABOLITES

(eg. 5α-DHP; 3α,5α-THP)

TARGET CELL

UPTAKE

& / or

NO METABOLISM   CONVERSION TO

ACTIVE METABOLITES
i.e. 5α-DHP; 3α,5α-THP, ETC.

1 →   → 2

VIA HORMONE RECEPTORS, NUCLEAR INTERACTIONS,
NON - GENOMIC EFFECTS, DIRECT EFFECTS, ETC.

MODIFICATION OF CELLULAR PROCESSES

BIOLOGICAL EFFECTS

e.g; synthesis / release of LH /FSH, lordosis behavior,
anesthesia, modulation of GABA receptors, etc.

1. OTHER HORMONES, ETC. FOR NECESSARY INTERACTIONS OR PERMISSIVE EFFECTS.

2. TERMINATION OF EFFECT:—→ DEGRADATION (INACTIVE METABOLITES, ETC.) —→ EXIT.

FIG. 3.   Diagram of a suggested model of the effects on progesterone target cells of
either progesterone itself or metabolites such as 5α-dihydroprogesterone (5α-DHP) and
3α,5α-tetrahydroprogesterone (3α,5α-THP). (Adapted from Karavolas et al 1979.)

by the anterior pituitary was lower on Days 15 and 21 of pregnancy than it
was on Day 1. Progesterone metabolism was also quantitatively different in
the anterior pituitary of aged rats during three stages of reproductive senescence
(constant oestrus, repeated pseudopregnancy and anoestrus) (Marrone &
Karavolas 1982). No such difference was observed in hypothalamic metabolism.
5α-Reduction and 3α-oxidoreduction in the anterior pituitary in pseudopregnant
or anoestrous rats was twice that of young cycling rats or rats exhibiting constant
oestrus. Both anterior pituitary and hypothalamic metabolism of progesterone
fluctuated during the oestrous cycle (Karavolas et al 1984). 5α-Reduction was
greatest on the mornings of dioestrus 2 and oestrus and lowest on the mornings
of dioestrus 1 and pro-oestrus.

Characteristics of anterior pituitary and
hypothalamic progesterone-metabolizing enzymes

In both the anterior pituitary and the hypothalamus, the formation of 5α-DHP and 3α,5α-THP (Fig. 1) is catalysed in turn by an irreversible progesterone 5α-reductase and by one of two distinct 5α-DHP 3α-hydroxysteroid oxidoreductases (3α-HSOR). Because the 5α- and 3α-reductions of progesterone appeared to be key steps in the processing of progesterone in the anterior pituitary and the hypothalamus, we studied the characteristics, regulation and hypothalamic regional distribution of the enzymes that catalyse these conversions (Table 5 and Figs. 4 and 5).

The progesterone 5α-reductases (Table 5) from both tissues have a dependence for NADPH and exhibit a K_m for progesterone (≈ 100 nM) that is consistent with reported plasma progesterone concentrations (Bertics & Karavolas 1984, 1985). The specificity of this enzyme in both tissues requires the steroid substrate to possess a conjugated ketone (Δ^4-3-oxo). Of the natural steroid hormones tested, only the ovarian Δ^4-3-oxo steroids (20α-DHP and 17α-OH-P) competitively inhibited 5α-reduction of progesterone within the range of their physiological plasma concentrations. The hypothalamic 5α-reductase may be regulated, at least in part, by metal ions; its activity is inhibited by Zn^{2+} and Cu^{2+}, but enhanced by K^+ and Li^+. Alterations in membrane composition may modulate progesterone 5α-reduction in the anterior pituitary because here the enzyme is stimulated by specific phospholipids. Progesterone 5α-reductases in both the anterior pituitary and the hypothalamus have ordered-sequential kinetic mechanisms (Campbell & Karavolas 1989). NADPH binding preferentially precedes the binding of progesterone. These results suggest that the formation of 5α-reduced metabolites is a function of available progesterone (not NADPH) during times of changing progesterone levels because the K_m for progesterone (≈ 100 nM) is in the range of circulating progesterone levels (10–200 nM), and the intracellular concentrations of NADPH (≈ 10–400 μM) are greater than the K_m for NADPH.

There are at least two different 5α-DHP 3α-HSOR activities in both the hypothalamus and the anterior pituitary; these two activities differ in their subcellular location, cofactor requirement, pH and temperature optima, and in various kinetic parameters (Table 5). In both tissues, an NADPH-linked activity is located in the cytosol, whereas an NADH-dependent activity is found in particulate fractions. The NADH and NADPH-linked 3α-HSORs from both anterior pituitary and hypothalamus appear to be reversible and exhibit K_m values for their various substrates that suggest they may operate *in situ* in opposite directions; that is, in the case of the NADPH-linked 3α-HSORs, the K_m for 5α-DHP is much less than that for 3α,5α-THP, indicating that this enzyme may preferentially catalyse the conversion of 5α-DHP to 3α,5α-THP. This direction of catalysis is supported by the fact that cytosolic NADPH/NADP ratios are generally greater than unity, thus favouring the reductive reaction.

TABLE 5   Properties of the anterior pituitary and hypothalamic progesterone 5α-reductases and 5α-DHP 3α-hydroxysteroid oxidoreductases

Progesterone 5α-reductase	Anterior pituitary[a]	Hypothalamus[a]
Subcellular location	Microsomes	Microsomes
Cofactor	NADPH	NADPH
K_m (progesterone)	117 ± 12 nM	113 ± 11 nM
K_m (testosterone)	ND	16 µM
Competitive inhibitors (substrates)	20α-DHP; 17α-OH-P	20α-DHP; 17α-OH-P
Specificity	Δ⁴-3-Oxosteroids	Δ⁴-3-Oxosteroids

5α-DHP 3α-hydroxy-steroid oxidoreductases	Anterior pituitary[b]		Hypothalamus	
	NADPH-linked	NADH-linked	NADPH-linked	NADH-linked
Subcellular location	Cytosol	Microsomes	Cytosol	Cell membranes
Reductive reaction				
K_m (cofactor)	0.71 µM	8.9 µM	0.71 µM	29 µM
K_m (5α-DHP)	0.083 µM	0.23 µM	0.083 µM	0.40 µM
Oxidative reaction				
K_m (cofactor)	1.6 µM	18.7 µM	21 µM	84 µM
K_m (3α,5α-THP)	1.4 µM	0.058 µM	2.3 µM	0.11 µM

[a]The progesterone 5α-reductases are also influenced by sulphydryl reagents and flavins (both anterior pituitary and hypothalamus), phospholipids (anterior pituitary) and metal ions (hypothalamus). These and other details of this table can be found in the papers cited in the text.
[b]The anterior pituitary 3α-hydroxysteroid oxidoreductases are sensitive to sulphydryl reagents and prefer C_{21} progestin substrates over the C_{19} androgen substrates. Both 5α-dihydrotestosterone (5α-DHT) and 5α-androstane-3α,17β-diol are competitive inhibitors (alternative substrates). The purified anterior pituitary NADPH-linked 3α-HSOR has an M_r of 36 000 and a 250-fold lower K_m for 5α-DHT (21 µM) than for 5α-DHP (J. Campbell & H. J. Karavolas, unpublished).
ND, not done.

Conversely, the NADH-linked 3α-HSORs possess K_m values for 3α,5α-THP that are less than that for 5α-DHP, suggesting that the conversion *in vivo* may proceed in the oxidative direction; that is, this enzyme may primarily catalyse the conversion of 3α,5α-THP *back* to 5α-DHP. Again, this direction is supported by the observation that cellular NADH/NAD ratios are generally less than unity. These 3α-HSORs, along with the 5α-reductase activity, may therefore differentially regulate the concentrations of the two progesterone metabolites 5α-DHP and 3α,5α-THP, depending on the tissue and compartment. These progesterone metabolites in turn may differentially affect LH and FSH secretion, or other effects of progesterone. There is also a difference in inhibition of the 3α-HSORs by indomethacin (J. Campbell & H. J. Karavolas, unpublished observations). Specificity studies indicate that the anterior pituitary 3α-HSORs prefer C_{21} (progestin) substrates over C_{19} (androgen) analogues.

Ovarian regulation of progesterone-metabolizing enzymes in the anterior pituitary and hypothalamus

The role of the ovary in the regulation of the hypothalamic and anterior pituitary enzymes that catalyse 5α- and 3α-reductions of progesterone was examined in the studies summarized in Figs. 4 and 5 (Krause et al 1981, Bertics et al 1987). In those studies we determined the hypothalamic and anterior pituitary levels of progesterone 5α-reductase and the two distinct 5α-DHP 3α-HSORs (NADH- and NADPH-linked) during various stages of the oestrous cycle and in the OVX rats treated with oestrogen or vehicle. Levels of the anterior pituitary 5α-reductase fluctuated significantly over the oestrous cycle (Fig. 4, left). Peak levels were observed at pro-oestrus, oestrus and metoestrus; these were significantly higher (about two-fold) than the lowest levels that were seen on dioestrus Days 1 and 2 of five-day cycling rats. The anterior pituitary NADH-linked 3α-HSOR also fluctuated significantly during the oestrous cycle (2–3-fold); the fluctuations observed were parallel to those of the 5α-reductase. When the changing oestrous cycle levels of anterior pituitary 5α-reductase and NADH-linked 3α-HSOR were viewed in relation to endogenous hormone levels, the changes appeared to be inversely correlated with plasma oestradiol concentration. We used an OVX rat model to exaggerate the ovarian impact and to assess oestrogen replacement modalities. The effect of ovariectomy on progesterone processing in the anterior pituitary was considerable (Fig. 4, right); after ovariectomy, levels of anterior pituitary 5α-reductase increased 10–12-fold relative to mean levels in intact rats, and levels of NADH-linked 3α-HSOR increased 4–5-fold. The anterior pituitary cytosolic NADPH-linked 3α-HSOR activity was unaffected by ovariectomy. Partial, to nearly complete, restorations of anterior pituitary 5α-reductase and NADH-linked 3α-HSOR activities occurred after particular replacement oestrogen treatments (Fig. 4). Replacement treatments of progesterone or progesterone plus oestrogen suggest that a biphasic response to progesterone occurs and that progesterone may antagonize the effects of oestrogen. Interestingly, the observed increases in anterior pituitary 5α-reductase and NADH-linked 3α-HSOR activities during the oestrous cycle and after ovariectomy appear to parallel the increased secretory activity of the gonadotropin-producing cell during these times. Furthermore, at a time when circulating progesterone levels are low (after ovariectomy), it is of interest that the two anterior pituitary activities that are presumably responsible for increasing 5α-DHP levels by catalysing the conversion of progesterone to 5α-DHP and of 3α,5α-THP back to 5α-DHP should be so drastically elevated. This suggests that there are possible correlations of increased gonadotropin secretory activity with 5α-DHP levels.

Levels and distribution of progesterone-metabolizing enzymes in discrete hypothalamic regions

The above studies of progesterone processing in the hypothalamus used a block

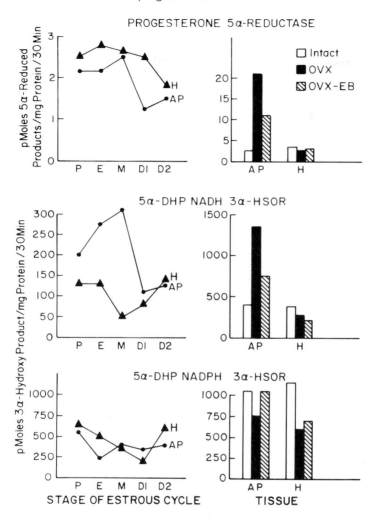

FIG. 4. *Left panels*: Anterior pituitary (AP) and hypothalamic (H) levels of the progesterone 5α-reductase and the two 5α-DHP (NADH- and NADPH-linked) 3α-hydroxysteroid oxidoreductase (HSOR) activities during the rat oestrous cycle. P, pro-oestrus; E. oestrus; M, metoestrus; D1, dioestrous Day 1; D2, dioestrous Day 2. *Right panels*: The effect of ovariectomy and oestrogen treatment on anterior pituitary (AP) and hypothalamic (H) progesterone 5α-reductase and the two 5α-DHP (NADH- and NADPH-linked) 3α-HSOR activities. Intact, data from intact cycling rats selected at random; OVX, 10-day ovariectomized rats; OVX-EB, ovariectomized rats treated on Days 7, 8 and 9 after ovariectomy with oestradiol benzoate (10 μg/day). Details of this data display and statistical comparisons can be found in the original publications cited in the text.

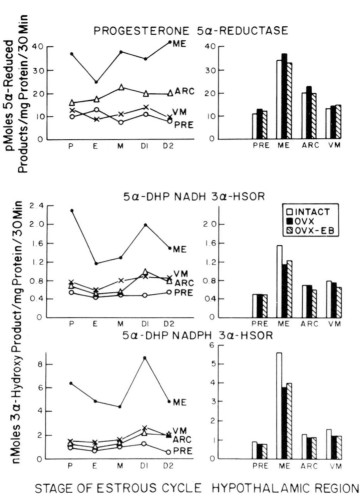

STAGE OF ESTROUS CYCLE   HYPOTHALAMIC REGION

FIG. 5. *Left panels*: Levels of the progesterone 5α-reductase and the two 5α-DHP (NADH- and NADPH-linked) 3α-hydroxysteroid oxidoreductase (HSOR) activities in various hypothalamic regions during the rat oestrous cycle. P, pro-oestrus; E, oestrus; M, metoestrus; D1, dioestrous Day 1; D2, dioestrous Day 2; ME, median eminence; VM, ventromedial nuclei; ARC, arcuate nuclei; PRE, medial preoptic area. *Right panels*: The effect of ovariectomy and oestrogen treatment on the levels of the progesterone 5α-reductase and NADH- and NADPH-linked 5α-DHP 3α-HSOR in various hypothalamic regions. INTACT, data taken from the intact cycling rats presented in the left panel; OVX, 10-day ovariectomized rats; OVX-EB, ovariectomized rats treated on Days 7, 8 and 9 after ovariectomy with oestradiol benzoate (10 μg/day). Details of this data display and statistical comparisons can be found in the original publication cited in the text.

of medial basal hypothalamic tissue that included the arcuate (ARC) and ventromedial (VM) nuclei in addition to the median eminence (ME). As a consequence of this, differences between various regions may have gone undetected: changes in enzyme levels within one hypothalamic region may have been masked by changes in other regions, or diluted by the size of unresponsive areas. Using similar protocols, we measured progesterone 5α-reductase and the two 5α-DHP 3α-HSOR levels in these three hypothalamic areas separately, and also in the medial preoptic area (PRE). ME levels of all three enzymes were significantly higher (two- to four-fold) than their mean levels in the PRE, VM and ARC areas (Fig. 5). These three regions had similar levels of the two 3α-HSOR activities. The arcuate nuclei, however, had intermediate 5α-reductase levels. There were appreciable fluctuations in some enzyme levels (as much as two-fold) during the oestrus cycle (Fig. 5, left half), but the variability observed meant that none were significant. After ovariectomy, there was a significant decrease (35%) in median eminence NADPH-linked 3α-HSOR levels as compared to those in intact animals. This change would presumably increase 5α-DHP levels. Replacement oestrogen treatments did not alter enzyme levels relative to OVX groups. These results suggest that the median eminence possesses a greater capacity for progesterone metabolism than the other hypothalamic regions tested, and that the NADPH-linked 3α-HSOR in this region may be under ovarian control. This high metabolic capacity of female rat ME for progesterone contrasts with the testosterone-metabolizing capacity of male rat ME (Melcangi et al 1985); it may be a sex-specific effect.

MAPD: a high affinity potent inhibitor of progesterone 5α-reductase

As one approach to assessing the role of progesterone 5α-reduction, we characterized a potent and selective inhibitor of the anterior pituitary and hypothalamic progesterone 5α-reductases (Bertics et al 1984). This is the 4-azasteroid analogue of 5α-DHP, 4-methyl-4-aza-5α-pregnane-3,20-dione (MAPD), which was kindly provided by Merck. By using a specific progesterone 5α-reductase inhibitor in combination with progesterone it may be possible to determine whether progesterone 5α-reduction generates metabolites that are either requisite, duplicative, or not involved in mediating progesterone's effects. One could examine progesterone's effects on processes such as gonadotropin regulation in the presence and absence of this inhibitor and compare them to the effects of 5α-DHP.

Can these ubiquitous progesterone-processing steps generate progesterone-specific target tissue responses in neuroendocrine tissues?

The widespread presence of the described progesterone-processing activities in body tissues might appear to argue against the idea that the *in situ* formation of these metabolites can provide specific target tissue mechanisms for the mediation of some of progesterone's neuroendocrine actions, unless, of course, the biological role of this hormone is greater than is presently envisaged. Many widespread enzymes such as adenylate cyclases, protein kinases and testosterone 5α-reductases, however, do produce tissue-specific effects because of (*inter alia*) tissue differences in the properties of these enzymes and in the levels of product(s) formed, and differences in the responsive cellular processes taking place in specific targets. Similarly, these ubiquitous progesterone-processing steps in neuroendocrine target tissues could generate specificity in their modes of action. Earlier, we reviewed several lines of evidence indicating (1) tissue differences in levels of the various metabolites that could affect subsequent intracellular events in a concentration-dependent manner, (2) relative tissue differences in enzyme activity, and (3) tissue differences in the catalytic and regulatory properties of the three progesterone-processing enzymes. Furthermore, specificity could be endowed by the differentiated function of a particular target tissue wherein only certain progesterone-sensitive processes are being expressed by the genetic machinery of its differentiated cells.

These and other results support the schematic model of progesterone action suggested earlier (Fig. 3), whereby the diverse effects of progesterone may result from the action of progesterone itself or of its metabolites, or from combinations. Processing of progesterone to some of these metabolites could thus provide a means for dissociating the control of progesterone's non-integrative biological functions—for example, effects on erythropoiesis (Karavolas & Nuti 1976, Karavolas et al 1984) as compared to effects on gonadotropin regulation or anaesthesia.

The results also suggest that these neuroendocrine conversions of progesterone may be important mechanisms not only for reducing or ending progesterone's effects but also for generating active metabolites that can mediate or duplicate some of those effects. A number of these metabolites, by duplicating certain effects of progesterone, may also provide a means of prolonging some of the effects of progesterone while others are terminated.

Acknowledgements

Our experimental work was supported by USPHS grants No. HD-05414 and AG 03429 in addition to a Research Career Development Award to H. J. K. (HD 70,006). We acknowledge the valuable contributions to this work made by the following colleagues in addition to those cited: R. Bleier, Y. Cheng, A. E. Colas, J. A. Czaja, D. Goldfoot, R. W. Goy, S. Herf, C. J. Mapletoft, R. K. Meyer, F. Nowak, J. Robinson, D. Smith and B. Sridharan.

References

Bertics PJ, Karavolas HJ 1984 Partial characterization of the microsomal and solubilized hypothalamic progesterone 5α-reductase. J Steroid Biochem 21:305–314

Bertics PJ, Karavolas HJ 1985 Pituitary progesterone 5α-reductase: solubilization and partial characterization. J Steroid Biochem 22:795–802

Bertics PJ, Edman CF, Karavolas HJ 1984 Potent inhibition of the hypothalamic progesterone 5α-reductase by a 5α-dihydroprogesterone analog. J Biol Chem 259:107–111

Bertics SJ, Bertics PJ, Clarke JL, Karavolas HJ 1987 Distribution and ovarian control of progestin-metabolizing enzymes in various rat hypothalamic regions. J Steroid Biochem 26:321–328

Campbell J, Karavolas HJ 1989 The kinetic mechanism of the hypothalamic progesterone 5α-reductase. J Steroid Biochem 32:283–289

Celotti F, Massa R, Martini L 1979 Metabolism of sex steroids in the central nervous system. In: De Groot LJ et al (eds) Endocrinology. Grune & Stratton, New York, vol 1:41–53

Gilles PA, Karavolas HJ 1981 Effect of 20α-dihydroprogesterone, progesterone and their 5α-reduced metabolites on serum gonadotropin levels and hypothalamic LHRH content. Biol Reprod 24:1088–1097

Gorzalka BB, Whalen RE 1977 The effects of progestins, mineralocorticoids, glucocorticoids and steroid solubility on the induction of sexual receptivity in rats. Horm Behav 8:94–99

Hanukoglu I, Karavolas HJ, Goy RW 1977 Progesterone metabolism in the pineal, brain stem, thalamus and corpus callosum of the female rat. Brain Res 125:313–324

Holzbauer M 1976 Physiological aspects of steroids with anaesthetic properties. Med Biol 54:227–242

Karavolas HJ, Nuti KM 1976 Progesterone metabolism by neuroendocrine tissues. In: Naftolin F et al (eds) Subcellular mechanisms in reproductive neuroendocrinology. Elsevier, Amsterdam, p 305–326

Karavolas HJ, Hodges DR, O'Brien DJ 1979 In vivo uptake and metabolism of [^{3}H]progesterone and [^{3}H]5α-dihydroprogesterone by rat CNS and anterior pituitary: tissue concentration of progesterone itself or metabolites? J Steroid Biochem 11:863–872

Karavolas HJ, Bertics PJ, Hodges D, Rudie N 1984 Progesterone processing by neuroendocrine structures. In: Celotti F et al (eds) Metabolism of hormonal steroids in the neuroendocrine structures. Raven Press, New York, p 149–170

Karavolas HJ, Hodges D, Normand N, O'Brien D 1988 Conversion of 17α-hydroxyprogesterone to 5α, 3α and 20α-reduced metabolites by female rat anterior pituitary and hypothalamus. Steroids 51:527–541

Krause JE, Bertics PJ, Karavolas HJ 1981 Ovarian regulation of hypothalamic and pituitary progestin-metabolizing enzyme activities. Endocrinology 108:1–7

Kubli-Garfias C 1984 Physiological role of 5α- and 5β-progesterone metabolites on the CNS. Trends Pharmacol Sci 5:439–442

Lloyd RV, Karavolas HJ 1975 Uptake and conversion of progesterone and testosterone to 5α-reduced products by enriched gonadotropic and chromophobic rat anterior pituitary cell fractions. Endocrinology 97:517–526

Majewska MD 1987 Steroids and brain activity. Biochem Pharmacol 36:3781–3788

Marrone BL, Karavolas HJ 1981 Progesterone metabolism by the hypothalamus, pituitary, and uterus of the rat during pregnancy. Endocrinology 109:41–45

Marrone BL, Karavolas HJ 1982 Progesterone metabolism by the hypothalamus, pituitary, and uterus of the aged rat. Endocrinology 111:162–167

Martini L 1982 The 5α-reduction of testosterone in the neuroendocrine structures. Biochemical and physiological implications. Endocr Rev 3:1–25

Melcangi RC, Celotti F, Negri-Cesi P, Martini L 1985 Testosterone 5α-reductase in discrete hypothalamic nuclear areas in the rat: effect of castration. Steroids 45:347–356

Nuti KM, Karavolas HJ 1977 Effect of progesterone and its 5α-reduced metabolites on gonadotropin levels in estrogen-primed ovariectomized rats. Endocrinology 100:777–781

Rommerts F, Van der Molen HJ 1971 Occurrence and localization of 5α-steroid reductase, 3α- and 17-β-hydroxysteroid dehydrogenases in hypothalamus and other brain tissues of the male rat. Biochim Biophys Acta 248:489–502

Zanisi M, Messi E, Martini L 1984 Physiological role of the 5α-reduced metabolites of progesterone. In: Celotti F et al (eds) Metabolism of hormonal steroids in the neuroendocrine structures. Raven Press, New York, p 171–183

DISCUSSION

Simmonds: The question of a glial or neuronal site for progesterone metabolism is an interesting one. Is there any information on whether glial cells are involved in these metabolic pathways, or is the metabolism all neuronal?

Majewska: Canick and colleagues (1986) showed that most of the 5α-reductase activity is localized in glial cells in rat hypothalamus and Krieger & Scott (1989) identified 3α-hydroxysteroid oxidoreductase also in the glia. Hence, I believe the steroid reduction takes place in the glial compartment, but I would like to know if this process is also neuronal.

Karavolas: When we examined progesterone conversion in separated cell fractions from rat hypothalamus and cerebral cortex (Lloyd et al 1979), we saw no significant differences between fractions enriched with glial cells or neurons. Both fractions converted progesterone to 5α- and 3α-reduced metabolites. I recall Dr Martini published studies relevant to this question; perhaps he can tell us about those results?

Martini: In our experiments we have used adult rats and have measured 5α-reductase activity by evaluating the conversion of labelled testosterone to dihydrotestosterone (DHT); because of the difference in substrates, our results may differ from those of Dr Karavolas. Our experiments were based on the observation that there is more 5α-reductase activity in the subcortical white matter than in the hypothalamus or the cerebral cortex (Melcangi et al 1987). This has been confirmed in the brain of the mouse (Melcangi et al 1987).

In further experiments we looked at different regions of the brain mainly composed of white matter; these were prepared using the microdissection technique of Palkovits. It was found that the 5α-reductase activity was present in practically all white matter structures examined. Particularly high levels of this enzymic activity were present in the hippocampal fimbria, in the cerebellar medulla, in the corticospinal tract and in pontine fibres (Melcangi et al 1988). All the white matter structures studied also possessed relatively low 3α-hydroxysteroid dehydrogenase activity; consequently, low amounts of 5α-androstane-3α,17β-diol (3α-diol) were also recovered.

The next step was to identify the cellular components of the brain that contain the 5α-reductase. This was important in view of the fact that myelin (the major component of the white matter) is manufactured mainly by glial cells. Two different approaches have been used. In the first, neurons and glial components (oligodendrocytes and astrocytes) were isolated from the brain and incubated *in vitro* with testosterone as the substrate. It was found that all three kinds of cells are able to convert testosterone into DHT; neurons appeared to be more active than either oligodendrocytes or astrocytes (R.C. Melcangi, F. Celloti, M. Ballabio, P. Castano, R. Massarelli, A. Poletti & L. Martini, unpublished results). The second approach utilized tissue cultures of neurons and glial cells; it was again found that neurons are much more effective than glial cells in transforming testosterone to DHT. However, active conversion has also been found in glial cells (R. C. Melcangi, F. Celotti, M. Ballabio, P. Castano, R. Massarelli, A. Poletti & L. Martini, unpublished results).

Finally, it has been found that myelin, the major constituent of the white matter, is extremely rich in 5α-reductase activity. This was shown using purified myelin membranes prepared from the whole brain of adult male rats (Melcangi et al 1988). Surprisingly, in the rat, a conspicuous amount of 5α-reductase activity was also found in the sciatic nerve, which is a highly myelinated structure but belonging to the peripheral rather than the central nervous system. The sciatic nerve also formed significant amounts of 3α-diol. When sciatic nerve preparations were obtained from old male rats (20 months), a decrease in both the 5α-reductase and the 3α-hydroxysteroid dehydrogenase activities was recorded (R. C. Melcangi, F. Celotti, M. Ballabio, A. Poletti & L. Martini, unpublished results).

Majewska: What is known about progesterone metabolism in male brains?

Karavolas: I could not cite all the studies in this area, but many other workers have observed similar neuroendocrine conversions of progesterone to 3α-, 5α- and 20α-reduced products as we reported, using not only female but also male rats. In many other species, including humans, these neuroendocrine 3α-, 5α and 20α conversions also occur in both males and females. In addition, there are reports of 5β- and 3β-reduced products in neuroendocrine structures of dogs, hens, and male and female rats. However, in some other body tissues, especially the liver, there is a gender difference, with males producing more of the β isomers.

Majewska: But would the level of progesterone in males be sufficient to satisfy the K_m values for some of these enzymes? Some of them are quite high.

Karavolas: Yes, some of the K_m values for these enzymes for C_{21} substrates in the oxidative direction are in the μM range, as compared to the K_m values in the nM range for substrates in the reductive direction. This may indicate a preferred direction. However, both sets of values are within the range of reported plasma concentrations of these steroids. If these kinetic parameters are similar for the enzymes from males, I believe the levels of progesterone and $3\alpha,5\alpha$-THP secreted by the adrenals (Holzbauer et al 1985) are within these ranges, especially for the reductive direction.

The question of the K_m and relevant physiological levels is, of course, very important. For example, on some progesterone-sensitive biological endpoints, the 5β- and 3β-reduced derivatives appear to be more potent than the 5α-reduced derivatives, but these effects may not be physiologically relevant if the β derivatives are not present, or they are not substrates, or they are present at concentrations that are not relevant. In terms of comparative K_m values or threshold dose responses, a metabolite could be more potent than progesterone (and/or have a lower K_m), but *if* there is always more than enough progesterone present to satisfy its K_m and/or to bring about the effect, it doesn't matter that the K_m for progesterone (or its threshold dose response) is higher than that for the metabolite, because you will always see the effect. In other words, depending upon available levels of these steroids, the differences in K_m values or relative potencies may not matter if adequate levels are present.

Ramirez: The issue of sex difference is an important one. We have shown that progesterone has different effects in the male and in the female. In the female rat and rabbit, progesterone stimulates the luteinizing hormone releasing hormone apparatus, causing release of LHRH, but it does not do so in the male rabbit (Lin & Ramirez 1988). We have also found—and I disagree with Harry Karavolas about this—that the 5β-reduced metabolite of progesterone, 5β-pregnan-3β-ol-20-one, is very effective in releasing LHRH in the female rat and rabbit (Lin & Ramirez 1990).

Karavolas: You are raising an important point in terms of the 5β- and 3β-reduced compound, as compared to 5α- and 3α-reduced compounds. Besides their thresholds for particular effects, we need to consider the metabolites in terms of the amounts being generated—that is, are there sufficient levels present to attain a threshold level? I have followed your work with the 3β,5β-reduced compound with interest and I think there are several possibilities that may explain the situation. First, as you just heard in our paper, we did not see production of 5β-reduced metabolites. This may indicate that none were generated or that the amounts generated were very small and beyond our detection. So it is possible, as with the very small conversion of androgens to oestrogens in brain tissues, that this low conversion, if present, could generate compounds with potent effects and/or different effects.

Secondly, there may be species differences. You may be using a hormone that works in one species (and is normally produced in that species), but, in addition, that steroidal derivative also works in another species although it is not usually produced in that second species. For example, we know that millions of women, for various reasons, are taking, as oestrogen therapy, a preparation of conjugated equine oestrogens: equilin and equilenin (Premarin). Humans, of course, don't produce these oestrogens, yet they are very potent oestrogens in humans.

Thirdly, there are many modified steroid hormones (such as synthetic analogues and isomers) that have been used as pharmacological agents—for example, diethylstilboestrol.

On the question of gender differences, these do exist and there are numerous examples. In addition, the male median eminence has a low capacity to metabolize testosterone, whereas the female median eminence has a very high capacity to metabolize progesterone to these 3α- and 5α-reduced metabolites.

I have no quick, easy answer to this whole problem. We do need to distinguish the effects of pharmacological agents from the effects of physiological levels of natural endogenous substances. We also need to establish whether particular metabolites are present and whether they are being produced *in situ* or are being created elsewhere; for example, the 5α- and 3α-reduced metabolites are produced by the adrenal cortex (Holzbauer et al 1985) and also by the ovary (Ichikawa et al 1974).

Ramirez: You said you considered that there was less than 0.05% conversion of progesterone to the 5β-reduced metabolite. A dose of 10 000 pg of progesterone per ml can stimulate LHRH release in the rabbit. However, although we don't yet know the minimal dose of 5β-pregnan-3β-ol-20-one required, 1 pg has the same effect as 10 000 pg of progesterone. This means that even if less than 0.01% of progesterone has been converted to 5β-pregnan-3β-ol-20-one, it still could exert the effect.

Karavolas: We did not say we had 0.05% conversion to 5β, but that, in those experiments, *if* there were any conversion to the 5β isomer, it would be less than 0.05% of the metabolized radioactivity (see p 24).

Ramirez: The problem is that we see an effect at a concentration below your detection level. With 10 000 pg of progesterone, even with less than 0.05% 5β-reduction, we would still produce 5β-pregnan-3β-ol-20-one in the range 1–10 pg and we get very effective LHRH release with 1 pg of 5β-pregnan-3β-ol-20-one. So I think this matter has not been resolved, because this substance is extremely potent.

Another point is that perhaps the function of 5α-reductase in the brain may be not to generate active metabolites, but to control the production of inactive substances at a specific site in the brain, particularly in the median eminence or the hypothalamus, for example. So instead of 5α-reductase being an element that generates bioactive compounds, it might really provide very fine tune control of the production of inactive metabolites to avoid having high levels of active compounds.

Karavolas: On the second point, as we stated, the generation of inactive metabolites of course is one possibility with all of these metabolites with respect to each of the diverse effects of progesterone. However, in your instance, it may be that you are prejudiced in considering a metabolite to be active on the sole basis of its ability to affect LHRH release with your system. Apparently in your system the 3α- and 5α-reduced metabolites of progesterone are not active, or not as active on LHRH release as the 3β- and 5β-reduced derivatives of progesterone. The point I tried to make is that some of these metabolites of progesterone are inactive metabolites on some parameters but active on others;

that is to say, they share some but not all of the diverse effects of progesterone. In your particular system, 5α-DHP or 3α,5α-THP may be inactive metabolites, but someone else examining a different endpoint will report that these are active metabolites in their test system. We must consider the broad and diverse range of all the effects of progesterone and its metabolites. We are not saying that these progestin-metabolizing enzymes generate only active metabolites with all of progesterone's actions. I stated that an array of metabolites are generated that are active on some but not all of the different biological effects ascribed to progesterone. To put it another way, there is an array of metabolites produced and some may be inactive on a particular biological effect.

Martini: Can you suggest a role for the 5α-reductase present in the uterus?

Karavolas: As you know, in these same *in vivo* studies with progesterone, we also obtained conversion to 5α- and 3α-reduced metabolites in the uterus. However, 5α-DHP was not selectively accumulated when compared to muscle tissue levels. Progesterone itself was selectively accumulated only after oestrogen treatment. Some 3α,5α-tetrahydroprogesterone was also selectively accumulated by the uterus. Neither 5α-DHP nor 3α,5α-THP has any of the classical uterine progestational effects, such as pregnancy maintenance, decidual reactions or inhibition of parturition. However, the selective accumulation of 3α,5α-THP may be linked to some of the effects that it reportedly has on uterine motility. In these same studies, there was no selective accumulation of 5α-DHP by the uterus when 5α-DHP was given intravenously. All in all, these results on the selective accumulation of progesterone, 5α-DHP and 3α,5α-THP by the uterus agree quite well with what we know about the uterine effects of progesterone and its metabolites and the need for oestrogen priming.

As you know, the 5α-reductase enzyme is widely distributed and present in a number of non-target tissues. Consequently, it is important to correlate these types of results with biological effects of progesterone and metabolites relevant to particular tissues.

Martini: You may be right; but what evidence have you to suggest that the 5α-reductase in the uterus physiologically converts progesterone to dihydroprogesterone and not testosterone to DHT?

Karavolas: That's a good question which we can approach by looking at the characteristics of the enzymes. To use an analogy, enzymes such as aldose reductase and sorbitol dehydrogenase, when presented with high glucose levels well within the range of their K_m values, can catalyse the formation of significant amounts of compounds such as sorbitol that can be harmful to some membranes. However, glucose levels are seldom high enough to be in range of their K_m values, except in diabetes. In the case of the steroid 5α-reductase, the K_m values clearly show that progesterone is the favoured substrate by two orders of magnitude over testosterone and by three orders of magnitude over glucocorticoids. Of course, if there is sufficient testosterone, there will be competition with progesterone. In addition, 17α-hydroxyprogesterone and

20α-dihydroprogesterone are effective competitors for 5α-reductase, acting as alternative substrates. Thus these progestins would not only generate their own 5α-reduced metabolites, but they could also (by competition) influence the 5α-reduction of testosterone or progesterone.

Martini: I agree. Even in the prostate, the affinity of the 5α-reductase for progesterone is twice as high as that for testosterone.

Makriyannis: It seems to me that the 3α-hydroxysteroid oxidoreductase activity causes drastic changes in the molecular features of the steroids involved. I would expect the conversion of the ketone group to a hydroxyl group to have some impact on the uptake of the steroid. Is there any information about differences in uptake profiles?

Karavolas: We have no information on the *in vivo* neuroendocrine uptake of 3α,5α-THP. We have always wanted to look at that in order to assess back-conversion of 3α,5α-THP to 5α-DHP in neuroendocrine target tissues.

In terms of classical *in vitro* sequestration mechanisms, we have observed binding of 5α-DHP to cytosolic progesterone receptors in the anterior pituitary and hypothalamus, but not binding of 3α,5α-THP, or the corresponding 5β- and 3β-reduced compounds.

Makriyannis: I am not aware how much is known about the transport of these steroids into cells through the membrane, but I would expect to see differences, depending on their chemical structures.

Karavolas: There are differences, of course; but, in addition, because of the lipophilic nature of steroids, tissues with high lipid content such as neural and adipose tissues can non-selectively accumulate high levels of steroids such as progesterone. Because of this, we did not use muscle as a non-target comparison tissue. To obtain a fair comparison with neural target tissues, we used cerebral cortex as a putative non-target tissue, since there could be high non-specific associations of these steroids with the high lipid containing neural tissues.

Simmonds: The uptake of those steroids will be complicated by the fact that the 3-hydroxy group is a site for conjugation with sulphate or acetate groups, for example. That is bound to affect their uptake. Is there any information on the ratios of conjugated forms, as compared to the free steroid?

Karavolas: There can be many such problems with *in vivo* use of 3α-reduced compounds. Passage through the liver is a special problem. Selye (1942) used hepatectomized rats to eliminate the complicating influence of the liver where several hydroxylations can take place and where these conjugated forms are produced.

The 3α- and 3β-reduced metabolites do not appear to have much affinity for the progesterone receptor. I think Dr Baulieu and Dr McEwen would both agree on that?

Baulieu: Yes.

McEwen: I agree that they don't bind to the intracellular progesterone receptor very well.

Majewska: If the 5α,3α-reduced steroid metabolites are synthesized in neurons, perhaps their cellular uptake may not be essential for their putative actions on neurons, because these steroids may be neuronal internal modulators.

Karavolas: Yes, exactly.

Majewska: According to Kraulis and colleagues (1975) there is very little or no 5β-reductase in the CNS, but I think the enzyme is quite active in the liver, so the 5β-reduced metabolites in the CNS may originate from the periphery.

Karavolas: That is an important point. Also, as previously mentioned, there is a sex difference in the rat liver with regard to production of the α- versus β-reduced metabolites (For example, see Crane et al 1970).

Baulieu: There is also a sex difference in steroid metabolism in humans (Baulieu et al 1963).

McEwen: Luciano Martini's data on the high levels of testosterone metabolism in myelin suggest that perhaps some steroid hormone conversion may be external and therefore the metabolites can more easily bind to membrane receptors.

Baulieu: Like Harry Karavolas, we could not demonstrate the formation of C_{19} steroids (androgens) from C_{21} steroids in brain preparations. I think that conjugation of hydroxylated 5α-reduced compounds may be important in your experiments. I imagine that the values you showed were obtained after simple extraction with only organic solvents. Did you do hydrolysis, which would allow you to recover larger amounts of steroids?

Karavolas: We did not lose any product(s). We extracted with 80% ethanol and we accounted for all the incubated radioactivity.

Baulieu: You alluded to some unidentified, polar metabolites. We have some evidence for 7α-hydroxysteroid hydroxylase activity in brain, though I don't know what effects 7α-hydroxylated compounds have in the brain.

Martini: We have also found 7α- and 6α-hydroxy triols in the brain.

Majewska: What is known about *de novo* synthesis of progesterone in the brain? Is it synthesized to some extent, or does it have to come from peripheral tissues?

Baulieu: We find progesterone in the brain, at a concentration of about 1 ng/g of total male rat brain tissue. So, is there steroid synthesis in neural cells in the brain? Cholesterol is the steroid precursor. We have demonstrated that C_{27} cholesterol can be converted to the C_{21} steroid pregnenolone in the CNS, using immunocytochemistry to identify, in the white matter of the caudate nucleus and other parts of the brain, the three enzymes which form the complex that transforms cholesterol to pregnenolone (LeGoascogne et al 1987, Robel & Baulieu 1990). Studies using cells in culture suggest that this metabolism may occur in oligodendrocytes, but not in astrocytes. So, mevalonate can be converted to cholesterol in oligodendrocytes and then cholesterol can be transformed to pregnenolone. In oligodendrocytes, pregnenolone can be transformed to 20α-hydroxypregnenolone. We have isolated pregnenolone from the brain as free, sulphated and fatty ester forms.

Pregnenolone was identified and quantified by mass spectrometry and radioimmunoassay (Corpéchot et al 1983, Jo et al 1989). We have found progesterone synthesis from pregnenolone in oligodendrocytes in culture, and also in astrocytes, but not in neurons (Jung-Testas et al 1989), but we do not know if this occurs *in vivo*.

We have found dehydroepiandrosterone (3-hydroxyandrost-5-en-17-one) in the rat brain, but we do not know how it occurs there (Corpéchot et al 1981). We find it even in adrenalectomized and castrated animals, so we don't think it comes from the periphery. There is some evidence that dehydroepiandrosterone and its sulphate ester have an effect on the GABA receptor (Mienville 1988). So I think we should not concentrate only on the production of reduced metabolites of progesterone; there are other compounds that may be important in the brain. We call 'neurosteroids' those steroids which are synthesized in the brain, in contrast to 'imported' steroids.

Karavolas: We also have looked at the neuroendocrine metabolism of cholesterol (unpublished). We were interested in this problem many years ago because some neuroendocrinologists were using implants of cholesterol as a control reference in implant studies with progesterone and oestrogen. In our studies we observed a large array of unidentified metabolites, other than those Etienne Baulieu described. After incubation with radioactive cholesterol, the recovered radioactivity was associated with compounds other than pregnenolone and progesterone. These unidentified metabolites could be other yet-to-be determined potent modulators or inactive degradation products. Of course, cholesterol is an important component of membranes and needs to be synthesized *in situ* to maintain functional membranes and cell growth.

In short, there is extensive steroid processing in the brain, and our studies of the neuroendocrine processing are only part of the steroid metabolism picture.

Majewska: We have to remember that there are very high concentrations of cholesterol and its sulphate in the synaptic regions in the brain. For example, Iwamori et al (1976) reported that there is about 15 µg/g of cholesterol sulphate in rat brain. Moreover, the highest level of cholesterol sulphate was found in the subcellular fraction of nerve endings, being about 10 times higher than the level in the mitochondrial fraction. Hence, it is likely that these steroids have a function in the CNS.

Baulieu: There is approximately 10 µg per gram of cholesterol sulphate in the rat brain, which is a very high concentration.

Bäckström: I would like to add to the discussion about production of steroids in the brain. We have looked at concentrations of steroid in different areas of the rat brain, using a pregnant mare serum gonadotropin (PMSG) model in which there is high oestradiol production from the ovary before ovulation but very low production of progesterone; after ovulation there is high progesterone production by the ovary but very low production of oestradiol. When progesterone concentrations in the rat brain were studied, all areas had a significantly higher progesterone concentration during the time of high production of the hormone by the ovary. In the cerebral cortex, the progesterone concentration during the period of high progesterone production by the ovary was very high, 300 times the concentration found before ovulation (Bixo et al 1986). As Harry Karavolas used the cerebral cortex as a reference area in his studies, perhaps these findings could be of importance.

We have also looked at progesterone levels in human brain tissue obtained from women who were killed as a result of accidents during the luteal phase. We studied 17 brain areas and found a significantly higher concentration of progesterone in all these brain areas in comparison to control tissue from post-menopausal women (M. Bixo, B. Winblad & T. Bäckström, unpublished). So the peripheral production of progesterone, and also oestradiol, certainly does have an impact on concentrations in the brain.

Turner: The anterior pituitary 3α-hydroxysteroid oxidoreductase enzyme that Harry Karavolas described is cytosolic, NADPH dependent, and has a relative molecular mass of 36 000. These are characteristics of the family of aldo/keto reductases. The functions of these enzymes are rather unclear, but they metabolize a wide range of aromatic aldehydes. Does this enzyme belong to that family? I believe these enzymes are inhibited by barbiturates and certain other anti-convulsants. Do you know whether this enzyme is inhibited by barbiturates?

Karavolas: I don't know if barbiturates inhibit the cytosolic 3α-hydroxysteroid oxidoreductase but indomethacin does. As you know, liver 3α-hydroxysteroid oxidoreductase also has dihydrodiol activity. Penning et al (1984, 1985) have looked at the liver and brain enzymes, but the brain enzyme does not have dihydrodiol dehydrogenase activity. We, too, found that the pituitary 3α-hydroxysteroid oxidoreductase was different from the liver enzyme in this respect. The enzymic activity in the liver and its regulation is very different from the pituitary and hypothalamic enzymes.

Turner: It might be worth looking to see if barbiturates and other anticonvulsants do affect the anterior pituitary enzyme.

Karavolas: Yes; that is a very important point that needs to be examined. On a related point, some years ago R.K. Meyer examined phenobarbitone blockade of ovulation using a rat model treated with PMSG (Ying & Meyer 1969). One of his ideas to explain this blockade of ovulation was that phenobarbitone, besides affecting the neuroendocrine ovulation process, might also have an effect on steroidogenesis. We did a collaborative project and there appeared to be an inhibition of 3β-hydroxysteroid dehydrogenase in the ovary and adrenal (Gupta & Karavolas 1973a,b).

Smith: You mentioned that phosphatidylcholine altered the activity of the 5α-reductase enzyme. Do you think variations in phospholipids in different CNS areas might account for some of the variations in localization of the various progesterone metabolites that you saw? Also, how does phosphatidylcholine actually inhibit the enzyme?

Karavolas: Yes, it is possible that phospholipids could account for these variations, but I don't know how phosphatidylcholine inhibits the enzyme.

de Kloet: The issue of ovarian control of the steroid-metabolizing enzyme activity is very interesting. You showed that ovariectomy actually increased 5α-reductase activity; yet when you treated with oestradiol you only partially reversed this effect. You also showed changes in the amount of the same enzyme activity during the oestrous cycle. Do you have any clues about the mechanism by which oestrogens have this effect? Is it a genomic effect involving intracellular receptors, or does oestradiol affect a membrane mechanism? Is the amount of enzyme protein increased, or are the cofactors affected?

Karavolas: That's a very important question. Because we found only partial restoration of normal levels of enzymic activity, we followed up some observations that Dr Martini had published on the 5α-reduction of progesterone (Stupnicka et al 1977). As with those studies, we also administered higher doses of oestradiol for longer periods of time. However, higher doses were not effective in further reducing the elevated activity. On the other hand, longer periods of oestrogen administration (7–8 days) did lower the elevated activity even further, but not completely to the levels observed in intact animals. We then examined other ovarian factors that might fully restore 5α-reductase activity to the levels in intact rats and we found progesterone had some effects.

Is it a genomic effect? I don't know if there is a change in the number of enzyme molecules or if an active form of the enzyme is being converted to an inactive form. Another possibility is that the enzyme is deactivated by phosphorylation or dephosphorylation schemes. When we directly examined the effects of oestradiol we found that high, non-physiological doses of oestradiol could inhibit enzyme activity.

These are all good questions that need to be investigated. The elevation of 5α-reductase activity after ovariectomy takes several days, so the time scale would suggest that genomic processes are being affected, but I have no definitive data.

de Kloet: I thought the 5α-reductase activity decreased after treatment with oestradiol, and increased after ovariectomy.

Karavolas: That's right. Oestradiol could be initiating an inactivating process (e.g., generating a competitor for the 5α-reductase), or it could be generating a protease that breaks down the enzyme. Ovariectomy could thus be eliminating an inhibitory factor(s). All of these are possible explanations.

References

Baulieu EE, Robel P, Mauvais-Jarvis P 1963 Différences du métabolisme des androgènes chez l'homme et chez la femme. CR Hebd Seances Acad Sci Ser D Sci Nat 256:1016–1018

Bixo M, Bäckström T, Winblad B, Selstam G, Andersson A 1986 Comparison between pre- and postovulatory distribution of oestradiol and progesterone in the brain of the PMSG-treated rat. Acta Physiol Scand 128:241–246

Canick JA, Vaccaro DE, Livingston E, Leeman SE, Ryan KJ, Fox TO 1986 Localization of aromatase and 5α-reductase to neuronal and non-neuronal cells in the fetal rat hypothalamus. Brain Res 372:277–283

Corpéchot C, Robel P, Axelson M, Sjovall J, Baulieu EE 1981 Characterization and measurement of dehydroepiandrosterone sulfate in the rat brain. Proc Natl Acad Sci USA 78:4704-4707

Corpéchot C, Synguelakis M, Talha S et al 1983 Pregnenolone and its sulfate ester in the rat brain. Brain Res 270:119-125

Crane M, Loring J, Villee CA 1970 Progesterone metabolism in regenerating rat liver. Endocrinology 87:80–83

Gupta C, Karavolas HJ 1973a Lowered ovarian conversion of ^{14}C-pregnenolone to progesterone and other metabolites during phenobarbital (PB) block of PMS-induced ovulation in immature rats: inhibition of 3β-hydroxysteroid dehydrogenation. Endocrinology 92:117–124

Gupta C, Karavolas HJ 1973b Adrenal steroid biosynthesis from 4–^{14}C-cholesterol (*in vitro*) during phenobarbital block of PMS-induced ovulation in immature rats. Endocrinology 92:1200–1207

Holzbauer M, Birmingham MK, De Nicola AF, Oliver JT 1985 In vivo secretion of 3α-hydroxy-5α-pregnan-20-one, a potent anaesthetic steroid, by the adrenal gland of the rat. J Steroid Biochem 22:97–102

Ichikawa S, Sawada T, Nakamura Y, Morioka H 1974 Ovarian secretion of pregnane compounds during the estrous cycle and pregnancy in rats. Endocrinology 94:1615–1620

Iwamori M, Moser HW, Kishimoto Y 1976 Cholesterol sulfate in rat tissues. Tissue distribution, developmental change and brain subcellular localization. Biochim Biophys Acta 441:268–279

Jo DH, Ait Abdallah M, Young J, Baulieu EE, Robel P 1989 Pregnenolone, dehydroepiandrosterone, and their sulfate and fatty acid esters in the rat brain. Steroids 54:287–297

Jung-Testas I, Hu ZY, Baulieu EE, Robel P 1989 Neurosteroids: biosynthesis of pregnenolone and progesterone in primary cultures of rat glial cells. Endocrinology 125:2083–2091

Kraulis I, Foldes G, Traikov H, Dubrovsky B, Birmingham MK 1975 Distribution, metabolism and biological activity of deoxycorticosterone in the central nervous system. Brain Res 88:1–14

Krieger NR, Scott RG 1989 Nonneuronal localization for steroid converting enzyme: 3α-hydroxysteroid oxidoreductase in olfactory tubercle of rat brain. J Neurochem 52:1866–1870

LeGoascogne C, Robel P, Gouézou M, Sananès N, Baulieu EE, Waterman M 1987 Neurosteroids: cytochrome P450$_{scc}$ in the rat brain. Science (Wash DC) 237:1212–1214

Lin WW, Ramirez VD 1988 Effect of pulsatile infusion of progesterone on the *in vivo* activity of the luteinizing hormone-releasing hormone neural apparatus of awake unrestrained female and male rabbits. Endocrinology 122:868–876

Lin WW, Ramirez VD 1990 Infusion of progestins into the hypothalamus of female New Zealand white rabbits: effect on *in vivo* luteinizing hormone-releasing hormone release as determined with push-pull perfusion. Endocrinology 126:261–272

Lloyd RV, Gilles P, Karavolas HJ 1979 Uptake and metabolism of female sex steroids by isolated small neurons and other cell fractions from the rat medial basal hypothalamus. Steroids 33:97–113

Melcangi RC, Celotti F, Poletti A, Negri-Cesi P, Martini L 1987 The 5alpha-reductase activity of the subcortical white matter, the cerebral cortex, and the hypothalamus of the rat and of the mouse: possible sex differences and effect of castration. Steroids 49:259–270

Melcangi RC, Celotti F, Ballabio M, Poletti A, Castano P, Martini L 1988 Testosterone 5alpha-reductase activity in the rat brain is highly concentrated in white matter structures and in purified myelin sheaths of axons. J Steroid Biochem 31:173–179

Mienville JM 1988 Pregnenolone sulfate and anionic currents. PhD dissertation, Georgetown University, Washington DC, USA

Penning TM, Mukharji I, Barrows S, Talalay P 1984 Purification and properties of a 3α-hydroxysteroid dehydrogenase of rat liver cytosol and its inhibition by anti-inflammatory drugs. Biochem J 222:601–611

Penning TM, Sharp RB, Krieger NR 1985 Purification of 3α-hydroxysteroid dehydrogenase from rat brain cytosol: inhibition by nonsteroidal anti-inflammatory drugs and progestins. J Biol Chem 260:15266–15272

Robel P, Baulieu EE 1990 Les neurostéroides: une nouvelle fonction du cerveau? Médecine Sciences 6:252–260

Selye H 1942 Correlations between the chemical structure and pharmacological actions of the steroids. Endocrinology 30:437–453

Stupnicka E, Massa R, Zanisi M, Martini L 1977 Role of anterior pituitary and hypothalamic metabolism of progesterone in the control of gonadotropin secretion. Prog Reprod Biol 2:88–95

Ying SY, Meyer RK 1969 Effect of steroids on neuropharmacologic blockade of ovulation in pregnant mare's serum (PMS) primed immature rats. Endocrinology 84:1466–1474

Steroid modulation of the GABA$_A$ receptor complex: electrophysiological studies

Jeremy J. Lambert, John A. Peters, Nicholas C. Sturgess and Tim G. Hales

Neuroscience Research Group, Department of Pharmacology & Clinical Pharmacology, Ninewells Hospital & Medical School, Dundee University, Dundee DD1 9SY, UK

Abstract. The effect of some endogenous and synthetic steroids on the operation of inhibitory and excitatory amino acid neurotransmitter receptors was examined. Anaesthetic pregnane steroids (e.g. alphaxalone, 5α-pregnan-3α-ol-20-one, 5α-pregnane-3α,21-diol-20-one) potentiated GABA$_A$ receptor-mediated whole-cell currents recorded from bovine chromaffin cells. The threshold concentration for enhancement was 10–30 nM. Potentiation was stereoselective and was mediated by a steroid-induced prolongation of the burst duration of the GABA-activated channel. Additionally, the pregnane steroids directly activated the GABA$_A$ receptor. Both the potentiation and activation appear to be mediated through a site(s) distinct from the well-known barbiturate and benzodiazepine allosteric sites of the GABA$_A$ receptor. Intracellularly applied alphaxalone and 5β-pregnan-3α-ol-20-one had no discernible effects on the GABA$_A$ receptor, suggesting that the steroid binding site can only be accessed extracellularly. Unlike behaviourally depressant barbiturates, which modulate GABA$_A$ receptor function in a manner similar to that of the pregnane steroids, alphaxalone and 5β-pregnan-3α-ol-20-one show striking pharmacological selectivity. Voltage-clamp recordings from rat central neurons in culture indicate that pentobarbitone exerts its potentiating and GABA-mimetic effects over a range of concentrations which also depress currents mediated by glutamate receptor subtypes. In contrast, alphaxalone and several endogenous steroids greatly enhance responses to GABA, but have no direct effect on glutamate receptors. Such pharmacological selectivity, coupled with appropriate stereoselectivity of action, suggests that the GABA$_A$ receptor mediates some of the behavioural effects of synthetic and endogenous pregnane steroids.

1990 Steroids and neuronal activity. Wiley, Chichester (Ciba Foundation Symposium 153) p 56–82

A number of steroid hormones are known to act in the central nervous system to exert marked behavioural effects. Many of these effects are thought to be mediated by an interaction with intracellular receptors that results in gene-controlled changes in protein synthesis (McEwen 1985). However, a number of pregnane steroids are potent, rapidly acting, general anaesthetics (Gyermek

& Soyka 1975). The fast onset of the central depressant actions of these steroids seems inconsistent with a genomic mechanism.

A more plausible hypothesis, that steroids may induce anaesthesia by enhancing inhibitory transmission within the central nervous system, has recently received considerable support. Electrophysiological experiments using the rat cuneate nucleus slice preparation demonstrated that the synthetic steroid alphaxalone (5α-pregnan-3α-ol-11,20-dione), which is a potent general anaesthetic, selectively potentiates extracellularly recorded responses to the inhibitory neurotransmitter GABA and GABA$_A$ receptor agonist muscimol (Harrison & Simmonds 1984). Interestingly, the behaviourally inactive isomer betaxalone (5α-pregnan-3β-ol-11,20-dione) was without effect (Harrison & Simmonds 1984). Consistent with these observations is the finding that alphaxalone potentiates GABA-evoked chloride currents recorded under voltage-clamp conditions from rodent central neurons and bovine adrenomedullary chromaffin cells maintained in cell culture (Barker et al 1987, Cottrell et al 1987). This effect is not restricted to synthetic steroids, because endogenous metabolites of progesterone and deoxycorticosterone are also active (Majewska et al 1986).

In the study reported here and in previous studies (Cottrell et al 1987, Callachan et al 1987, Lambert et al 1987, Peters et al 1988, Lambert & Peters 1989) we have used the voltage-clamp technique to investigate the effects of some synthetic and endogenous steroids on the GABA$_A$ receptors of bovine chromaffin cells and rat hippocampal neurons. The results demonstrate that some steroids are potent and highly selective modulators of the GABA$_A$ receptor, such modulation being likely to contribute to the central actions of these agents.

Methods

Bovine adrenomedullary chromaffin cells and rat hippocampal neurons were isolated and maintained in culture as previously described (Cottrell et al 1987, Halliwell et al 1989). Mouse spinal neurons were prepared using the method of Ransom et al (1977) with minor modifications. Agonist-activated currents were recorded under voltage-clamp conditions from whole cells and outside-out membrane patches using standard techniques (Hamill et al 1981). The extracellular solution routinely employed in recordings from chromaffin cells and central neurons consisted of (in mM): NaCl 140, KCl 2.8, MgCl$_2$ 2.0, CaCl$_2$ 1.0 and Hepes 10 (pH 7.2). Currents evoked by N-methyl-D-aspartate (NMDA) on central neurons were recorded in the nominal absence of Mg^{2+}, and were potentiated by the inclusion of glycine (1 μM) in the perfusate. Tetrodotoxin (100–300 nM) was used to suppress spontaneous synaptic currents in spinal and hippocampal neuron cultures. In most recordings cells were dialysed with a patch pipette solution containing (in mM): CsCl 140, MgCl$_2$ 2.0, CaCl$_2$ 0.1, EGTA 1.1 and Hepes 10 (pH 7.2). When the effects of barbiturate and steroid compounds on membrane currents evoked by glutamate receptor agonists were studied, a pipette solution containing (in mM) K gluconate 132, KCl 11, $MgCl_2$ 2.0, $CaCl_2$ 0.1, EGTA 1.1 and Hepes 10 (pH 7.2) was used. By clamping the membrane potential close to the theoretical Cl^- equilibrium potential of -58 mV, Cl^- currents evoked by the direct agonist action of barbiturates and steroids were minimized, allowing currents mediated by glutamate receptors to be recorded in relative isolation. Agonists were applied locally by pressure ejection (1.4×10^5 Pa) from modified patch pipettes or by ionophoresis. All experiments were conducted at room temperature (17–21 °C). Data were stored and analysed essentially as described previously (e.g. Peters et al 1988).

Results and discussion

Steroids modulate the GABA_A receptor in a stereoselective manner

Our initial investigations, performed on voltage-clamped bovine adreno-medullary chromaffin cells in culture, confirmed that alphaxalone potentiates the GABA-evoked chloride current that underlies the effect of $GABA_A$ receptor agonists on the membrane potential of central and peripheral neurones (cf. Harrison & Simmonds 1984). In brief, bath application of alphaxalone (30 nM–1 µM) produced a rapid, dose-dependent, and fully reversible potentiation of the amplitude and duration of submaximal chloride currents evoked by locally applied GABA (100 µM) (Cottrell et al 1987). Subsequently, structurally related endogenous steroids derived from the reductive metabolism of progesterone were found to mimic the effect of alphaxalone on GABA-induced currents in chromaffin cells (Callachan et al 1987). The pregnane steroids 5α-pregnan-3α-ol-20-one, 5β-pregnan-3α-ol-20-one (Fig. 1A) and the deoxycorticosterone metabolite 5α-pregnane-3α,21-diol-20-one were particularly potent in this respect, producing threshold enhancement of GABA responses in the concentration range 10–30 nM (Callachan et al 1987, Lambert & Peters 1989).

The enhancement by pregnane steroids of responses to GABA shows marked stereoselectivity. The possession of a hydroxyl group in the α-configuration at C–3 of the steroid A ring is an important determinant of potency . Unlike their corresponding 3α-ol isomers, 5β-pregnan-3β-ol-20-one (Fig. 1A), 5α-pregnan-3β-ol-20-one and betaxalone (the 3β-ol isomer of alphaxalone) are inactive at nanomolar concentrations and act as either weak potentiators or antagonists of GABA-evoked currents at higher doses (1–100 µM) (Cottrell et al 1987, Peters et al 1988). The importance of the hydroxyl group at C–3 is further emphasized by the finding that its oxidation, as in 5β-pregnane-3,20-dione, results in a dramatic loss of potency (Callachan et al 1987).

5α-Pregnan-3α-ol-20-one and 5β-pregnan-3α-ol-20-one, each applied to chromaffin cells at concentrations of 30 and 100 nM, enhanced GABA-evoked currents in a concentration dependent manner; at each concentration tested, the degree of potentiation produced by the two steroids was similar (Peters et al 1988). This indicates that pregnane steroids with *cis* or *trans* A/B ring conformations are equally effective in enhancing the actions of GABA. Electrophysiological studies on rat hippocampal neurons maintained in culture substantiate the above conclusions and additionally demonstrate that a reduced pregnane skeleton and a C–20 ketone moiety are essential for potent enhancement of GABA-evoked currents (Harrison et al 1987a). Such structural criteria are also apparent in radioligand binding studies examining the steroid-induced displacement of [^{35}S] *t*-butylbicyclophosphorothionate (TBPS) from rat brain synaptosomal membranes (Harrison et al 1987a). However, the structure–activity relationship determined in chromaffin and neuronal cell cultures does not entirely agree with that found in rat brain slice preparations. Extracellularly recorded depolarizing responses to muscimol in the cuneate slice are potentiated by 3β-hydroxy pregnane steroids which are either inactive or very weakly active in isolated cell preparations (Turner & Simmonds 1989). Additionally, although alphaxalone is reported to be equally effective as (Harrison et al 1987a) or less effective (Lambert & Peters 1989) than either 5α- or 5β-pregnan-3α-ol-20-one in culture systems, its potency in potentiating muscimol in the cuneate slice greatly exceeds that of any other from a broad range of steroids examined (Turner & Simmonds 1989). Methodological differences may contribute to these discrepancies.

Mechanism of steroid-induced potentiation of the GABA$_A$ receptor

The mechanism by which the active pregnane steroids potentiate GABA$_A$ receptor-mediated events has been addressed directly by observing their influence on single-channel currents activated by GABA on outside-out membrane patches excised from bovine chromaffin cells. Figure 1B illustrates representative data segments of channel activity evoked by 1 μM GABA alone, and by GABA applied with 5β-pregnan-3α-ol-20-one (300 nM). The predominant effect of the steroid was to prolong the burst duration of channel currents elicited by GABA (Callachan et al 1987). 5α-Pregnan-3α-ol-20-one (100 nM–1 μM) shares this effect (Lambert et al 1987), and fluctuation analysis of macroscopic currents elicited by GABA in mouse spinal neurons in culture suggests that alphaxalone also greatly prolongs the burst duration of channels activated by GABA (Barker et al 1987). Attempts to analyse in detail the kinetic behaviour of channel events evoked by GABA in the presence or absence of pregnane steroids have been hindered by the occurrence of multiple conductance states, and also by an apparent direct agonist action of the steroids at the GABA$_A$ receptor (see Callachan et al 1987, Lambert & Peters 1989, and below). A simple analysis of the data indicates that the channel-open state probability is dramatically enhanced by steroids and that this effect might be largely accounted for by the increased burst duration of single-channel currents (Lambert & Peters 1989).

60

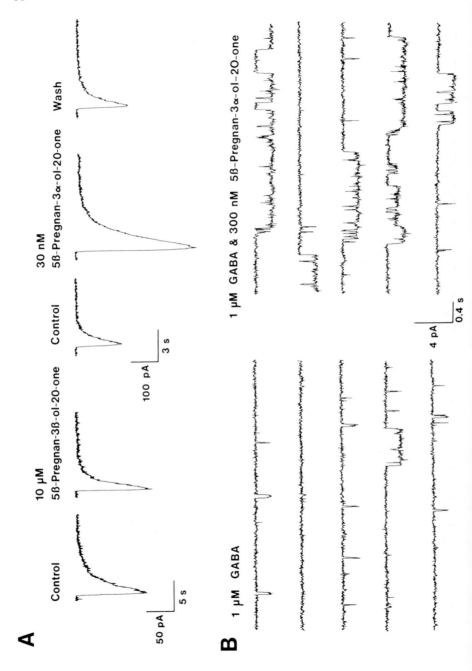

The increased burst duration presumably underlies the ability of alphaxalone (Harrison et al 1987b) and endogenous pregnane steroids (Harrison et al 1987a) to prolong $GABA_A$ receptor-mediated inhibitory postsynaptic currents in hippocampal neurons in culture.

Steroids directly activate the GABA_A receptor

At concentrations higher than those required for threshold enhancement of GABA-evoked currents, alphaxalone and some other pregnane steroids apparently directly activate the $GABA_A$ receptor. Figure 2A illustrates inward currents recorded from bovine chromaffin cells in response to locally applied alphaxalone (100 µM). Such currents were reversibly antagonized by the $GABA_A$ receptor antagonist bicuculline (3 µM) and markedly enhanced by barbiturates such as phenobarbitone. Additionally, alphaxalone elicited currents which reversed in sign at the chloride equilibrium potential, and evoked single-channel currents on outside-out membrane patches which displayed a mainstate conductance ($\approx 30 \, pS$) close to that of GABA-evoked channels (Cottrell et al 1987). Similar results have been obtained with 5β-pregnan-3α-ol-20-one and 5β-pregnane-3,20-dione (Callachan et al 1987). Although these initial studies used relatively high steroid concentrations (10–100 µM), we have also observed single-channel activity on patches excised from bovine chromaffin cells in response to far lower concentrations of these compounds ($\approx 300 \, nM$; Fig. 2B). Additionally, in experiments on rat hippocampal neurons in culture, alphaxalone elicited substantial and dose-dependent inward currents over the same range of concentrations (100 nM–1 µM) that were effective in potentiating GABA (J. A. Peters & J. J. Lambert, unpublished work 1989). However, it should be borne in mind that such effects might, at least in part, reflect a potentiating action of alphaxalone on background levels of GABA in CNS cultures, where GABAergic synapses can readily be demonstrated (e.g. Harrison et al 1987b). Results obtained from chromaffin cells, and particularly from membrane patches excised from them, may prove more reliable in this respect.

FIG. 1. *(opposite)*   The stereoselectivity and mechanism of steroid action. (A) Inward currents in response to locally applied GABA (100 µM) recorded from a voltage-clamped bovine chromaffin cell. Each trace is the computer-generated average of five consecutive responses recorded at a holding potential of $-60 \, mV$. Bath-applied 5β-pregnan-3β-ol-20-one (10 µM) has little effect on the response to GABA, whereas the corresponding 3α-hydroxy isomer, at a concentration of 30 nM, more than doubles response amplitude. (B) Single channels recorded from an outside-out membrane patch in the presence of 1 µM GABA alone and during co-perfusion of 5β-pregnan-3α-ol-20-one (300 nM). Note that the steroid primarily acts to increase the burst duration of GABA-activated channel currents. The five traces illustrated in each panel are consecutive. Channel activity was recorded at a holding potential of $-60 \, mV$.

A

Alphaxalone Currents

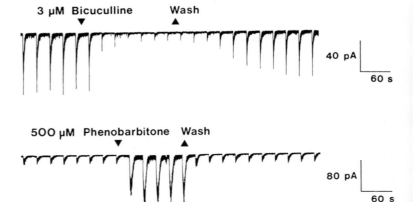

3 μM Bicuculline   Wash

40 pA
60 s

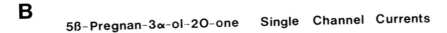

500 μM Phenobarbitone   Wash

80 pA
60 s

B

5ß-Pregnan-3α-ol-2O-one   Single Channel Currents

Control

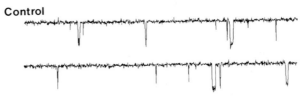

500 μM Phenobarbitone

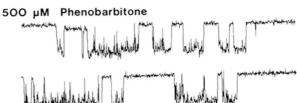

Wash

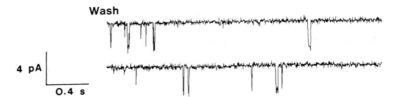

4 pA

0.4 s

The site of steroid action

Several lines of evidence suggest that the pregnane steroids do not potentiate GABA-induced currents by interacting with the allosteric benzodiazepine recognition site of the GABA$_A$ receptor–channel complex. Firstly, the potentiation observed with alphaxalone, 5β-pregnan-3α-ol-20-one or 5β-pregnane-3,20-dione is unaffected by the benzodiazepine receptor antagonist flumazenil (Ro 15-1788). Secondly, currents elicited by high concentrations (10–100 μM) of these steroids are greatly potentiated by the benzodiazepine agonist diazepam (Cottrell et al 1987, Callachan et al 1987, J. A. Peters & J. J. Lambert, unpublished work 1988).

The evidence excluding the barbiturate recognition site associated with the GABA$_A$ receptor as the locus of steroid action is less direct. Electrophysiological studies have demonstrated that membrane currents evoked by alphaxalone (100 μM; Fig. 2A) and 5β-pregnan-3α-ol-20-one (30 μM) are enhanced by phenobarbitone (Callachan et al 1987, Cottrell et al 1987). As with barbiturate enhancement of responses to GABA, a prolongation of the open-time of agonist-evoked channels by phenobarbitone appears to be responsible (Fig. 2B). The interaction between barbiturates and steroids is reciprocal, in that membrane currents elicited by pentobarbitone (1 mM) can be greatly enhanced by 5β-pregnan-3α-ol-20-one (Peters et al 1988). Radioligand binding assays provide further, and perhaps more compelling, evidence that steroid and barbiturate modulatory sites are distinct. The levels of binding of [^{3}H]muscimol, [^{3}H]flunitrazepam and [^{35}S]TBPS to the GABA$_A$ receptor–channel complex are all affected by combinations of barbiturates and steroids in a manner that is inconsistent with a common site of action (Peters et al 1988, Gee et al 1988).

The above results might indicate that steroids interact with a novel regulatory site on the GABA$_A$ receptor protein, but it is equally plausible that the effects described result from a steroid-induced perturbation of membrane structure. The stereoselectivity and apparent potency of steroid action are not inconsistent with the latter possibility. Because of their lipophilic nature, the concentrations of steroids in the membrane will greatly exceed those in the aqueous phase. Furthermore, the stereoselectivity observed in electrophysiological and

---

FIG. 2. *(opposite)* Direct agonist actions of pregnane steroids. (A) Chart recorder traces illustrating inward currents evoked from voltage-clamped chromaffin cells by locally applied alphaxalone (100 μM). Bicuculline (3 μM) antagonizes, whereas pheno-barbitone (500 μM) potentiates, alphaxalone-induced currents. The two compounds were tested on separate cells, both clamped at −60 mV. (B) Single-channel currents evoked by 300 nM 5β-pregnan-3α-ol-20-one (in the absence of GABA) on an outside-out membrane patch. Phenobarbitone (500 μM) reversibly increases the burst duration of the steroid-activated channels. Channel activity was recorded at a holding potential of −100 mV.

radioligand binding studies correlates with the selectivity which steroids show in disordering lipid membranes (Fesik & Makriyannis 1985). In an attempt to distinguish between a membrane or an extracellularly located receptor protein site of action of the steroids, we have recently performed experiments in which chromaffin cells were internally dialysed for at least 15 minutes with a solution containing high concentrations of either alphaxalone (3 μM) or 5β-pregnan-3α-ol-20-one (1 μM). These compounds were subsequently applied extracellularly, at a 10-fold lower concentration, to such 'steroid pre-loaded' cells and their effect upon GABA-evoked currents was assessed. We reasoned that if the steroids potentiate GABA-induced currents by perturbing membrane structure, or by binding to a hydrophobic region of the GABA$_A$ receptor bounded by membrane lipid, intracellularly applied steroid should be effective in modulating GABA$_A$ receptor function (see Fig. 3). An excess of intracellular steroid would thus be expected to dramatically reduce the effect of extracellularly applied steroid.

Our results are contrary to this prediction. The degree of potentiation produced by extracellularly applied alphaxalone or 5β-pregnan-3α-ol-20-one in steroid pre-loaded cells was not statistically different from that observed in cells dialysed wih steroid-free solution (Fig. 4A, B and Table 1). Similar results were obtained with the barbiturate secobarbitone (Fig. 4C and Table 1). Moreover, chromaffin cells dialysed with either alphaxalone (3 μM) or 5β-pregnan-3α-ol-20-one (1 μM) did not display a noticeably greater level of membrane noise than untreated control cells, but did demonstrate a large increase in membrane current

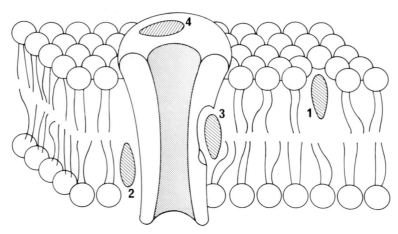

FIG. 3. Schematic diagram illustrating the possible sites of steroid action at the membrane. Steroids are envisaged as acting: (1) in the bulk of the lipid bilayer; (2) at the interface between lipid molecules and the GABA$_A$ receptor protein; (3) within a membrane-bounded hydrophobic pocket on the GABA$_A$ receptor itself; or (4) at an extracellular site on the GABA$_A$ receptor.

TABLE 1 Potentiation of GABA-evoked currents by extracellular anaesthetics is unaffected by their presence intracellularly

	Mean GABA-evoked current amplitude (% of control)	
Extracellularly applied anaesthetic	*Control intracellular solution*	*Intracellular solution containing a high concentration of anaesthetic*[a]
Alphaxalone (300 nM)	260 ± 27 $(n = 15)$	296 ± 39 $(n = 6)$
5β-Pregnan-3α-ol-20-one (100 nM)	254 ± 29 $(n = 9)$	289 ± 47 $(n = 6)$
Secobarbitone (30 μM)	377 ± 41 $(n = 9)$	322 ± 15 $(n = 12)$

[a]The intracellular concentration of anaesthetic was 3 μM for alphaxalone, 1 μM for 5β-pregnan-3α-ol-20-one and 100 μM for secobarbitone.
There was no significant difference in the potentiation of GABA-gated currents produced by bath application of the test anaesthetic between control and anaesthetic-containing pipette solutions (unpaired Student's t-test; $P > 0.28$ in all cases), n, the number of cells investigated.

fluctuation when the concentrations of steroid present internally were applied extracellularly (Fig. 4D). In the study, care was taken to provide a good diffusional exchange between the contents of the pipette and the cell, ensuring that substantial intracellular concentrations of the modulating agent were achieved (Pusch & Neher 1988). These results suggest that steroids and barbiturates can only access their binding site(s) from the extracellular surface. Although we cannot exclude the possibility that these drugs exhibit asymmetry in their membrane solubility, the most probable site of binding is to the GABA$_A$ receptor protein itself. Nevertheless, further work is required to substantiate this conclusion.

The selectivity of steroid action

Several reports in which voltage changes in response to glutamate and other excitatory substances have been recorded from neuronal populations or single neurons, using extra- and intracellular recording techniques respectively, have suggested that pregnane steroids and depressant barbiturates reduce glutamate receptor-mediated responses (e.g. Richards & Smaje 1976, Sawada & Yamamoto 1985, Smith et al 1987). We have recently assessed the pharmacological selectivity of a pregnane steroid, in comparison with that of pentobarbitone, in voltage-clamp recordings from rat hippocampal and mouse spinal neurons maintained in culture. In hippocampal neurons, alphaxalone (30 nM–1 μM) and pentobarbitone (10–300 μM) enhanced inward currents elicited by locally applied GABA in a dose-dependent manner (Fig. 5). In contrast, strychnine-sensitive, glycine-induced currents recorded from mouse spinal neurons were minimally

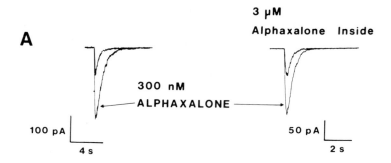

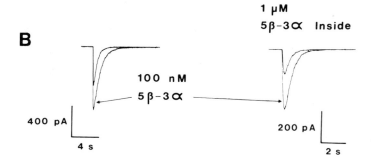

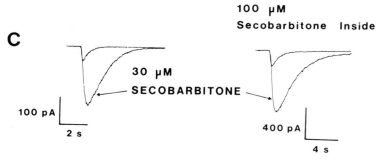

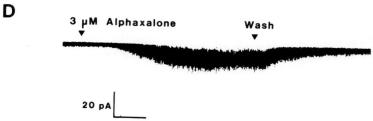

affected by 100 μM pentobarbitone (response = $97.5 \pm 5\%$ of control [mean $\pm$ SEM], $n = 7$), or by 10 μM alphaxalone (response = $113.0 \pm 7\%$ of control, $n = 6$). In rat hippocampal neurons, pentobarbitone antagonism of currents evoked by locally applied quisqualate, kainate and NMDA was reversible and concentration dependent, with IC_{50} values of 60, 69 and 690 μM respectively. Alphaxalone (10 μM) had no appreciable effect on currents evoked by these compounds. However, depolarizing responses to ionophoretically applied glutamate were depressed by alphaxalone (10 μM). The reduction in the excitatory response was sufficient to abolish the glutamate-induced action potential discharge (Fig. 5). The dissimilar influence of alphaxalone on glutamate receptor-mediated currents and depolarizations, recorded under voltage- and current-clamp respectively, could be explained by the direct agonist action of alphaxalone at the GABA_A receptor. Whereas an increase in membrane chloride conductance would not influence agonist-evoked currents (membrane potential being constant), depolarizing responses would be depressed by the decreased input resistance of the neuron.

Future directions

The electrophysiological results reported here, together with those of previous work, demonstrate that some synthetic and endogenous steroids are potent, stereoselective and specific modulators of the GABA_A receptor. Whether these effects are mediated via membrane pertubation or by binding to the GABA_A receptor protein itself is still not clear. Preliminary evidence discussed here shows that intracellularly applied steroids are inactive, supporting an interaction with the receptor protein. However, the results described are open to alternative

---

FIG. 4. *(opposite)*   The potentiation of GABA-evoked whole-cell currents by pregnane steroids and a barbiturate exhibits membrane asymmetry. On the *left* are illustrated GABA-evoked membrane currents in control and after bath application of (A) 300 nM alphaxalone, (B) 100 nM 5β-pregnan-3α-ol-20-one and (C) 30 μM secobarbitone. Currents illustrated on the *right* demonstrate that the potentiation of GABA-evoked whole-cell currents by bath application of (A) 300 nM alphaxalone, (B) 100 nM 5β-pregnan-3α-ol-20-one and (C) 30 μM secobarbitone is not influenced by intracellular dialysis with 3 μM alphaxalone (A), 1μM 5β-pregnan-3α-ol-20-one (B) and 100 μM secobarbitone (C) for 15-60 minutes. Each trace depicts the computer-generated average of at least four responses to GABA, each recorded at a holding potential of -60 mV. Each pair of current traces represents recordings from two chromaffin cells. (D) A trace obtained from a chromaffin cell 40 minutes after establishing the whole-cell recording mode with a pipette containing 3 μM alphaxalone. Visual inspection of the membrane current record at this time indicates low baseline noise with no obvious single-channel events. Subsequent bath application of 3 μM alphaxalone to this cell induced an inward current, associated with an increase in membrane noise, which reversed upon washout. The current was recorded at a holding potential of -60 mV.

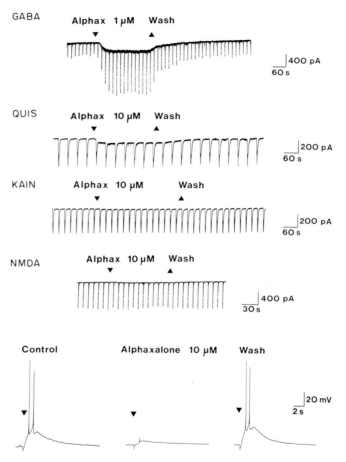

FIG. 5.   Effect of alphaxalone on GABA$_A$ and glutamate receptor-mediated responses in rat hippocampal neurons. *Top trace:* currents elicited by ionophoretically applied GABA are reversibly potentiated by bath-applied alphaxalone (1 µM). The cell was dialysed with a pipette solution containing 144 mM Cl⁻ and voltage-clamped at a holding potential of − 60 mV. The large inward current during alphaxalone application is thus likely to be due to the direct agonist action of this steroid on the GABA$_A$ receptor (see text for fuller details). Traces labelled QUIS, KAIN and NMDA show currents evoked by repetitive pressure application of quisqualate (100 µM), kainate (100 µM) and *N*-methyl-D-aspartate (100 µM) respectively. Bath-applied alphaxalone (10 µM) had no consistent effect on responses elicited by any of these agonists. The recordings illustrated were obtained from different hippocampal neurons, each dialysed with a pipette solution containing 15 mM Cl⁻ and voltage-clamped at a holding potential of − 60 mV. *Bottom trace:* current-clamp recording from a hippocampal neuron showing membrane depolarizations and associated action potential discharge in response to pressure-applied glutamate (100 µM). Alphaxalone (10 µM) reversibly depressed the glutamate-induced depolarization and blocked spike initiation. The cell was dialysed with a pipette solution containing 15 mM Cl⁻ and had a resting potential of − 61 mV.

interpretations. Further experimentation is required to resolve this fundamental question.

In contrast to steroids such as alphaxalone which potentiate the actions of GABA on GABA$_A$ receptors, others, such as the endogenous steroid pregnenolone sulphate, act as antagonists, albeit at relatively high (10 μM–1 mM) concentrations (Kirkness 1989). Adding further complexity, a recent study investigating the actions of pregnane steroids on chloride uptake into rat cortical synaptoneurosomes demonstrated that the progesterone metabolite 5α-pregnane-3α,20α-diol behaves like a 'partial agonist' (Belleli & Gee 1989). In support of these observations, preliminary voltage-clamp experiments show that 5α-pregnane-3α,20α-diol (10 μM) produces only a small increase in the magnitude of GABA-evoked whole-cell currents (H. Callachan & J. J. Lambert, unpublished work 1988). The concept of a more subtle modulation by steroids is reminiscent of the interactions of benzodiazepines with the GABA$_A$ receptor (Simmonds & Turner 1987). Investigations of this kind may lead to the development of novel pharmacological agents with a high therapeutic index.

Recent molecular biological studies have revealed a level of complexity of the GABA$_A$ receptor merely hinted at by pharmacological investigations (Schofield 1989). Rapid advances are being made in relating the subunit composition to the physiological and pharmacological properties of the receptor. Future electrophysiological experiments investigating the influence of steroids on GABA$_A$ receptors of known subunit composition, and indeed known amino acid composition, should yield important information on their mechanism and site of action.

The demonstration by Harrison & Simmonds (1984) that alphaxalone potentiates the actions of GABA for the first time provided a logical mechanism which could explain the rapid, central depressant effects of pregnane steroids. This study was the impetus for a variety of electrophysiological, biochemical and behavioural investigations that have further characterized the interaction and have strongly suggested that GABA$_A$ receptors may be modulated endogenously by steroids. Future investigations should allow a better understanding of the influence of steroids on the central nervous system and may lead to the development of novel anticonvulsants and anaesthetics.

Acknowledgements

The work reported here was supported by grants from the Medical Research Council, The Scottish Hospitals Endowments Research Trust and Organon Teknika (Turnhout, Belgium).

References

Barker JL, Harrison NL, Lange GD, Owen DG 1987 Potentiation of γ-aminobutyric-acid-activated chloride conductance by a steroid anaesthetic in cultured rat spinal neurones. J Physiol (Lond) 386:485–501

Belelli D, Gee KW 1989 5α-Pregnan-3α,20α-diol behaves like a partial agonist in the modulation of GABA-stimulated chloride ion uptake by synaptoneurosomes. Eur J Pharmacol 167:173–176

Callachan H, Cottrell GA, Hather NY, Lambert JJ, Nooney JM, Peters JA 1987 Modulation of the GABA$_A$ receptor by progesterone metabolites. Proc R Soc Lond B Biol Sci 231:359–369

Cottrell GA, Lambert JJ, Peters JA 1987 Modulation of GABA$_A$ receptor activity by alphaxalone. Br J Pharmacol 90:491–500

Fesik SW, Makriyannis A 1985 Geometric requirements for membrane perturbation and anesthetic activity. Mol Pharmacol 27:624–629

Gee KW, Bolger MB, Brinton RE, Coirini H, McEwen BS 1988 Steroid modulation of the chloride ionophore in rat brain: structure–activity requirements, regional dependence and mechanism of action. J Pharmacol Exp Ther 246:803–812

Gyermek L, Soyka LF 1975 Steroid anaesthetics. Anaesthesiology 42:331–344

Halliwell RF, Peters JA, Lambert JJ 1989 The mechanism of action and pharmacological specificity of the anticonvulsant NMDA antagonist MK-801: a voltage clamp study of neuronal cells in culture. Br J Pharmacol 96:480–494

Hamill OP, Marty A, Neher E, Sakmann B, Sigworth FJ 1981 Improved patch clamp techniques for high resolution current recordings from cells and cell-free membrane patches. Pflügers Arch Eur J Physiol 391:85–100

Harrison NL, Simmonds MA 1984 Modulation of the GABA receptor by a steroid anaesthetic. Brain Res 323:287–292

Harrison NL, Majewska MD, Harrington JW Barker JL 1987a Structure–activity relationships for steroid interaction with the γ-aminobutyric acid$_A$ receptor complex. J Pharmacol Exp Ther 241:346–353

Harrison NL, Vicini S, Barker JL 1987b A steroid anesthetic prolongs inhibitory postsynaptic currents in cultured rat hippocampal neurons. J Neurosci 7:604–609

Kirkness EF 1989 Steroid modulation reveals further complexity of GABA$_A$ receptors. Trends Pharmacol Sci 10:6–7

Lambert JJ, Peters JA 1989 Steroidal modulation of the GABA$_A$–benzodiazepine receptor complex: an electrophysiological investigation. In: Barnard E, Costa E (eds) Allosteric modulation of amino acid receptors: therapeutic implications. Raven Press, New York, p 139–155

Lambert JJ, Peters JA, Cottrell GA 1987 Actions of synthetic and endogenous steroids on the GABA$_A$ receptor. Trends Pharmacol Sci 8:224–227

Majewska MD, Harrison NL, Schwartz RD, Barker JL, Paul SM 1986 Steroid hormone metabolites are barbiturate-like modulators of the GABA receptor. Science (Wash DC) 232:1004–1007

McEwen BS 1985 Steroids and brain function. Trends Pharmacol Sci 6:22–26

Peters JA, Kirkness EF, Callachan H, Lambert JJ, Turner AJ 1988 Modulation of the GABA$_A$ receptor by depressant barbiturates and pregnane steroids. Br J Pharmacol 94:1257–1269

Pusch M, Neher E 1988 Rates of diffusional exchange between small cells and a measuring patch pipette. Pflügers Arch Eur J Physiol 411:204–211

Ransom BR, Neale EA, Henkart M, Bullock PN, Nelson PG 1977 Mouse spinal cord in cell culture. I. Morphology and intrinsic neuronal electrophysiological properties. J Neurophysiol (Bethesda) 40:1132–1150

Richards CD, Smaje JC 1976 Anaesthetics depress the sensitivity of cortical neurones to L-glutamate. Br J Pharmacol 58:347–357

Sawada S, Yamamoto C 1985 Blocking action of pentobarbital on receptors for excitatory amino acids in the guinea pig hippocampus. Exp Brain Res 59:226–231

Schofield PR 1989 The GABA$_A$ receptor: molecular biology reveals a complex picture. Trends Pharmacol Sci 10:476–478

Simmonds MA, Turner JP 1987 Potentiators of responses to activation of γ-aminobutyric acid (GABA$_A$) receptors. Neuropharmacology 26:923–930

Smith SS, Waterhouse BD, Chapin JK, Woodward DJ 1987 Progesterone alters GABA and glutamate responsiveness: a possible mechanism for anxiolytic actions. Brain Res 400:353–359

Turner JP, Simmonds MA 1989 Modulation of the GABA$_A$ receptor complex by steroids in slices of rat cuneate nucleus. Br J Pharmacol 96:409–417

DISCUSSION

de Kloet: Experiments have now been performed in which cells were transfected with gene expression vectors for the different subunits of the GABA$_A$ receptor. These cell systems may be ideal for testing whether the steroids act on the membrane or on the GABA$_A$ receptor protein subunits.

Gee: In collaboration with Dr Peter Seeburg at the University of Heidelberg, Dr Nancy Lan in our laboratory has expressed subunits of the GABA$_A$ receptor in human embryonic kidney cells and has indeed found the steroid site on the expressed receptor to have structure–activity relationships the same as those seen in brain (Lan et al 1990). We have expressed the $\alpha 1$, $\beta 1$ and $\gamma 2$ subunits together in human embryonic kidney 293 cells which do not normally have GABA receptors or GABA. This allows us to look at heterotropic cooperativity between the steroid site and the benzodiazepine site, because when the γ subunit is expressed with α and β subunits we can measure [^{3}H] flunitrazepam binding, so we can measure potentiation of that binding by steroids. We have obtained a dose–response relationship for enhancement of [^{3}H] flunitrazepam binding by 5α-pregnan-3α-ol-20-one, with an EC$_{50}$ in the nanomolar range, which agrees with results from *in vitro* binding studies using brain synaptosomal membranes. We find that the structure–activity requirements are the same as in brain; 5α-pregnan-3α-ol-20-one is the most potent steroid and the second most potent is 5β-pregnan-3α-ol-20-one. Progesterone is inactive, which suggests that where effects of progesterone are observed it is being metabolized to an active form. 3β-Hydroxylated compounds have no activity. So basically what we see in brain is also found in the expressed receptor.

Majewska: What about the GABA receptor subunits expressed in *Xenopus* oocytes?

Gee: E. Costa and co-workers may be doing that.

Majewska: It is important to know whether the properties of the cell membrane play a role in this effect. The kind of phospholipids which are present in *Xenopus* oocytes may be different from those in mammalian tissues.

Gee: I think we have shown that the heterotropic cooperativity that is seen is all within the same protein complex. This implies that the two sites are closely related and the steroid site is almost certainly on the protein complex itself, because all the predicted heterotropic cooperative interactions are observed.

Simmonds: Is there a subunit combination that does not respond to steroids?

Lambert: Professor Eric Barnard and his co-workers, using expression in *Xenopus* oocytes, have demonstrated that with only α subunits or with β subunits you can still get a barbiturate effect (Blair et al 1988).

Gee: With the α subunit by itself, steroids have no effect on benzodiazepine binding.

Majewska: Reports from Seeburg's lab. suggest that co-expression of the γ subunit together with the α and β subunits is required for the formation of the benzodiazepine binding site (Pritchett et al 1989). Hence you may not see potentiation of flunitrazepam binding by the steroids in the configuration of subunits which does not express the benzodiazepine site.

Gee: Unfortunately, we don't know the cooperative interactions between the different subunits that are needed to observe steroid binding. You may need one subunit to induce some conformational difference in another subunit for the steroid effect to be shown as an increase in [^{3}H] flunitrazepam binding; it doesn't necessarily mean that the steroid site is not there if [^{3}H] flunitrazepam binding is not observed.

Olsen: I was wondering if Jerry Lambert saw any quantitative differences in steroid sensitivity between the two cell preparations used.

Lambert: No, we get potentiation of GABA over the same dose range, but the problem is that usually we are applying unknown doses of agonists from a puffer pipette; we don't necessarily know where we are on the GABA dose-response curve, and this complicates quantitative comparisons. We have looked at rat hippocampal neurons and bovine chromaffin cells, and also rat dorsal root ganglion cells and cortical neurons. The effective concentration ranges for alphaxalone and 5β-pregnan-3α-ol-20-one seem to be similar in all these cells. These steroids are effective from 10 nm to 1 μM; then the response starts to decrease at higher concentrations. Thus, in conclusion, we have no evidence for receptor differences between the cell types that we have investigated.

Johnston: Have you ever seen any GABA antagonist actions of steroids?

Lambert: Yes. The dose–response curve for potentiation of GABA by alphaxalone is bell-shaped (Cottrell et al 1987). We don't know the reason for this but the most obvious explanation is that alphaxalone enhances receptor desensitization. In our experiments we apply the agonist GABA every 10 seconds. Sometimes when you apply high concentrations of steroid you get a massive potentiation of the first response to GABA but the next response is much reduced; the degree of potentiation depends on when you apply the steroid in relation to when you apply GABA. So the steroids that potentiate responses to GABA have the opposite effect at high doses. I don't know if they would do that *in vivo*, of course, because our techniques of agonist application are rather crude in comparison with a functioning synapse.

On the question of steroids which might work as specific antagonists, like Dorota Majewska (Majewska et al 1988) we see antagonist effects of pregnenolone sulphate, but the concentrations required for those effects tend to be much higher than those required for the anaesthetic steroids to potentiate GABA. This doesn't necessarily mean they're not important, but you have to work at a concentration of about 10 µM and above, and you may have noticed that the behaviourally inactive steroid betaxalone at that sort of dose also starts to suppress the response to GABA (Cottrell et al 1987). So we have not seen an antagonist that has equivalent potency to the potentiating steroids. There is the steroid RU5135 that Michael Simmonds looked at some time ago (Simmonds & Turner 1985), which we have also used (Callachan et al 1987). This has a potent GABA$_A$ receptor antagonist effect, but I think the steroid structure there may be partly incidental to the effect.

Simmonds: Yes; nitrogens have been inserted into the D ring and a substituent on that ring. You can actually see a GABA backbone there.

Johnston: This compound acts as an antagonist?

Simmonds: Yes, and it is competitive (Simmonds & Turner 1985).

Johnston: In our structure–activity investigations we have found quite a few compounds that are pure antagonists and they work at picomolar levels.

Simmonds: Are you sure they are antagonists and not good desensitizers?

Johnston: No, but functionally that's the same thing in our system. They're not classic antagonists because they will drop the response to GABA to about 50%, but no further.

Lambert: Which steroids were those?

Johnston: One example is cortisone, which reduced responses to GABA by about 50%.

Baulieu: At what concentration?

Johnston: 10^{-11} M.

Lambert: In which assay?

Johnston: In a gut preparation from guinea pig.

Lambert: We went from that sort of concentration up to about 1 µM and saw no effect on GABA-induced currents recorded from bovine chromaffin cells, so perhaps it's a different receptor in the gut.

Johnston: The gut wall receptor may be special.

Simmonds: You mentioned some direct effects of steroids on the GABA receptor. Do you think that to exert these direct effects the steroids bind at a recognition site different from the site for potentiation of responses to GABA?

Lambert: We don't have any data on that point. What I can say is that the steroids that are potent in enhancing responses to GABA tend to be the ones that can also directly activate the receptor. The most active steroids tend to potentiate GABA-evoked currents at around about 30 nM, and at a concentration about 3–10-fold higher the 'agonist type' effect begins. As with the barbiturates, there seems to be first of all, at low concentrations, a potentiation of responses to GABA, and then a direct activation at higher concentrations.

McEwen: I don't understand how you distinguish it from the indirect effect. Why do you call it a *direct* effect?

Johnston: There is no agonist present.

Lambert: This is why you can't do these sorts of studies in neurons where a lot of GABA is present. We don't think the chromaffin cell contains GABA; we cannot measure any by HPLC. Furthermore, we can take a patch of membrane from a chromaffin cell that has $GABA_A$ receptors, fill the bath with saline, and move the electrode up well away from all the cells, just in case they do release GABA, and look at the activity of the patch. It can be silent, though not always. You then apply the steroid to a system that has never seen GABA and it will induce single-channel currents that have a reversal potential dictated by the chloride ion concentration and a distribution of single-channel amplitudes similar to that of GABA-activated single-channel amplitudes. The whole-cell currents induced by steroids can be blocked by bicuculline and are potentiated by barbiturates. There are many anaesthetic compounds with very little obvious structural similarity to one another that seem to be able to exert a 'direct effect'. Presumably they're not working through the same agonist recognition site as GABA does, but perhaps they act to perturb the channels.

Simmonds: The way I see this is that receptor theory does not preclude the possibility of the unliganded receptor being able to open the channel, albeit at a very low frequency. If what the barbiturates or the steroids do is to increase the duration of opening associated with either the GABA-liganded or the unliganded receptor, it is possible that the steroids could act at the same site for both potentiation and the so-called direct effects; but I don't know how you could prove this.

Johnston: You need a steroid antagonist.

Smith: Everything that I have seen in *in vivo* experiments agrees with the idea that progestins enhance GABA action at the $GABA_A$ receptor (Smith et al 1987a,b). I have looked at effects of both locally and intravenously administered progesterone. Over a range of doses that includes some physiological doses I found enhanced responses to GABA in rat cerebellar Purkinje cells recorded extracellularly from an intact circuit. I also observed these modulatory effects of progesterone over the oestrous cycle, which would suggest that endogenously fluctuating hormones may be capable of altering GABA function under physiological conditions in the whole animal. I do however see a latency of about 10 minutes after injecting progesterone before GABA responses are significantly augmented, which would certainly give time for conversion of progesterone to the 3α-hydroxy-DHP metabolite. I also see immediate effects with locally applied 3α-hydroxy-DHP, which would indicate that it is the metabolite and not the parent compound that affects responses to GABA (Smith et al 1987b). Preliminary results from my lab. also indicate that blocking the conversion of progesterone to the 5α-reduced metabolite with a 5α-reductase blocker prevents the modulatory effect of a physiological dose of intravenously injected progesterone on responses to GABA (S. S. Smith, unpublished work). This further suggests that endogenous progesterone must be metabolized before it can alter GABAergic function.

I have also looked at the effects of steroid on responses to excitatory amino acids, and found that progesterone tends to diminish responses to NMDA, quisqualate and kainate (Smith 1990). I gave the GABA$_A$ receptor blocker, bicuculline, when administering quisqualate and found that progesterone is still able to decrease responses to quisqualate. This suggests that progesterone may be able to alter excitatory amino acid responses as an action separate from its GABA-enhancing ability.

I noticed, Dr Lambert, that in your progestin effects on excitatory amino acid responses you saw a slight decrease in the excitatory amino acid-induced current. Is that a significant response, do you think, or an artifact?

Lambert: The slight decrease shown in Fig. 5 is not significant. You may have noticed that for that particular cell I hadn't got the holding potential set exactly at the Cl$^-$ equilibrium potential. Hence I saw a slight inward current induced by the steroid, which may complicate the interpretation of the trace. We don't see any effect of alphaxalone on inward current responses to excitatory amino acids at the concentrations we tested.

Baulieu: Do you see an effect of progesterone in males, Dr Smith?

Smith: I haven't tried this in male rats.

Baulieu: Do you work in oestrogen-primed animals?

Smith: Progesterone has an effect in ovariectomized rats without oestrogen priming, but oestrogen priming appears to make a difference. In the oestrogen-primed animals I don't see as great an effect of progesterone on excitatory amino acid responses in general as I do in controls and the effect on responses to NMDA appears to be reversed; if I give enough oestrogen, progesterone actually increases the responses to NMDA (S. S. Smith, unpublished work). When tested in normally cycling rats, progesterone also increases responses to NMDA on days of the cycle when oestradiol is increased (dioestrus$_2$, pro-oestrus), whereas decreases in response to this excitatory amino acid after progesterone administration are observed when circulating oestradiol levels are lower (oestrus, dioestrus$_1$). This suggests that in normally cycling animals the background steroid milieu determines the effect of progesterone on excitatory amino acid function. These effects are reminiscent of classical neuroendocrine effects of steroids, when oestrogen priming can allow progesterone to exert facilitative effects on reproductive function (for example, LHRH release and lordosis behaviour) and may thus be indicative of more conventional steroid receptor mechanisms.

Majewska: I have also tested the steroids that are very potent modulators of the GABAergic system to see if they affect the NMDA receptor. Using various ligands, including glutamate, phencyclidine (PCP), and TCP (*N*-(1-[2-thienyl]cyclohexyl)-3,4-piperidine) I haven't seen any direct interaction of these steroids with any of the ligands that label the NMDA receptor. This agrees with Jeremy Lambert's results. Nevertheless, it is still possible that the biological effects of progesterone which you observe *in vivo* may be partially due to the activation by tetrahydroprogesterone of GABA$_A$ receptors, located on the same neuron as glutamergic receptors, resulting in the alteration of responses to excitatory amino acids.

Smith: It is also possible that other mediating factors may allow progesterone to exert these effects on excitatory amino acid responses. Perhaps monoamines are involved *in vivo*, because serotonin is also able to decrease responses to excitatory amino acids in the cerebellum (Hicks et al 1989).

Lambert: An indirect effect of progesterone acting through the GABA$_A$ receptor, which I thought might explain the decreased response to excitatory amino acids that you observe, may not be a possible explanation if progesterone's effect is not bicuculline sensitive.

Smith: With quisqualate, a dose of bicuculline that completely abolishes responses to GABA doesn't abolish the effect of progesterone on responses to quisqualate. So, at least in this situation, if there is another factor involved, it is not the GABA receptor. As background oestradiol levels influence the ability of progesterone to modulate excitatory amino acid function, perhaps conversion of progesterone to an as yet undefined active metabolite depends on circulating levels of other ovarian steroids.

I have also looked at the effect of 17β-oestradiol on responses to glutamate, recorded from cerebellar Purkinje cells *in vivo* using extracellular and iontophoretic techniques (Smith et al 1988, Smith 1989). I was interested in the cerebellum because sex steroids have very dramatic effects on locomotion, gait and coordination. Oestradiol in particular has been associated with increases in locomotion and coordination, in humans and in animal models (Becker et al 1987), and the cerebellum is a brain region that might mediate some of these effects. There is also evidence that sex steroids affect learning and the cerebellum is known to play a role in certain types of learning (such as the vestibulo-ocular reflex and eyeblink reflex) (McCormick & Thompson 1984).

In my paradigm I looked at responses to iontophoretic pulses of glutamate and the effect on those responses produced by i.v. administration of physiological levels of oestradiol or locally applied oestradiol. Several minutes after the onset of continuous pressure ejection of oestradiol in the vicinity of the Purkinje cell you begin to see an increase in response to glutamate which continues to increase over the next 6–9 min (Fig. 1; Smith et al 1988).

When the pressure ejection is turned off the cells do not recover to control levels of glutamate response. I have consistently seen an increase in response to glutamate after both i.v. injection and local application of oestradiol. In neither case does the response recover to control levels, but I can't record for more than a couple of hours, so the response to glutamate might return to control levels over a longer time course. The effect is relatively fast, which suggests a non-genomic action.

Neither anisomycin, a protein synthesis inhibitor, nor tamoxifen, an anti-oestrogen, blocks the effect, which again suggests a non-genomic action of oestradiol. The background oestrogen level also has an effect, because oestrogen priming appears to reduce the latency of the increased response to glutamate after i.v. administration of oestradiol. In intact rats oestradiol has a greater effect on the days of the cycle following increases in endogenous oestradiol, namely pro-oestrus and oestrus, and less effect when oestrogen levels are lower, such as on dioestrus Day 1.

I looked at the effect of oestradiol on quisqualate-, NMDA- and kainate-sensitive excitatory amino acid receptor subtypes and found a differential effect (Smith 1989). Several minutes after i.v. administration of 100 ng/kg oestradiol there was an increase in response to quisqualate (Fig. 2). Unlike the response to glutamate, the quisqualate response recovered to approximately control levels about 15 min after oestradiol injection. Oestradiol also potentiated responses to NMDA in Purkinje cells (Fig. 2) but the effect was more prolonged than this steroid's effect on quisqualate responses. The non-NMDA receptor blocker 6,7-dinitro-quinoxaline-2,3-dione (DNQX) did not prevent the effect of oestradiol on responses to NMDA, suggesting that NMDA acts at the NMDA receptor rather than at another subtype of excitatory amino acid receptor.

These data suggested that perhaps oestradiol acts initially at the quisqualate receptor and then has a prolonged effect at the NMDA receptor, to increase neuronal excitability. I don't yet know whether oestrogen acts intracellularly or at the membrane, but preliminary results suggest that oestradiol may produce increases in quisqualate-induced phosphatidylinositol turnover (S. S. Smith, unpublished results), and this effect could conceivably lead to an increase in responses to quisqualate.

These results are consistent with some of the reported activating effects of oestradiol on locomotion and other sensorimotor activities (Becker et al 1987), and with the reported convulsant effects of oestradiol (Marcus et al 1966). In addition, because increases in NMDA function have been implicated in learning mechanisms (Morris et al 1986), potentiating effects of oestradiol on neuronal responses to this excitatory amino acid are consistent with reports of facilitative effects of oestradiol on certain avoidance and maze-learning tasks.

McEwen: Quisqualate and NMDA receptors have different roles in long-term potentiation (LTP). Do you think the effects of oestrogen that you saw might have some relationship to that?

Smith: The effects of oestrogen in producing persistent effects on NMDA excitability are reminiscent of LTP in terms of NMDA involvement, duration and initial latency to effect.

McEwen: Am I right in thinking that quisqualate initiates LTP and then NMDA maintains it?

Smith: Quisqualate is important initially in producing the depolarization that relieves the Mg^{2+} blockade and allows NMDA to initiate LTP. This sequence

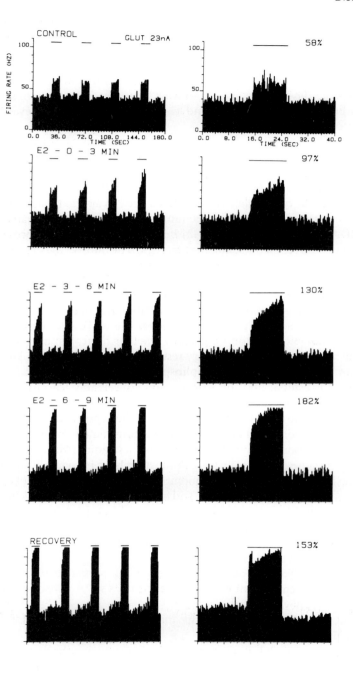

of excitatory amino acid action is similar to that seen after oestradiol administration. However, continued sensitivity to quisqualate postsynaptically, and possible presynaptic events, are important for maintaining LTP. The potentiation of NMDA-induced increases in quisqualate sensitivity by oestradiol (Smith 1989) is, thus, also similar to the excitatory amino acid mechanisms underlying LTP (Davies et al 1989).

McEwen: Has anyone looked at the effects of oestrogen on LTP?

Smith: Not that I know of. However, Teyler found that oestradiol potentiates evoked responses to afferent stimulation in the hippocampus (Teyler et al 1980).

Dubrovsky: The evidence suggests that LTP is not related to a rapid increase in expression of receptors. Davies et al (1989) showed that the sensitivity of CA1 rat neurons in hippocampal slices to iontophoretically applied quisqualate receptor ligands increases slowly after the induction of LTP, reaching a maximum level two hours after induction. Most synapses that exhibit LTP use an excitatory amino acid neurotransmitter that acts on the two types of receptor already mentioned (the NMDA and quisqualate receptors). The quisqualate receptor mediates the fast synaptic response evoked by low frequency stimulation, whereas the NMDA receptor system is activated transiently by tetanic stimulation, leading to the induction of LTP. Whether LTP is maintained by pre- or postsynaptic mechanisms is controversial. The demonstration that sensitivity changes in postsynaptic membranes are usually slow to develop (15–30 min) (Davies et al 1989) suggests that presynaptic mechanisms contribute to the maintenance of LTP but do so earlier than postsynaptic ones.

Kordon: Have you looked at the effect of oestrogen on K$^+$-induced depolarizations rather than on amino acid-evoked responses? In some of our preparations, in particular pituitary gonadotropes in primary culture, oestradiol alters the opening frequency of L-type voltage-dependent calcium channels (Drouva et al 1988). This amplifies any response to transmitters connected to

---

FIG. 1 *(opposite)* *(Smith).* Locally applied oestradiol (E$_2$) augments Purkinje cell responses to glutamate. Strip chart records *(left)* and corresponding peri-event histograms *(right)* indicate changes in Purkinje cell responses to glutamate before (upper records), during (middle three lines of records) and after (lower records) continuous pressure ejection of E$_2$ (0.5 µM in 0.01% propylene glycol-saline) at 1–2 pounds/in^2. Each histogram sums activity from 4–5 glutamate pulses (solid bar, 23 nA) of 10 s duration, occurring at 40 s intervals. The degree of glutamate-induced excitation is indicated as % change in firing rate relative to spontaneous discharge (numbers next to bars). Control records were collected for 20 min, after which E$_2$ was locally applied by continuous pressure for 10 min. Unit activity of the cell was monitored for 20–30 min after termination of E$_2$ application. Peak glutamate augmentation was noted by 6–9 min after the onset of continuous E$_2$ application. Vehicle alone did not alter glutamate responses ($n = 12$ cells, four rats). Recovery was not attained by 30 min after cessation of E$_2$ application. These results are representative of 18 out of 20 cells tested in eight rats. (From Smith et al 1988 with permission of Elsevier Science Publishers.)

that channel. This however does not involve direct actions on the transmitter receptor, but an effect at the transduction level.

Smith: I have not looked at the effect of oestrogen on depolarization, but oestradiol has no effect on responses to kainate, so oestrogen's effect does seem to be somewhat specific, at least for certain excitatory amino acid agonists. An effect on calcium influx could be a mechanism for the potentiation of responses to NMDA, because increases in calcium influx are seen after NMDA and oestradiol administration.

Lambert: When you talk about rapid effects seen after local application of oestradiol, exactly how quick are they?

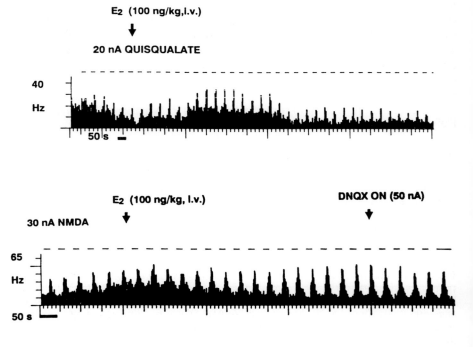

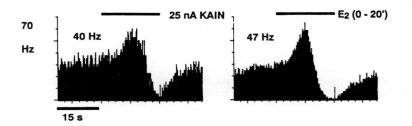

Smith: You begin to see increased response to glutamate almost immediately, within 60 seconds, but the effect may not be significant until several minutes later. There is a slow, constant increase in the effect, but the initial action may be very fast. Therefore it is possible that a metabolite of oestradiol may be the active agent, as has been shown for progesterone modulation of GABAergic function.

Ramirez: You inject at least 10 µg oestradiol intravenously, whereas oestradiol levels in rat blood are of the order of ng per ml. Have you tried injecting lower concentrations?

Smith: No, but the pharmacokinetics of oestradiol indicates that its levels decrease rapidly in the circulation ($t_{1/2} = 2.5$ min), and the oestradiol in my experiments is injected slowly over a three-minute period. Thus the concentration of the steroid would be within physiological limits very quickly. I have also examined the effect of subcutaneously injected oestradiol at a dose of 40 ng/kg which results in peak levels of the circulating steroid that are physiological within 10–15 min after injection. This paradigm also results in significant enhancement of excitatory amino acid responses.

References

Becker JB, Snyder PJ, Westgate SA, Jenuwine MJ 1987 The influence of estrous cycle and intrastriatal estradiol on sensorimotor performance in the female rat. Pharmacol Biochem Behav 27:53–59

Blair LAC, Levitan ES, Marshall J, Dionne VE, Barnard EA 1988 Single subunits of the GABA$_A$ receptor form ion channels with the properties of the native receptor. Science (Wash DC) 242:577–579

FIG. 2 *(opposite)* *(Smith)*. Oestradiol (E$_2$) potentiates excitatory responses of cerebellar Purkinje cells to quisqualate (QUIS) and NMDA but not to kainate. Rate-meter records (upper two traces) and peri-event histograms (lower trace) demonstrate Purkinje cell responses to iontophoretic application of QUIS (20 mM), NMDA (100 mM) or kainic acid (50 mM) delivered as 20 s pulses (solid bars) at 50 s intervals over a two-hour period. Each amino acid-induced excitation (numbers next to bars) is indicated as % increase in firing rate relative to background discharge and was evaluated before and for 5–6 min intervals after i.v. administration of E$_2$ (100 ng/kg) to adult female rats, anaesthetized with urethane (1.2 g/kg, i.p.). *Top panel*: potentiation of excitatory responses to QUIS was achieved by 5–10 min after E$_2$ ($n = 60$ cells in 25 rats). *Middle panel*: significant augmentation of NMDA excitation was observed by 5–11 min after steroid. Local application of the specific non-NMDA receptor blocker DNQX (3 mM) did not alter the observed neuromodulatory effects of the sex steroid ($n = 17$ neurons from six rats). *Lower panel*: unlike its effects on QUIS and NMDA excitability, E$_2$ did not produce significant changes in responses of Purkinje cells to kainate. Histograms averaging excitatory amino acid responses from control and post-steroid epochs are presented ($n = 10$ cells). (From Smith 1989, with permission of Elsevier Science Publishers.)

Callachan H, Lambert JJ, Peters JA 1987 The actions of the steroidal convulsant RU5135 on glycine and GABA$_A$ receptors. Br J Pharmacol 90:120P

Cottrell GA, Lambert JJ, Peters JA 1987 Modulation of GABA$_A$ receptor activity by alphaxalone. Br J Pharmacol 90:491–500

Davies SN, Lester RAJ, Reymann KG, Collingridge GL 1989 Temporally distinct pre- and postsynaptic mechanisms maintain long-term potentiation. Nature (Lond) 338:500–503

Drouva SV, Rérat E, Bihoreau et al 1988 Dihydropyridine sensitive calcium channel activity related to prolactin, growth hormone and luteinizing hormone release from anterior pituitary cells in culture: interactions with somatostatin, dopamine and estrogens. Endocrinology 123:2762–2773

Hicks TP, Krupa M, Crepel F 1989 Selective effects of serotonin upon excitatory amino acid-induced depolarizations of Purkinje cells in cerebellar slices from young rats. Brain Res 492:371–376

Lan NC, Chen J-S, Belelli D, Pritchett DB, Seeburg PH, Gee KW 1990 A steroid recognition site is functionally coupled to an expressed GABA-benzodiazepine receptor. Eur J Pharmacol (Mol Pharmacol Sect), in press

Majewska MD, Mienville J-M, Vicini S 1988 Neurosteroid pregnenolone sulphate antagonizes electrophysiological responses to GABA in neurons. Neurosci Lett 90:279–284

Marcus EM, Watson CW, Goldman PL 1966 Effects of steroids on cerebral electrical activity. Arch Neurol 15:521–531

McCormick DA, Thompson RF 1984 Cerebellum: essential involvement in the classically conditioned eyelid response. Science (Wash DC) 223:296–299

Morris RGM, Anderson E, Lynch GS, Baudry M 1986 Selective impairment of learning and blockade of long-term potentiation by an N-methyl-D-aspartate receptor antagonist, AP5. Nature (Lond) 319:774–776

Pritchett DB, Sontheimer H, Shivers BD et al 1989 Importance of a novel GABA$_A$ receptor subunit for benzodiazepine pharmacology. Nature (Lond) 338:582–585

Simmonds MA, Turner JP 1985 Antagonism of inhibitory amino acids by the steroid derivative RU5135. Br J Pharmacol 84:631–635

Smith SS 1989 Estrogen administration increases neuronal responses to excitatory amino acids as a long-term effect. Brain Res 503:354–357

Smith SS 1990 Progesterone administration attenuates excitatory amino acid responses of cerebellar Purkinje cells. Neuroscience, in press

Smith SS, Waterhouse BD, Chapin JK, Woodward DJ 1987a Progesterone alters GABA and glutamate responsiveness: a possible mechanism for its anxiolytic action. Brain Res 400:353–359

Smith SS, Waterhouse BD, Woodward DJ 1987b Locally applied progesterone metabolites alter neuronal responsiveness in the cerebellum. Brain Res Bull 18:739–747

Smith SS, Waterhouse BD, Woodward DJ 1988 Locally applied estrogens potentiate glutamate-evoked excitation of cerebellar Purkinje cells. Brain Res 475:272–282

Teyler TJ, Vardaris RM, Lewis D, Rawitch AB 1980 Gonadal steroids: effects on excitability of hippocampal pyramidal cells. Science (Wash DC) 209:1017–1018

Steroid regulation of the GABA$_A$ receptor: ligand binding, chloride transport and behaviour

Maria Dorota Majewska

Addiction Research Center, National Institute on Drug Abuse, P. O. Box 5180, Baltimore, MD 21224, USA

Abstract. Certain endogenous steroids are modulators of GABA$_A$ receptors. Tetrahydroprogesterone (THP, 5α-pregnan-3α-ol-20-one) and tetrahydrodeoxy-corticosterone (THDOC, 5α-pregnane-3α,21-diol-20-one) behave as allosteric agonists of GABA$_A$ receptors whereas pregnenolone sulphate acts as an antagonist. THP and THDOC modulate ligand binding to GABA$_A$ receptors like barbiturates; they potentiate binding of the GABA$_A$ receptor agonist muscimol and the benzo-diazepine flunitrazepam and they allosterically inhibit binding of the convulsant *t*-butylbicyclophosphorothionate. THP and THDOC also stimulate chloride uptake and currents in synaptoneurosomes and neurons. Pregnenolone sulphate acts principally as an allosteric GABA$_A$ receptor antagonist; it competitively inhibits binding of [^{35}S]TBPS and blocks GABA agonist-activated Cl$^-$ uptake and currents in synaptoneurosomes and neurons. In behavioural experiments the GABA-agonistic steroid THDOC shows anxiolytic actions whereas the GABA-antagonistic steroid pregnenolone sulphate antagonizes barbiturate-induced hypnosis. Changes in physiological levels of GABAergic steroids may alter GABA$_A$ receptor function, influencing neuronal excitability and CNS arousal. For example, pregnancy and the puerperium are associated with alterations in GABA$_A$ receptor binding which might be attributable to steroid actions.

1990 Steroids and neuronal activity. Wiley, Chichester (Ciba Foundation Symposium 153) p 83–106

GABA (γ-aminobutyric acid), the principal inhibitory neurotransmitter in the mammalian CNS, activates two types of receptor, the ionotropic GABA$_A$ receptor and the metabolotropic (G protein-coupled) GABA$_B$ receptor. The GABA$_A$ receptor is a tetra- or pentameric protein (Schofield et al 1987) whose activation by agonists opens an associated Cl$^-$ channel, leading to an increase in Cl$^-$ transport that results in membrane hyperpolarization. The activity of this receptor can be modified by several psychotropic drugs, including benzodiazepines, barbiturates and convulsants, which act at distinct but interacting domains of the receptor. Benzodiazepines and barbiturates potentiate the effects of $GABA_A$ receptor agonists whereas convulsants, such as picrotoxin or t-butylbicyclophosphorothionate (TBPS), inhibit receptor activity.

We have recently shown that some endogenous steroids interact with the $GABA_A$ receptor and modulate the function of the associated Cl^- channel. Some steroids behave as allosteric agonists of the receptor, others as antagonists (for review see Majewska 1987a). The finding that steroids can modulate $GABA_A$ receptors explains earlier observations of rapid alterations by steroids of neuronal excitability. Such reports first appeared in the 1920s, when Cashin and Moravek described the anaesthetic effects of intravenously injected cholesterol (Cashin & Moravek 1927). Subsequently, Selye demonstrated rapid and reversible hypnotic effects of progesterone and deoxycorticosterone (Selye 1942). These and other findings led to the development of a class of steroidal anaesthetics (Gyermek & Soyka 1975, Kraulis et al 1975).

Since the steroid concentrations in the plasma and CNS undergo physiological changes, the modulation of $GABA_A$ receptors by steroids may be vital for appropriate CNS activity and behaviour. This article summarizes our research on GABA receptor–steroid interactions and discusses theoretical concepts which stem from it.

Effects of steroids on ligand binding to the $GABA_A$ receptor

Our studies on possible interactions between steroids and the $GABA_A$ receptor were prompted by my original observation that cholesterol changes the binding of GABA to the $GABA_A$ receptor *in vitro*. Subsequent studies have shown that other steroids, such as pregnenolone sulphate and corticosterone, also alter the binding of the $GABA_A$ receptor agonist muscimol to rat synaptosomal membranes and that the interaction between steroids and $GABA_A$ receptors is observed in various brain regions (Majewska et al 1985).

Subsequent investigations disclosed complex types of interaction between steroids and $GABA_A$ receptors. Steroids with reduced A rings and hydroxyl groups at 3α positions, such as tetrahydroprogesterone (THP, 5α-pregnan-3α-ol-20-one; originally termed 3α-OH-dihydroprogesterone, 3α-OH-DHP) and tetrahydrodeoxycorticosterone (THDOC, 5α-pregnane-3α,21-diol-20-one) interact with the $GABA_A$ receptor in a manner similar to that of anaesthetic/hypnotic barbiturates. These steroids, at nanomolar concentrations, potentiate the binding of muscimol and benzodiazepines to the $GABA_A$ receptor and allosterically inhibit the binding of the convulsant TBPS (Majewska et al 1986, Harrison et al 1987). Figure 1 (panel A) shows potentiation of [^{3}H]muscimol binding by THP (3α-OH-DHP); panel C shows the increase in [^{3}H]flunitrazepam binding caused by THP and THDOC, with Scatchard analysis demonstrating that the increase results from a change in affinity of binding; and panel B demonstrates inhibition of [^{35}S]TBPS binding by THP

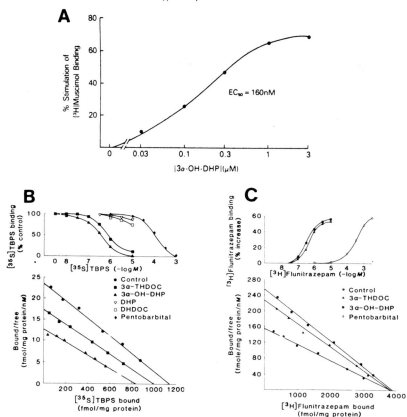

FIG. 1.   Effects of THP and THDOC on ligand binding to GABA$_A$ receptor in rat brain synaptosomal membranes. (A) Effect of THP (tetrahydroprogesterone; 5α-pregnan-3α-ol-20-one, 3α-OH-DHP) on [^{3}H]muscimol binding. (B) Effect of THP (5α-pregnan-3α-ol-20-one), THDOC (3α-THDOC; tetrahydrodeoxycorticosterone) and pentobarbitone on [^{35}S]TBPS binding; lower panel shows the Scatchard plots made from the THP and THDOC binding data. (DHP refers to dihydroprogesterone and DHDOC to dihydrodeoxy-corticosterone.) (C) Effect of THP, THDOC and pentobarbitone on [^{3}H]flunitrazepam binding; lower panel shows Scatchard plots. Data shown are representative of a single experiment, performed in triplicate, that was reproduced with similar results at least three times. (Panels (B) and (C) are reproduced from Majewska et al 1986 by permission of *Science*. ©1986 by the American Association for the Advancement of Science.)

and THDOC, with Scatchard analysis showing a decrease in the receptor density by steroids, which suggests an allosteric type of interaction. Qualitatively, the effects of these steroids resemble those of barbiturates, but steroids are about 1000 times more potent than pentobarbitone. Partially reduced metabolites such as dihydroprogesterone (DHP) and dihydrodeoxycorticosterone (DHDOC) did not alter TBPS binding at concentrations at which THP and THDOC completely inhibited TBPS binding (panel B).

Pregnenolone, dehydroepiandrosterone and their sulphates are synthesized locally in the CNS, and have therefore been termed 'neurosteroids' (Baulieu et al 1987). Pregnenolone sulphate interacts with the $GABA_A$ receptor in a mixed GABA-agonistic/antagonistic fashion. At nanomolar concentrations, pregnenolone sulphate increases [^{3}H]muscimol binding in brain synaptosomal membranes prepared from adrenalectomized rats, but decreases the binding at micromolar concentrations (Fig. 2A) (Majewska et al 1985). Although pregnenolone sulphate increases [^{3}H]flunitrazepam binding (Fig. 2B, top panel), it can also abolish pentobarbitone potentiation of the binding of this benzodiazepine (Fig. 2B, bottom panel), thus demonstrating its mixed GABA-agonistic/antagonistic features. At micromolar concentrations pregnenolone sulphate also inhibits binding of the convulsant [^{35}S]TBPS in an apparently competitive manner (Fig. 2C), suggesting that this steroid interacts with the GABA-gated Cl^- channel.

In contrast to THP, THDOC or pregnenolone sulphate, which all inhibit [^{35}S]TBPS binding, the glucocorticoids cortisol (hydrocortisone) and cortisone increase [^{35}S]TBPS binding. This effect resembles the action of the $GABA_A$ antagonist bicuculline (Majewska 1987b) and suggests that glucocorticoids possess some GABA-antagonistic properties. Antagonistic effects of glucocorticoids were indeed observed in bioassays (Ong et al 1987) and are consistent with the reported excitatory actions of these steroids on neurons (Feldman 1983). However, since glucocorticoids also behave as allosteric GABA agonists, by increasing ligand binding to the $GABA_A$ receptor (Majewska et al 1985) and potentiating responses to GABA (Ong et al 1987), they may be considered as mixed-type modulators of the $GABA_A$ receptor. The manifestation of the GABA-agonistic or antagonistic features of glucocorticoids may depend on their concentration and on other factors determined by the internal biochemical milieu.

An additional insight into steroid–$GABA_A$ receptor interactions was gained by examining the binding of radiolabelled pregnenolone sulphate to brain membranes. Our studies show that [^{3}H]pregnenolone sulphate binds to two populations of sites in rat brain synaptosomal membranes. The higher affinity sites (K_d about 500 nM and B_{max} about 4.6 pmol/mg protein) seem to be associated with the $GABA_A$ receptor-coupled Cl^- channel (because binding to these sites is selectively inhibited by picrotoxin), whereas the lower affinity sites (K_d about 200 µM) may be associated with membrane lipids (Demirgoren et al 1989). Although equilibrium binding data indicated that there is a competitive interaction between pregnenolone sulphate and TBPS, the sites of binding of these molecules may not be identical, because [^{3}H]pregnenolone sulphate binding is inhibited by the neurosteroid dehydroepiandrosterone sulphate whereas binding of [^{35}S]TBPS is not (Majewska & Schwartz 1987). Thus there

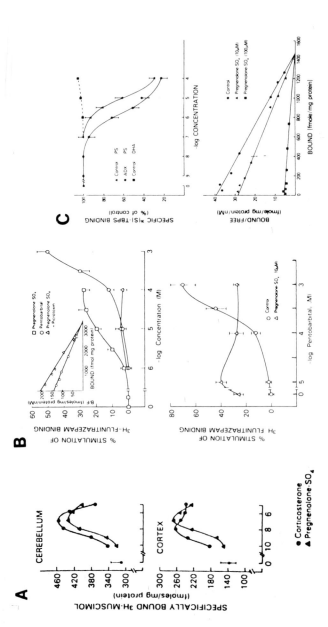

FIG. 2. Effect of pregnenolone sulphate (PS) on ligand binding to the GABA$_A$ receptor complex. (A) Effect of PS and corticosterone on [^{3}H] muscimol binding in cerebral cortex and cerebellum of the rat. (B) Effect of PS on [^{3}H] flunitrazepam binding: upper panel shows that PS increases binding in a dose-dependent manner; lower panel shows that it inhibits the pentobarbitone-stimulated enhancement of [^{3}H] flunitrazepam binding. (C) Inhibitory effect of PS on [^{35}S]TBPS binding; lower panel shows Scatchard analysis. ADX stands for adrenalectomized rats and DHA for dehydroepiandrosterone sulphate. Data represent means from triplicate samples in a representative experiment ± SEM; the experiments were reproduced at least three times. (Reproduced from *Brain Research* by permission of Elsevier Science Publishers.)

may be a number of distinct but interacting steroid-binding sites associated with the $GABA_A$ receptor complex; some of these sites may be located at the interface between the phospholipid cell membrane and the receptor protein (Fig. 3).

Effects of steroids on Cl^- transport via the $GABA_A$ receptor complex

The difference between the effects that THP/THDOC and pregnenolone sulphate have on ligand binding to $GABA_A$ receptors suggested that these steroids should alter receptor function in different ways. The effects of these steroids on Cl^- transport in synaptoneurosomes were therefore examined. THP potentiated Cl^- uptake in a dose-dependent manner, resembling the actions of muscimol or pentobarbitone. Its effect could be annulled by the Cl^- channel blocker picrotoxin (Fig. 4A; Majewska et al 1986). Pregnenolone sulphate did not alter the basal Cl^- uptake, but it reduced muscimol-stimulated transport at micromolar concentrations (Fig. 4B) that also inhibit [^{35}S] TBPS

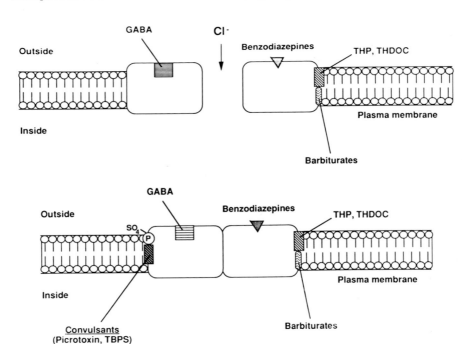

FIG. 3.   Possible sites of steroid interaction with the $GABA_A$ receptor. THP, tetrahydroprogesterone, 5α-pregnan-3α-ol-20-one; THDOC, tetrahydrodeoxycortico-sterone, 5α-pregnane-3α,21-diol-20-one; P-SO$_4$, pregnenolone sulphate. THP and THDOC affect the chloride channel like anaesthetic barbiturates (upper diagram) whereas P-SO$_4$ closes the channel, like the convulsant picrotoxin (lower diagram).

A

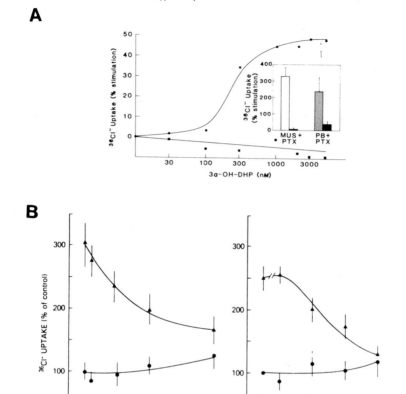

B

FIG. 4. Effect of steroids on Cl$^-$ uptake by synaptoneurosomes. (A) THP (3α-OH-DHP) stimulates basal Cl$^-$ uptake in a dose-dependent manner (circles) and its effect is blocked by picrotoxin (PTX, 200 μM; squares). Insets show that muscimol- (MUS; 20 μM; open bar) and pentobarbitone(PB; 500 μM; shaded bar)-stimulated Cl$^-$ uptake is also blocked by picrotoxin (black bars). Chloride uptake was measured over a period of five seconds. The method is described in Majewska et al (1986). (B) Inhibitory effect of pregnenolone sulphate (PS) on muscimol(10 μM)-stimulated Cl$^-$ uptake by synapto-neurosomes. Inhibition is dependent on time (minutes) of preincubation with the steroids and concentration of pregnenolone sulphate. The method is described in Majewska & Schwartz (1987). Circles represent basal uptake and triangles, the muscimol(10 μM)-stimulated uptake. Data are means ± SEM of quadruplicate samples from a representative experiment which was reproduced with similar results three times. In (B: *left*) concentration of PS was 30 μM and in (B: *right*) synaptoneurosomes were preincubated for 20 min with varying concentrations of PS. (Panel (A) is reproduced from Majewska et al 1986 by permission of *Science*. ©1986 by the American Association for the Advancement of Science. Panel (B) is reproduced from Brain Research by permission of Elsevier Science Publishers.)

binding. Hence the Cl⁻ transport data, in agreement with binding data, demonstrate that THP and THDOC behave, like barbiturates, as allosteric agonists of the $GABA_A$ receptor, whereas pregnenolone sulphate (at micromolar concentrations) behaves as a Cl⁻ channel antagonist.

Electrophysiological studies provide additional proof that steroids interact with $GABA_A$ receptors. They show that THP and THDOC potentiate Cl⁻ currents in neurons (Majewska et al 1986, Harrison et al 1987) in a manner like that of barbiturates or the synthetic anaesthetic steroid alphaxalone (Harrison & Simmonds 1984). Pregnenolone sulphate, however, inhibits GABA-induced currents (Majewska et al 1988). Thus electrophysiological studies demonstrate the allosteric, GABA-agonistic actions of THP and THDOC and the antagonistic effects of pregnenolone sulphate that were observed in biochemical studies.

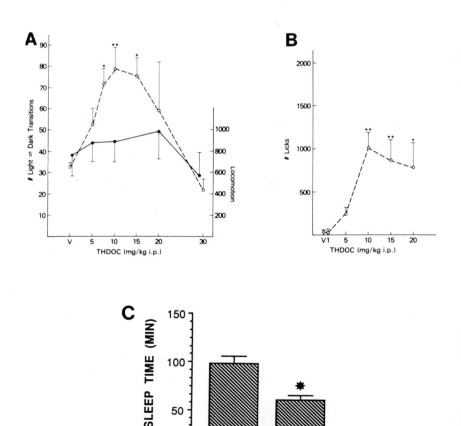

Behavioural aspects of THP, THDOC and pregnenolone sulphate activity

The GABAergic effects of THP, THDOC and pregnenolone sulphate, as observed *in vitro*, suggested that these steroids should alter animal behaviour in predictable ways. Indeed, THDOC behaves as a classical anxiolytic agent in behavioural tests for anxiety, such as tests of exploratory behaviour in mice (Fig. 5A) or of conflict behaviour in rats (Fig. 5B; Crawley et al 1986). THDOC also has potent sleep-inducing properties in rats (Mendelson et al 1987). In contrast, pregnenolone sulphate antagonizes barbiturate-induced sleep in rats (Fig. 5C) (Majewska et al 1989a). These behavioural responses closely follow the anticipated patterns, indicating that GABAergic steroids do modify the functioning of central GABA$_A$ receptors *in vivo* and therefore may participate in the physiological control of CNS excitability. The biochemical, electrophysiological and behavioural effects of THP, THDOC and pregnenolone sulphate which we observed are summarized in Table 1.

The origin of GABAergic steroids

The precursors of the GABA-enhancing steroids, THP and THDOC, are progesterone and deoxycorticosterone, respectively, which are the major hormones secreted by the ovaries and the adrenal cortex. Both organs contain the two enzymes, 5α-reductase and 3α-oxidoreductase, which reduce progesterone and deoxycorticosterone and thus are capable of synthesizing THP and THDOC

FIG. 5.   Behavioural consequences of the action of steroids that interact with the GABA$_A$ receptor. (A) Anxiolytic effect of THDOC on exploratory behaviour in mice. The experiments were performed using the two-chambered exploratory behavioural model of anxiety. Anxiolytics appear to enhance the natural tendencies of mice to explore the novel environment by reversing the behavioural inhibition observed when mice are exposed to a brightly lit open field; this is reflected in an increased number of passages from dark to light areas. THDOC (injected intraperitoneally) significantly increased the number of light–dark passages (broken line), but had no effect on general motor activity (solid line). (B) Anxiolytic effect of THDOC on conflict behaviour in rats. Suppressed water consumption was assessed in thirsty rats. Application of a mild electrical shock every few licks typically suppresses drinking, but anxiolytics reverse this process. THDOC (i.p.) significantly increased number of licks, suggesting that it had an anxiolytic action, but did not significantly lower motor activity until the concentration of > 10 mg/kg (results not shown). The methods are described in Crawley et al (1986). In (A) ($n = 6$; i.e. each point represents mean + SEM from six rats) and in (B) ($n = 8$), by Newman-Keuls comparison of individual means versus control, $*P < 0.05$, $**P < 0.01$. (C) Antagonistic effect of pregnenolone sulphate on pentobarbitone-induced sleep time in rats. Sleep time was measured after the i.p. injection of pentobarbitone-Na (45 mg/kg), starting from the moment of loss of righting reflex until its return. Pregnenolone sulphate (PS), injected intracerebroventricularly (lateral ventricle) in a dose of 8 µg/10 µl of 0.25% saline 15 minutes after pentobarbitone injection, decreased the sleep time by about 30%. The methods are described in Majewska et al (1989a). Data are mean values ± SEM from five animals. *, values statistically different from control ($P < 0.02$, Student's *t*-test).

via a process that is under strict physiological control. In female rats, secretion of THP from the ovaries follows closely after the release of progesterone during the oestrous cycle and is stimulated by luteinizing hormone (LH) (Ishikawa et al 1974). It is possible that ovarian secretion of THP in humans is also controlled by LH, and may therefore change during the menstrual cycle. The ovaries also secrete THDOC. In male rats, progesterone and THP, and deoxycorticosterone and THDOC, are secreted by the testes. THP and THDOC are also synthesized by the adrenal cortex (Holzbauer et al 1985). THDOC release from the adrenals is stimulated by adrenocorticotropic hormone (ACTH) (Schambelan & Biglieri 1972), which suggests that this steroid is a stress hormone.

CNS tissues and the pituitary gland also convert progesterone to THP and deoxycorticosterone to THDOC (Kraulis et al 1975, Karavolas et al 1984). In the CNS, steroid metabolism seems to take place primarily in the glia: 5α-reductase and 3α-oxidoreductase have been localized in glial cells (Canick et al 1986, Krieger & Scott 1989) and oligodendroglia have been reported to synthesize 3β-hydroxysteroids such as pregnenolone, dehydroepiandrosterone and their sulphates (Baulieu et al 1987, Hu et al 1987). The fast turnover of such steroids and the changes seen in their physiological levels suggest that they have an active role in CNS functions. The fact that conversion

TABLE 1 Summary of biochemical, electrophysiological and behavioural effects of tetrahydroprogesterone (THP), tetrahydrodeoxycorticosterone (THDOC) and pregnenolone sulphate (PS)

Effects	THP	THDOC	PS
[³H]Muscimol binding	↑	↑	↑↓
[³H]Flunitrazepam binding	↑	↑	↑↓
[³⁵S]TBPS binding	↓	↓	↓
Cl⁻ transport	↑	↑	↓
Cl⁻ current	↑	↑	↓
Hypnosis	↑	↑	↓
Anxiety	↓(?)	↓	↑(?)

Arrows show either potentiation (pointing up) or inhibition (pointing down) of the measured effects, which are described in the text.

of pregnenolone to progesterone also occurs in the brain indicates that this organ is capable of limited *de novo* synthesis of excitatory and inhibitory steroids.

Physiological and pathological aspects of steroid–GABA_A receptor interactions

Sexual functions, pregnancy and 'post-partum blues'

GABA facilitates sexual receptivity in female rats. Since progesterone and deoxycorticosterone, and their reduced metabolites, promote lordosis, it was proposed that they act by potentiating GABAergic inhibition in neurons involved in the expression of this behaviour (Schwartz-Giblin & Pfaff 1987). A role for pregnenolone sulphate in the expression of male sexual behaviour is suggested by the finding that the amount of this steroid becomes altered in some brain regions in male rats after exposure to females (Baulieu et al 1987). Pregnenolone sulphate has GABA-antagonistic properties, so a local change in its concentration might influence neuronal firing in brain regions that control male sexual behaviour.

During pregnancy in mammals, concentrations of THP and THDOC are high in the plasma as a result of increased activity of their synthesizing enzymes in the placenta and fetal tissues, and the extremely high levels of their precursor hormones, progesterone and deoxycorticosterone. Brain concentrations of THP and THDOC are also likely to be high, so these steroids might potentiate the functioning of GABA_A receptors. Indeed, the ligand binding affinity of GABA_A receptors in the brains of pregnant rats is increased in a way that suggests it might be influenced by THP or THDOC (Majewska et al 1989b). The observed post-partum decrease in the density of GABA_A receptors could also be steroid mediated (Majewska et al 1985). Analogous changes that take place in humans might be responsible for alterations in mood and psyche, such as the feelings of well-being and of depression that are typical of human pregnancy and the puerperium, respectively. Similar steroid-mediated modulation of the GABA_A receptor may occur during the menstrual cycle, to contribute to the symptoms of premenstrual tension.

Stress, depression and anxiety

According to Selye, who pioneered studies on the biological aspects of stress, reactions to stress develop in three stages, namely alarm reactions, resistance and exhaustion (Selye 1950). These reactions differ in their physiological manifestations, which include adrenal secretion of catecholamines and steroids. It was found recently in rats that the concentration of the GABA-antagonistic steroid pregnenolone sulphate in the brain also increases during stress (Baulieu et al 1987). It is conceivable that the elevated level of this steroid in the CNS, by suppressing the inhibitory action of GABA, contributes to the arousal that accompanies the early stages of stress, thus playing an analeptic role. On the other hand, ACTH stimulates secretion of the anxiolytic steroid THDOC (Crawley et al 1986) from adrenals (Schambelan & Biglieri 1972). THDOC may protect neurons from overstimulation by coming into play during the later phases of stress reactions, to preserve CNS homeostasis.

Different acute stressors have been reported to either diminish (Biggio et al 1987) or potentiate (Schwartz et al 1987) the function of $GABA_A$ receptors. Both phenomena could be mediated by stress steroids: glucocorticoids and pregnenolone sulphate, at concentrations that are achieved during stress, reduce the density of $GABA_A$ receptors in several brain regions (such as cerebral cortex, cerebellum, thalamus, hippocampus and hypothalamus) (Majewska et al 1985), whereas THDOC potentiates $GABA_A$ receptor function (Majewska et al 1986). Hence, activity in the CNS during stress may be shaped by an interplay between excitatory and inhibitory steroids which can modulate one another's actions. Diversity of reactions to particular stressors may be determined by a change in the predominant steroid(s). We may also predict that behavioural reactions to stress will be modified by a change in physiological state, such as puberty or pregnancy, or during phases of the menstrual cycle or menopause, where there is an alteration in plasma and CNS levels of neuroactive steroids.

Depression and anxiety are related to stress in terms of their biological and psychological manifestations and they both seem to be associated with inefficiency of GABAergic neurotransmission (Berrettini & Post 1984). Because these two states are typified by overactivity of the hypothalamo-pituitary-adrenal axis, a role for steroid–$GABA_A$ receptor interactions in mood disorders can be predicted. Hence, potential aberrations in these interactions should be examined as possible causative factors in anxiety and depressive disorders.

Feeding, seizures and blood pressure regulation

GABA influences feeding behaviour, acting primarily via hypothalamic $GABA_A$ receptors. Micro-injection of various $GABA_A$ receptor agonists (muscimol, benzodiazepines and barbiturates) into the ventromedial hypothalamus induces feeding by inhibiting the satiety centre (Matsumoto 1989). One can therefore predict that steroids with GABA-agonistic features will increase feeding by potentiating the function of hypothalamic $GABA_A$ receptors. Although this concept has yet to be tested experimentally, such a mechanism could explain the increased appetite and food consumption that are observed during pregnancy and the luteal phase of the menstrual cycle, which are physiological states in which levels of GABA-agonistic steroids are high.

Impairment of GABAergic neurotransmission is linked to seizure disorders. The frequency of seizures is altered in physiological states such as stress and pregnancy that are accompanied by changes in steroid hormone secretion. Since anaesthetic steroids are expected to increase the seizure threshold, and convulsant steroids lower it (Woodbury 1952, Peterson 1989), the profile of circulating steroids might affect the occurrence of seizures. Some anaesthetic steroids may prove to be useful anticonvulsants.

A role for GABA-enhancing steroids in the regulation of cardiovascular function is suggested by the correlation that is seen between hypertension and reduced adrenal secretion of THP (Holzbauer et al 1985). The presumed hypotensive effects of this steroid may be both central and peripheral in nature; THP could potentiate GABA$_A$ receptors in neural and vascular tissues, both of which are involved in the regulation of heart rate and blood pressure.

Defects in steroidogenesis

Because steroids modulate GABA$_A$ receptor function, thereby increasing or decreasing neuronal excitability, aberrant steroid synthesis could underlie certain CNS disorders. For example, Cushing's disease, which is characterized by oversecretion of adrenal steroids, is linked to severe neuropsychiatric manifestations, including mood lability, insomnia and agitation, which resemble symptoms of depression. Insufficiency of adrenal hormones in Addison's disease is also accompanied by psychiatric disturbances such as irritability, apathy, fatigue, somnolence, dulling of intellect and memory deficits. It is likely that some of these psychoneurological manifestations result from aberrant steroid–GABA receptor interactions. In addition to gross defects in steroid production, the physiologically important steroid balance may be disturbed by inborn errors in individual steroidogenic enzymes in the adrenal glands, gonads, liver or CNS (New & Levine 1984) and this might alter neuronal excitability.

Summary

Different steroids affect neuronal excitability by either positively or negatively modulating the functioning of GABA$_A$ receptors. This regulation may be a vital means of brain–body communication, essential for integrated responses to external stimuli or internal signals. Steroid–GABA receptor interactions may form the basis of numerous psychophysiological phenomena such as stress, anxiety and depression, among others. Disturbances in the synthesis of centrally active steroids may contribute to the defects in neurotransmission that underlie a variety of neural and affective disorders.

Acknowledgements

I gratefully acknowledge the collaboration of the following colleagues at different stages of this work: Drs Neil Harrison, Rochelle Schwartz, Jeffery Barker, Jackie Crawley, John Glowa, Serdar Demirgoren and Edythe D. London.

References

Baulieu E-E, Robel P, Vatier O, Haug A, Le Goascogne C, Bourreau E 1987 Neurosteroids: pregnenolone and dehydroepiandrosterone in the rat brain. In: Fuxe K, Agnati LF (eds) Receptor–receptor interaction: a new intramembrane integrative mechanism. Macmillan, Basingstoke, p 89–104

Berrettini WH, Post RM 1984 GABA in affective illness. In: Post RM, Ballanger JC (eds) Neurobiology of mood disorders. Williams & Wilkins, Baltimore, p 673–685

Biggio G, Concas A, Mele S, Corda MG 1987 Changes in GABAergic transmission induced by stress, anxiogenic and anxiolytic β-carbolines. Brain Res Bull 19: 301–308

Canick JA, Vaccaro DE, Livingston EM, Leeman SE, Ryan KJ, Fox TO 1986 Localization of aromatase and 5α-reductase to neuronal and non-neuronal cells in the fetal rat hypothalamus. Brain Res 372:277–282

Cashin MF, Moravek V 1927 The physiological actions of cholesterol. Am J Physiol 82:294–298

Crawley JN, Glowa JR, Majewska MD, Paul SM 1986 Anxiolytic activity of endogenous adrenal steroid. Brain Res 339:382–386

Demirgoren S, Majewska MD, Wagner HN Jr, London ED 1989 Binding of pregnenolone sulfate to rat brain membranes: interaction with the GABA$_A$ receptor complex. Soc Neurosci Abstr 15:994 (#397.4)

Feldman S 1983 Neurophysiological changes in the limbic system related to adrenocortical secretion. In: Endröczi E et al (eds) Integrative neurohumoral mechanisms. Elsevier Science Publishers, Amsterdam, p 173–188

Gyermek L, Soyka LF 1975 Steroid anesthetics. Anesthesiology 42:331–344

Harrison NL, Simmonds MA 1984 Modulation of GABA receptor complex by a steroid anaesthetic. Brain Res 323:284–293

Harrison NL, Majewska MD, Harrington JW, Barker JL 1987 Structure–activity relationships for steroid interaction with the γ-aminobutyric acid$_A$ receptor complex. J Pharmacol Exp Ther 241:346–353

Holzbauer M, Birmingham MK, De Nicola AF, Oliver JT 1985 In vivo secretion of 3α-hydroxy-5α-pregnan-20-one, a potent anaesthetic steroid, by the adrenal gland of the rat. J Steroid Biochem 22:97–102

Hu Z-Y, Bourreau E, Jung-Testas I, Robel P, Baulieu E-E 1987 Neurosteroids: oligodendrocyte mitochondria convert cholesterol to pregnenolone. Proc Natl Acad Sci USA 84:8215–8219

Ishikawa S, Sawada T, Nakamura Y, Marioka T 1974 Ovarian secretion of pregnane compounds during estrous cycle and pregnancy in rats. Endocrinology 94:1615–1620

Karavolas HJ, Bertics PJ, Hodges D, Rudie N 1984 Progesterone processing by neuroendocrine structures. In: Celotti F et al (eds) Metabolism of hormonal steroids in the neuroendocrine structures. Raven Press, New York, p 149–169

Kraulis I, Foldes G, Traikov H, Dubrovsky B, Birmingham MK 1975 Distribution, metabolism and biological activity of deoxycorticosterone in the ventral nervous system. Brain Res 88:1–14

Krieger NR, Scott RG 1989 Nonneuronal localization for steroid converting enzyme: 3α-hydroxysteroid oxidoreductase in olfactory tubercle of rat brain. J Neurochem 52:1866–1870

Majewska MD 1987a Actions of steroids on neurons: role in personality, mood, stress, and disease. Integr Psychiatry 5:258–273

Majewska MD 1987b Antagonist-type interaction of glucocorticoids with the GABA receptor-coupled chloride channel. Brain Res 418:377–382

Majewska MD, Schwartz RD 1987 Pregnenolone-sulfate: an endogenous antagonist of the γ-aminobutyric acid receptor complex in brain? Brain Res 404:355–360

Majewska MD, Bisserbe JC, Eskay RE 1985 Glucocorticoids are modulators of GABA$_A$ receptors in brain. Brain Res 339:178–182

Majewska MD, Harrison NL, Schwartz RD, Barker JL, Paul SM 1986 Steroid hormone metabolites are barbiturate-like modulators of the GABA receptor. Science (Wash DC) 232:1004–1007

Majewska MD, Mienville JM, Vicini S 1988 Neurosteroid pregnenolone sulfate antagonizes electrophysiological responses to GABA in neurons. Neurosci Lett 90:279–284

Majewska MD, Bluet-Pajot M-T, Robel P, Baulieu E-E 1989a Pregnenolone sulfate antagonizes barbiturate-induced sleep. Pharmacol Biochem Behav 33:701–703

Majewska MD, Ford-Rice F, Falkay G 1989b Pregnancy-induced alterations of GABA$_A$ receptor sensitivity in maternal brain: an antecedent of post-partum 'blues'? Brain Res 482:397–401

Matsumoto RR 1989 GABA receptors: are cellular differences reflected in function? Brain Res Bull 14:203–225

Mendelson WB, Martin JV, Perlis M, Wagner R, Majewska MD, Paul SM 1987 Sleep induction by adrenal steroid in the rat. Psychopharmacology 93:226–229

New MI, Levine LS 1984 Inborn errors of steroid biosynthesis. In: Makin HLM (ed) Biochemistry of steroid hormones, 2nd edn. Blackwell Scientific Publications, Oxford, p 595–632

Ong J, Kerr DIB, Johnston GAR 1987 Cortisol: a potent biphasic modulator at GABA$_A$-receptor complexes in guinea pig isolated ileum. Neurosci Lett 82:101–106

Peterson SL 1989 Anticonvulsant profile of anaesthetic steroids. Neuropharmacology 28:877–887

Schambelan M, Biglieri EG 1972 Deoxycorticosterone production and regulation in man. J Clin Endocrinol & Metab 34:695–699

Schofield PR, Darlison MG, Fujita N et al 1987 Sequence and functional expression of the GABA$_A$ receptor shows a ligand-gated receptor super-family. Nature (Lond) 328:221–227

Schwartz-Giblin S, Pfaff DW 1987 Commentary. Integr Psychiatry 5:258–273

Schwartz RD, Weiss MG, Labarca R, Skolnick P, Paul SM 1987 Acute stress enhances the activity of the GABA receptor-gated chloride ion channel in brain. Brain Res 411:151–155

Selye H 1942 Correlations between the chemical structure and the pharmacological actions of the steroids. Endocrinology 30:437–452

Selye H 1950 Stress and the general adaptation syndrome. Br Med J 1:1387–1392

Woodbury DM 1952 Effect of adrenocortical steroids and adrenocorticotropic hormone on electroshock seizure threshold. J Pharmacol Exp Ther 105:27–36

DISCUSSION

Gee: I am interested in your results with pregnenolone sulphate. You were able to show specific binding of that steroid, which surprises me because we have been unable to achieve this. Under what conditions were you able to identify the two types of binding site for pregnenolone sulphate? What concentration of tritiated pregnenolone sulphate do you use to label the binding sites?

Majewska: We normally used a 5 nM concentration of the radiolabelled steroid. At this concentration we found that about 60% of total binding was specific binding—i.e., displaced by a maximal concentration of 1– 3 mM of the unlabelled pregnenolone sulphate.

Gee: You said that you found one binding site with a K_d of 500 nM and a second site with a K_d of about 200 µM on the basis of your analysis of the displacement curve.

Majewska: Yes; this is based on computer analysis of the curve of displacement of [^{3}H] pregnenolone sulphate binding by unlabelled pregnenolone sulphate. The 'LIGAND' program generates these numbers.

Gee: I was curious as to how you could detect a site with a K_d of 200 µM if you are using only a 5 nM concentration of the labelled ligand. The difference between this affinity and the concentration of labelled ligand that you are using is three orders of magnitude, and because of this difference you would probably detect very little if any of such low affinity binding.

Majewska: You have to remember that this site is very abundant; the density is of the order of 20 nmol per mg protein, so although [^{3}H] pregnenolone sulphate binds to only a small proportion of the sites, the density of these sites is high enough for one to detect the binding. I believe that the analysis of the ligand binding from the displacement curves is almost as good as the analysis of curves of saturation binding, generated with increasing concentrations of radioligand. Particularly in cases where the binding affinities are low, this is the only available method. In the case of 'homologous displacement' (with the same cold ligand used to compete with radioligand) you increase the total concentration of the ligand in the test tube, not by adding more of the 'hot' ligand, but by diluting its specific activity with the cold ligand. The computer curve-fitting program 'LIGAND' is designed to perform Scatchard analysis and to generate K_d and B_{max} values.

Gee: What concentration of pregnenolone sulphate did you use to define non-specific binding?

Majewska: The maximum concentration used was 1 mM. Using 600 µM the results were similar; there was about 6% more displacement when we used 1 mM pregnenolone sulphate than when we used 600 µM.

Glowinski: This is a very high concentration.

Majewska: Yes; we wanted to see the whole profile of pregnenolone sulphate binding. We do not believe that the low affinity site is associated with the GABA$_A$ receptor. In fact, the tremendous density of the low affinity sites, which is in nmol/mg protein, suggests that these sites are loci of steroid incorporation into membrane lipids. In contrast, the higher affinity sites may have some association with the GABA$_A$ receptor. These high affinity sites may mediate the GABA-antagonistic actions of pregnenolone sulphate, such as the inhibition of GABA-activated Cl$^-$ transport or Cl$^-$ currents, and the inhibition of [^{35}S] TBPS binding.

Gee: For the high affinity site, have you looked at both association and dissociation kinetics, to verify your K_d values?

Majewska: We would have liked to do this but we had only a limited amount of the radiolabelled ligand, so we couldn't. Our data are based purely on the results from displacement experiments.

Gee: Did you use filtration to separate bound from unbound ligand?

Majewska: Yes, the assay was done by filtration.

Gee: It is usually very difficult to characterize a binding site that has a K_d of 500 nM using filtration methods, because ligand dissociation typically is too rapid. Perhaps you should try to confirm your results by using a centrifugation assay.

Majewska: With centrifugation assays there are other problems. Steroids are lipids so they tend to bind to plastic, which increases non-specific binding. There are faults in whichever method you use.

I would like to say that the existence of this high affinity binding site for pregnenolone sulphate is compatible with our previous results on the interaction of this steroid with the GABA$_A$ receptor. The estimated density of the high affinity [^{3}H] pregnenolone sulphate binding sites is compatible with the density of GABA$_A$ receptors, and the affinity of [^{3}H] pregnenolone sulphate binding also corresponds to the potency of pregnenolone sulphate in relation to inhibition of the function of GABA$_A$ receptors.

Lambert: I would like to ask about [^{35}S] TBPS binding. I had thought that compounds that affect TBPS binding might be binding very close to the chloride channel. You have suggested that GABA itself or muscimol reduces [^{35}S] TBPS binding. Could you explain this? Because, as I understand it, TBPS binds to the ion channel only when you open the channel, so it's a use-dependent channel blocker (Van Renterghem et al 1987).

Majewska: TBPS, like picrotoxin, is a convulsant. The binding of these convulsants can be allosterically reduced by GABA, muscimol and other GABAergic agonists (Squires et al 1983, Majewska 1987). In addition, the GABA$_A$ receptor antagonist, bicuculline, increases TBPS binding (Majewska 1987). Hence, TBPS seems to be a good biochemical marker for measuring the functional state of the channel. Picrotoxin decreases TBPS binding to synaptosomal membranes in a competitive manner, which suggests that picrotoxin and TBPS may bind to the same site. GABA or barbiturates reduce TBPS binding in an allosteric manner, although both of them act at sites different from each other and also different from the convulsant site.

Lambert: So in electrophysiological experiments (Van Renterghem et al 1987) you need GABA for TBPS to block the channel, but in binding experiments you don't need GABA to promote TBPS binding?

Majewska: You need GABA to open the channel in order to see that picrotoxin can block it, but in binding experiments GABA allosterically inhibits TBPS binding. The work from Akaike's lab. (Yakushii et al 1987) and from Barnard's lab. (Van Renterghem et al 1987) suggests that picrotoxin or TBPS actually do not block the channel but, rather, stabilize a closed conformation of the ligand–receptor–channel complex; their effects are voltage independent. This evidence is from electrophysiological studies. In biochemical assays, TBPS seems to be a good probe for measurement of the functional state of the channel. (The neurosteroid pregnenolone sulphate manifests a pattern of inhibition of GABA-induced currents very similar to that shown by picrotoxin or TBPS; Majewska et al 1988.)

McEwen: Of all the various *in vitro* effects of pregnenolone sulphate, the one that is potentially most directly related to its convulsive effects is the competitive, or pseudocompetitive, effect on TBPS binding. Is that a distinct effect, with kinetics different from the kinetics of the effects of tetrahydroprogesterone, for example?

Majewska: Pregnenolone sulphate has a clear-cut effect in the sense that it inhibits TBPS binding in an apparently competitive manner, whereas the effect of tetrahydroprogesterone is allosteric. Further results suggest that pregnenolone sulphate does not really compete with TBPS for binding; the interaction is probably pseudocompetitive. In other words, this steroid may reduce the affinity of TBPS for its binding site, but in binding experiments this would give the same results as a competitive interaction would give. The interaction of pregnenolone sulphate with TBPS binding and the concentrations at which it inhibits this binding are consistent with the results from electrophysiological studies (Majewska et al 1988) and with the concentration of steroid required to block GABA-induced currents or GABA-induced chloride uptake; these concentrations are those at which pregnenolone sulphate behaves like an allosteric GABA antagonist.

Usually we observe inhibition of GABA$_A$ receptor functioning using 10–30 μM concentrations of pregnenolone sulphate, so the important question is whether such concentrations can be achieved in the synaptic region. The kinetics of the enzymes that metabolize pregnenolone sulphate and other steroid sulphates suggest that micromolar (about 10 μM) concentrations of these steroids could be present in some brain compartments. I don't know if anyone has measured the actual concentrations that exist in the synaptic cleft. The volume of the cleft is very small, so even if only a small amount of pregnenolone sulphate is secreted (probably from the oligodendroglia where it is formed), it could reach a concentration high enough to block GABA$_A$ receptor functioning and thus work as an endogenous antagonist of the receptor.

We have identified another steroid sulphate, dehydroepiandrosterone sulphate, which also acts as a GABA receptor antagonist, but operates at a site different from the pregnenolone sulphate site (Majewska et al 1990). There appear to be many different sites for steroid interaction with the GABA receptor, and I think these sites are located not on the receptor protein, but either at the interface between the receptor and the lipid milieu, or in the lipid part of the receptor. It is possible that it is this lipid portion of the receptor that is sensitive to steroids.

de Kloet: It would help to know the concentration of the steroids in the cerebrospinal fluid or in the extracellular space of the brain, because the concentrations you refer to are mostly based on the amount of steroid extracted from brain tissue. Would it be possible to measure these steroid concentrations in the extracellular space, using microdialysis?

Baulieu: We know a little about this, but one must distinguish between species, because steroid concentrations vary between rats and humans, for example. Levels of pregnenolone and its sulphate are much higher in rat blood than they are in human blood, whereas the dehydroepiandrosterone sulphate concentration is very high in human blood but almost undetectable in rat blood.

Also, steroids, but not steroid sulphates, enter the brain from the circulation; the blood–brain barrier is almost impermeable to steroid sulphates but free steroids can cross it. We have data from the rat and the human, but the human data have been collected from cadavers, so the values may be of questionable significance (Lanthier & Patwardhan 1986). Pregnenolone itself, pregnenolone sulphate and pregnenolone fatty acid esters are present at a concentration of 10–40 ng/g of total brain tissue. This gives a molarity of at least 10^{-7} M, so, if there is some compartmentalization, a concentration of 10^{-5} M is possible.

I think that some steroid metabolites have been termed endogenous before the evidence is conclusive. For instance, nobody has yet measured 5α-pregnan-3α-ol-20-one levels in the brain. We speak about compounds being endogenous, but we don't know if they definitely are present in the brain; the necessary synthetic enzymes are there, but we don't know if they work as we predict. Deoxycorticosterone is not a naturally circulating steroid in humans and we haven't found any evidence for the C-11 or C-21 hydroxylation of steroids in the rat brain, which means that corticosteroid-like compounds are probably not made in the brain.

We have measured pregnenolone in human cerebrospinal fluid: it's very low in most cases (<0.1 ng/ml). Interestingly, in patients with multiple sclerosis, where oligodendrocytes are altered, we saw elevated levels of pregnenolone in the cerebrospinal fluid (unpublished data). However, the CSF may not have the same composition as the intercellular fluid in the brain, and, in any case, connections between steroid-synthesizing cells like oligodendrocytes and astrocytes or neurons may be direct.

Bäckström: We have measured the concentration of oestradiol, progesterone and testosterone in the cerebrospinal fluid (CSF) of humans. The concentrations were similar to the concentrations of unbound steroids in blood. Oestradiol in CSF was about 3% of the total concentration in serum. The corresponding concentration for progesterone was 10% and for testosterone was 1–2% of the total concentration of the hormone in serum. Concentrations in cerebrospinal fluid are slightly higher than the unbound concentrations found in blood, because there is a smaller amount of albumin in the cerebrospinal fluid available to bind the steroids (Bäckström et al 1976).

de Kloet: What are the actual steroid concentrations in cerebrospinal fluid? I have calculated from your data that the progesterone concentration in the cerebrospinal fluid is about 1 nM.

Bäckström: I would agree with that value.

de Kloet: Perhaps this question of the actual levels of steroids in the extracellular space of the brain can be settled using microdialysis. On the basis of the levels you measured in tissue extracts, one can only guess what the local concentrations might have been.

Bäckström: I would say that we don't know whether it is the intracellular concentration, or the amount in the membranes, or the concentration in extracellular fluid, that is most interesting to know, because we don't know the exact location of the steroid action in all situations.

Karavolas: I would like to raise the issue of the solubility and bioavailability of the administered steroids. Some of these 5α-reduced steroids are poorly soluble in aqueous media. I wonder if you are exceeding the limits of their solubility in these aqueous media—especially with 10^{-5} M concentrations. These reduced steroids may not be in solution and may be giving unusual dose–response relationships. On another point: with pregnenolone sulphate, if esterase activity is present in your tissues, then unesterified pregnenolone, which is much less soluble, would be generated and could precipitate out of solution. This could, of course, contribute to your atypical dose–response curves. It is therefore important to know whether these steroids were completely in solution in your vehicles. It is also important to know whether you used aqueous vehicles, because of these problems of limited solubility. Also, if propylene glycol was used, there are nasty haemorrhagic effects.

Majewska: Pregnenolone sulphate is water soluble (up to 5 mM concentration), so we used aqueous solutions of this steroid. At room temperature we did not observe any precipitation of pregnenolone sulphate at concentrations used in our studies (usually $< 100 \mu$M, and never greater than 2 mM). Tetrahydroprogesterone (THP) and tetrahydrodeoxycorticosterone (THDOC) were dissolved in ethanol-containing solutions; the vehicle solutions were always tested for possible effects. When we used steroid (THP) concentrations below 10 μM we did not observe any vehicle effects; the active concentrations of this steroid *in vitro* were typically nanomolar. For *in vivo* experiments we dissolved pregnenolone sulphate in saline and THDOC in the vehicle containing 90% saline, 5% ethanol and 5% Emulphor (GAF Corporation, New York, NY); these vehicle solutions were inactive in our experimental paradigms.

de Kloet: You have observed some of your glucocorticoid effects *in vivo* only in adrenalectomized animals, Dr Majewska. I am puzzled by this, because your membrane preparations will be devoid of steroids after a certain period of incubation, whether you obtained these preparations from adrenalectomized or adrenally intact animals. It might be that you are dealing with long-term steroid effects that persist during the subsequent *in vitro* experiments. If so, you might be looking at the consequence of a long-term genomic effect, as Bruce McEwen discussed earlier.

Hall: I am interested in the biphasic dose–response curves which Dr Majewska found in a number of her studies. We have seen this type of dose–response curve in much of our work on the effects of glucocorticoids on neuronal electrical properties, and on the protective effects of steroids on the injured nervous system. To me, the biphasic dose–response curve suggests that a non-specific membrane action might be operating, or at least comes in at higher concentrations.

Olsen: I would like to describe the evidence that steroids modulate the binding of various ligands to the purified GABA$_A$ receptor.

We know that there are four or five different kinds of polypeptide subunits in the GABA$_A$ receptor which have very similar extracellular and membrane-spanning domains; the cytoplasmic domain varies between different subunits. These differences are probably involved in the intracellular regulation of function—for example, by phosphorylation—and in determining specificity of function. Differential gene expression could therefore generate tissue-specific forms of the GABA$_A$ receptor.

Many people have shown in brain homogenates and in tissue sections by autoradiography that there are brain regional variations in GABA receptor ligand binding densities (Olsen et al 1990) and in steroid modulation of binding of [^{35}S] TBPS, [^{3}H] flunitrazepam and [^{3}H] muscimol to the GABA$_A$ receptor (e.g. Gee et al 1988). In our studies for example, adding alphaxalone to tissue sections has no effect on muscimol binding in the granule cell layer of the cerebellum, but in the molecular cell layer the binding is more than doubled. This indicates heterogeneity of GABA$_A$ receptors. The variation in steroid modulation could be due to endogenous ligands for the various receptor sites on the GABA$_A$ receptor complex present in the tissue sections, such as GABA (Turner et al 1989), or it could be a result of region-specific gene expression. We feel that the variations are probably due to there being different proteins present, because there is heterogeneity of binding of many ligands and regional pharmacological heterogeneity of responses to GABA agonists and antagonists measured by electrophysiologists (Johnston 1986, Olsen & Tobin 1990).

To purify the GABA$_A$ receptor protein we solubilize membranes prepared from regions of the cow brain or whole fetal rat brain with Triton X-100 and purify the protein on a benzodiazepine affinity column. The reversible binding to both benzodiazepine and muscimol sites is enhanced by barbiturates and steroids in the purified receptor (King et al 1987, Bureau & Olsen 1990). We also found that covalent photoaffinity labelling of these sites at subsaturating ligand concentrations can be enhanced by steroids, and that different polypeptide bands in the purified receptor preparation showed different sensitivities to steroid modulation.

When we run the purified receptor on SDS–polyacrylamide gels we see two major bands, called α and β, but in fact these two bands are each composed of a heterogeneous mixture of polypeptides. We have reproducibly seen at least four, and probably six or eight polypeptides in the 50–60 kDa region of the gel. We have monoclonal antibodies specific for the α subunits or the β subunits (Schoch et al 1985, Stauber et al 1987), which each react with two of the polypeptide bands, two α bands at 51 and 53 kDa, and two β bands at 55 and 58 kDa. Thus there are at least four different polypeptides that we can identify by protein staining and antibody recognition.

When we photoaffinity label the purified receptor with [^{3}H] muscimol and run the sample on an SDS gel we see heavy labelling of two types of β subunit, 55 kDa and 58 kDa, and light labelling of two types of α subunits (51 kDa and 53 kDa). The covalent incorporation of [^{3}H] muscimol into these four different polypeptides was differentially inhibited by analogues of GABA such as 4,5,6,7-tetrahydroisoxazolo [5,4-c] pyridin-3-ol (THIP), or differentially enhanced by pentobarbitone, alphaxalone and other steroids such as dihydro-deoxyprogesterone (Bureau & Olsen 1990). Anaesthetic steroids and pento-barbitone markedly enhanced the binding of [^{3}H] muscimol to the 51 kDa α and 55 kDa β peptides but poorly enhanced binding to the 58 kDa β and 53 kDa α peptides. Photoaffinity labelling by [^{3}H] flunitrazepam of the 51 kDa and 53 kDa α peptides was also differentially enhanced by steroids, binding to the 51 kDa band being more enhanced.

In these experiments we are looking at a lipid-free protein, so there is no possibility that steroids are interacting within the membrane. (Although the protein is in a detergent micelle it has been in detergent for several days in the absence of added lipids, so there should be no lipids left in those micelles unless they are extremely tightly attached to the protein.) The relative molecular mass of the protein, as determined on a sizing column, indicates that there are very few lipids present but we cannot definitely say there are no molecules at all.

Deliconstantinos: How many lipids did you find after protein solubilization?

Olsen: We didn't measure that.

Deliconstantinos: As far as I know, it is virtually impossible to isolate receptors or membrane-bound enzymes without their annular lipids, even using Triton X-100. Even if as few as 10–15 lipid molecules per protein molecule remain, the fluidity of these annular lipids (Lee 1988) could be altered by steroids or barbiturates. There have been many reports that barbiturates increase membrane fluidity (Sweet & Schroeder 1986).

Olsen: As I said, we cannot rule out the possibility that there are tightly bound lipids remaining in the purified protein, but there is no intact membrane structure.

McEwen: The expression of different subunits of the $GABA_A$ receptor could explain the differential *in vivo* effects of oestrogens and progestins on the receptor. The reason we saw an elevation of [³H]muscimol binding in the hippocampus, but a suppression in the hypothalamus, may be that different subunits are being expressed in these tissues and these may be subject to different degrees of steroid regulation, perhaps by a genomic mechanism. In some cases, progesterone reverses the effect of oestrogen on [³H]muscimol binding and this effect is in the same direction that you would expect from an *in vitro* effect of the progestins, according to the work discussed by Dr Majewska. This might also be due to the differential expression of certain $GABA_A$ receptor subunits. It also suggests a way of seeing the link between the genomic action and the subsequent local membrane effects of progesterone.

Ramirez: To me, Richard Olsen's results argue against steroid effects on the $GABA_A$ receptor being due to lipid perturbation, because one would expect the same amount of lipid contamination in all the subunits.

Majewska: But the lipid may not be a contaminant; it may be part of the receptor. For example, as far as I know it's virtually impossible to remove all the lipid from nicotinic acetylcholine receptors; some lipids may be tightly (perhaps covalently) bound, and these lipids may play a role in the modulation of nicotinic receptor function (Heidmann et al 1983). We know that there is structural homology between the nicotinic acetylcholine receptor and the $GABA_A$ receptor (Barnard et al 1987), so the role of lipids in these receptors may be similar.

References

Bäckström T, Carstensen H, Södergord R 1976 Concentration of estradiol, testosterone and progesterone in cerebrospinal fluid, compared to plasma unbound and total concentrations. J Steroid Biochem 7:469–472

Barnard E, Darlison M, Seeburg P 1987 Molecular biology of the $GABA_A$ receptor: the receptor/channel superfamily. Trends Neurosci 10:502–509

Bureau M, Olsen RW 1990 Multiple distinct subunits of the γ-aminobutyric acid-A receptor protein show different ligand binding affinities. Mol Pharmacol 37:497–502

Gee KW, Bolger MB, Brinton RE, Coirini H, McEwen BS 1988 Steroid modulation of the chloride ionophore in rat brain: structure–activity requirements, regional dependence and mechanism of action. J Pharmacol Exp Ther 246:803–812

Heidmann T, Oswald RE, Changeux J-P 1983 Multiple sites of action of noncompetitive blockers of acetylcholine receptor rich membrane fragments from *Torpedo marmorata*. Biochemistry 22:3112–3127

Johnston GAR 1986 Multiplicity of GABA receptors. In: Olsen RW, Venter JC (eds) Benzo-diazepine/GABA receptors and chloride channels: structural and functional properties. ALan R Liss, New York (Receptor Biochemistry and Methodology vol 5) p 57–71

King RG, Nielsen M, Stauber GB, Olsen RW 1987 Convulsant/barbiturate activities on the soluble GABA/benzodiazepine receptor complex. Eur J Biochem 169:555–562

Lanthier A, Patwardhan VV 1986 Sex steroids and 5-en-3 hydroxysteroids in specific regions of the human brain and cranial nerves. J Steroid Biochem 25:445–449

Lee A 1988 Annular lipids and the activity of the calcium-dependent ATPase. In: Aloia RC et al (eds) Advances in membrane fluidity. Alan R Liss, New York, vol 2:111–139

Majewska MD 1987 Antagonist-type interaction of glucocorticoids with the GABA receptor-coupled chloride channel. Brain Res 418:337–382

Majewska MD, Mienville JM, Vicini S 1988 Neurosteroid pregnenolone sulfate antagonizes electrophysiological responses to GABA in neurons. Neurosci Lett 90:279–284

Majewska MD, Demirgoren S, Spivak CE, London ED 1990 The neurosteroid dehydroepiandrosterone sulfate is an allosteric antagonist of the GABA$_A$ receptor. Brain Res, in press

Olsen RW, Tobin AJ 1990 Molecular biology of GABA$_A$ receptors. FASEB (Fed Am Soc Exp Biol) J 4:1469–1480

Olsen RW, McCabe RT, Wamsley JK 1990 GABA$_A$ receptor subtypes: autoradiographic comparison of GABA, benzodiazepine, and convulsant binding sites in the rat central nervous system. J Chem Neuroanat 3:59–76

Schoch P, Richards JG, Häring P et al 1985 Co-localization of GABA$_A$ receptors and benzodiazepine receptors in the brain shown by monoclonal antibodies. Nature (Lond) 314:168–171

Squires RF, Casida JE, Richardson M, Seaderup E 1983 [^{35}S]t-butylbicyclophosphorothionate binds with high affinity to brain sites coupled to γ-aminobutyric acid-A ion recognition sites. Mol Pharmacol 23:326–336

Stauber GB, Ransom RW, Dilber AI, Olsen RW 1987 The γ-aminobutyric acid-receptor protein from rat brain: large-scale purification and preparation of antibodies. Eur J Biochem 167:125–133

Sweet WD, Schroeder F 1986 Charged anesthetics alter LM fibroblast plasma membrane enzymes by selective fluidization of inner or outer membrane leaflets. Biochem J 239:301–310

Turner DM, Ransom RW, Yang JS, Olsen RW 1989 Steroid anesthetics and naturally occurring analogs modulate the γ-aminobutyric acid receptor complex at a site distinct from barbiturates. J Pharmacol Exp Ther 248:960–966

Van Renterghem C, Bilbe G, Moss S, Smart TG, Brown DA, Barnard EA 1987 GABA receptors induced in *Xenopus* oocytes by chick brain mRNA: evaluation of TBPS as a use-dependent channel blocker. Mol Brain Res 2:21–31

Yakushii T, Tokutomi N, Akaike N, Carpenter DO 1987 Antagonists of GABA responses studied using internally perfused frog dorsal root ganglion neurons. Neuroscience 22:1123–1133

Steroid binding at σ receptors: CNS and immunological implications

Tsung-Ping Su*, Kenhiya Shukla† and Tamara Gund†

*National Institute on Drug Abuse, Addiction Research Centre, P.O. Box 5180, Baltimore, MD 21224 and †Departments of Chemistry, Chemical Engineering and Environmental Science, New Jersey Institute of Technology, Newark, NJ 07102, USA

Abstract. The σ receptor has been suggested to be the mediator of the psycho-mimetic effects induced by certain benzomorphan opioids and phencyclidine. Potent σ receptor ligands include haloperidol and other 'atypical' potential antipsychotic drugs. The σ receptor is found in the central nervous system and also in the immune and endocrine systems. Gonadal and adrenal steroids such as progesterone, testosterone, deoxycorticosterone and corticosterone were found to be competitive inhibitors of binding of the σ receptor ligand [^{3}H] d-SKF-10 047. The σ receptor is not the traditionally recognized cytosolic progesterone receptor and is found in crude membrane fractions. Results from molecular modelling using geometric fitting and electrostatic potential calculations suggested that the molecular skeleton of steroid hormones shares common features with prototypic σ ligands such as d-SKF-10 047 and that the oxygen of the C-20 carbonyl group on these steroids may represent a critical 'pharmacophore' for their interactions with σ receptors. Comparison of the affinities of steroids at σ receptors with their efficacies in an anti-inflammatory test yielded a striking qualitative correlation. Taken together these results suggest that σ receptors may mediate certain aspects of steroid-induced mental disturbances and alterations in immune function.

1990 Steroids and neuronal activity. Wiley, Chichester (Ciba Foundation Symposium 153) p 107–116

Steroid use in humans is known to induce psychiatric disturbances as well as alterations in immune function. The psychiatric disturbances induced by steroids are particularly evident in heavy users who abuse steroids to gain in body weight and strength. Typically, these people routinely use doses 10–100 times greater than those reported in clinical studies (Pope & Katz 1987). The symptoms of steroid-induced psychiatric disturbance may include depression, paranoia, euphoria, irritability, hyperactivity, feelings of guilt, and visual and auditory hallucinations (Ling et al 1981, Freinhar & Alvarez 1985, Wilson et al 1974, Pope & Katz 1987). Although steroid-induced psychiatric disturbances have been recognized for some time, the exact mechanism behind these disturbances, like that underlying the steroid-induced alterations in immune response, is largely unknown.

Certain benzomorphan opioids such as SKF-10 047 (*N*-allylnormetazocine) have long been known to have psychotomimetic effects in humans (Keats & Telford 1964). The dissociative anaesthetic phencyclidine (PCP) is well known to be psychogenic in humans (Luby et al 1959). Several animal studies have indicated that certain behavioural effects of SKF-10 047 and PCP are indistinguishable (Martin et al 1976, Vaupel & Janinski 1979, Shannon 1982). Attempts to demonstrate specific binding sites responsible for the psychotomimetic effects of these two drugs led to the discovery of two receptors, the σ receptor and the PCP receptor, each proposed as the mediator of the psychotomimetic responses (Vincent et al 1979, Zukin & Zukin 1979, Su 1982, Quirion et al 1987).

Although these two receptors are known to differ in their pharmacology and anatomical distribution and may mediate certain distinguishable behaviours, it is still unclear which receptor mediates the psychiatric disturbances in humans (Quirion et al 1987). Part of the problem is that no animal model definitively represents or mimics psychotomimetic disturbances in humans. It is likely that our understanding of the exact relationship between σ and PCP receptors and psychiatric disturbances in humans will be clarified only when results are obtained from current clinical trials using ligands selective for either receptor. One point worth noting, though, is that haloperidol, chlorpromazine, and several 'atypical' antipsychotic agents, proved to be efficacious in preclinical studies, were all effective ligands at σ receptors (Su 1982, Tam & Cook 1984, Taylor & Dekleva 1987, Snyder & Largent 1989), supporting the idea that σ receptors may be involved in psychiatric disturbances in humans. The structures of these potential antipsychotic agents are shown in Fig. 1.

In an attempt to isolate and examine endogenous brain substances that interact with σ receptors, we tentatively identified an active substance (Su & Vaupel 1988) which had several unusual characteristics: it was small, with a molecular mass of about 480 Da, it contained no nitrogen, and it potentiated electrically induced contractions in a guinea pig vas deferens preparation (a bioassay for σ receptor ligands; Su & Vaupel 1988). Steroids also have some of these properties. We therefore examined steroids and steroid analogues to assess their affinities of binding at σ receptors. Details of the σ receptor binding assay are described elsewhere (Su 1982, Su et al 1988a,b).

Among more than 40 steroids tested, only a few were able to inhibit binding of the σ receptor ligand [^{3}H] *d*-SKF-10 047 to guinea pig brain and spleen membrane preparations (Su et al 1988b, Table 1), namely progesterone, testosterone, deoxycorticosterone, 11β-hydroxyprogesterone, pregnenolone sulphate and corticosterone. (The endogenous substance was also active in this assay.) The Hill coefficients derived from the binding curves were all close to one, indicating absence of cooperativity. Furthermore, progesterone reduced

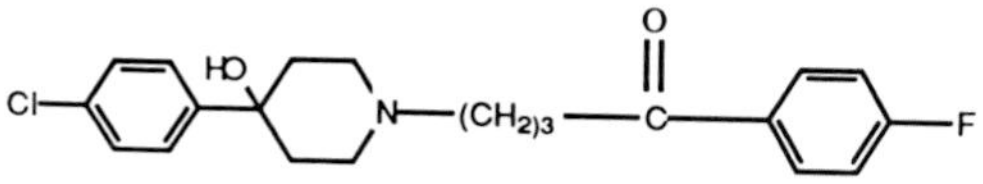

HALOPERIDOL

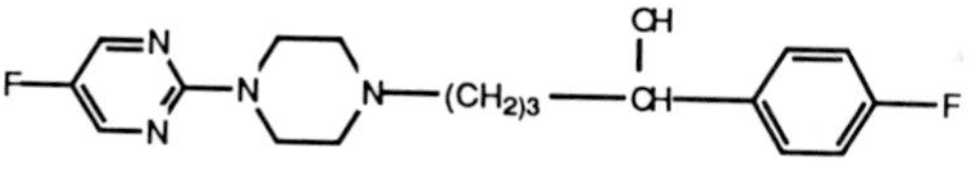

BMY 14802

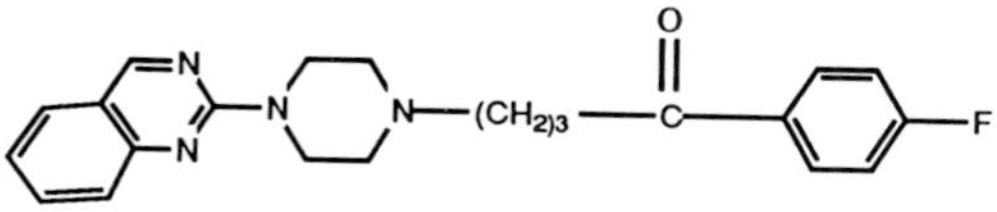

CINUPERONE

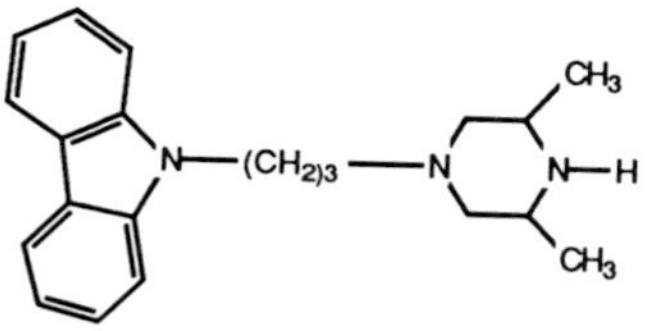

RIMCAZOLE (BW 234U)

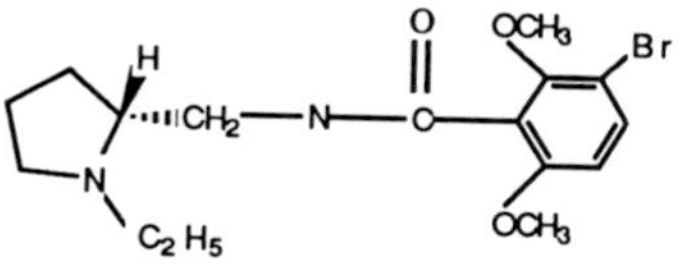

REMOXIPRIDE

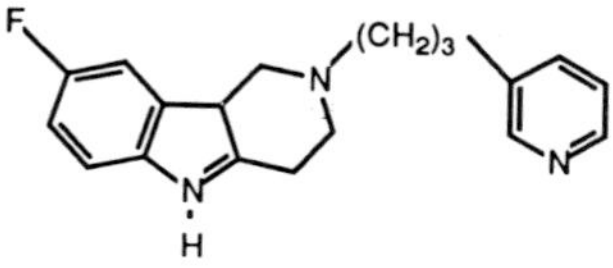

WY 47,384

FIG. 1. Structures of potential 'atypical' antipsychotic agents which are potent ligands at σ receptors. For details see Snyder & Largent (1989).

TABLE 1 Potencies of steroids in σ receptor binding assays in guinea pig brain and spleen homogenates

Steroid	Brain ($[^3H]$ d-SKF-10 047) (K_i, nm)	Spleen ($[^3H]$ haloperidol) (K_i, nM)
Progesterone*	268	376
Testosterone	1014	1715
Deoxycorticosterone*	938	2477
11β-Hydroxyprogesterone	1535	5384
Pregnenolone sulphate	3196	1272
Corticosterone*	4074	1698

K_i values reflect potency of inhibition of binding of 2 nM $[^3H]$ d-SKF-10 047 or 1 nM $[^3H]$ haloperidol to σ receptors in guinea pig brain and spleen crude membrane preparations (see Su et al 1988b). Asterisks indicate compounds active in an anti-inflammatory test (Siiteri et al 1977). Testosterone was inactive in the anti-inflammatory test; pregnenolone sulphate and 11β-hydroxyprogesterone were not tested. Steroids that were inactive in both the σ receptor binding assay and the anti-inflammatory test include oestriol, oestrone 3-hemisuccinate, 17β-oestradiol 17-hemisuccinate, hydrocortisone, 17α-hydroxyprogesterone, pregnenolone, 20α-hydroxyprogesterone, 20β-hydroxyprogesterone, 5α-dihydroprogesterone, 5β-dihydroprogesterone, 17α-hydroprogesterone, d-norgestrel, norethisterone, 19-nortestosterone, cortisol, 11-deoxycortisol, testosterone acetate, dihydrotestosterone acetate, androstenedione, oestrone, oestradiol, oestriol and diethylstilboestrol. Three potent cytosolic steroid receptor ligands were inactive in the σ receptor binding assay (promegestone, RU27987 and RU486).

the affinity of $[^3H]$ d-SKF-10 047 for σ receptors without affecting the total number of σ binding sites (Su et al 1988b).

Although steroids bind to the σ receptor, this receptor is not the traditionally recognized cytosolic steroid receptor. First, σ receptors must be membrane bound, because brain and spleen membrane preparations were used in the ligand binding assays. Second, several steroids that are good ligands for cytosolic steroid receptors, including promegestone, oestradiol, RU27987 and RU486, were almost inactive in the σ receptor binding assay (Su et al 1988b, T.-P. Su, unpublished observation); and, third, the K_d values of these steroids are in the range of 0.1 to 10 nM at cytosolic steroid receptors (Gorski & Gannon 1976), but are much higher (200 nM to 3 μM) at σ receptors.

Since the σ receptor is thought to mediate drug-induced psychiatric disturbances in humans, the interaction of steroids with this receptor suggests that the undesirable psychiatric disturbances induced by certain steroids may result from their action at the σ receptor. If this speculation is correct, putative antipsychotic agents with affinity for σ receptors may prove useful in the treatment of steroid-induced psychological disturbances.

Since almost all σ-active ligands contain nitrogen whereas steroids do not, steroid interactions with σ receptors raise the question of whether there is structural similarity between steroids and other σ receptor ligands, and what area of the steroid molecule mimics the nitrogen of other σ receptor ligands that appears to be an important 'pharmacophore' for interactions with σ

receptors. Using geometric fit and electrostatic potential calculations on the van der Waals surface of σ-active ligands, we found that the oxygen of the C-20 carbonyl group in these steroids may be critical in their interaction with the σ receptor. The oxygen may provide a lone pair of electrons to interact with an unknown site on the receptor molecule, just as the nitrogen does in other σ receptor ligands. According to the results of geometric fitting, ring B of progesterone should superimpose on the lipophilic moiety of other σ receptor ligands. Electrostatic potential calculations showed that the lipophilic moieties of such ligands and ring B of progesterone have a feature in common, namely possession of the highest electrostatic potential in the molecule. These results (unpublished) indicate that the interaction of steroids with σ receptors is structurally plausible.

The σ receptor has also been found in spleen (Su et al 1988a) and in lymphocytes (Wolfe et al 1988). The relative potencies of progesterone and testosterone in the spleen σ receptor binding assay correlated well with those in the brain σ receptor binding assay (Su et al 1988a). These observations raise several questions. Could σ receptors be involved in immune functions? And, further, do steroids modulate immune responses, at least in part, through an action at σ receptors? A review of the results of several studies, together with the evidence described here, suggests that σ receptors may mediate immune responses, including those involving steroids. For example, phencyclidine has been shown to be an immunosuppressive agent in a lymphocyte assay (Khansari et al 1984). This PCP-induced immunosuppression could operate through σ receptors, because lymphocytes contain many more σ receptors than PCP receptors (Wolfe et al 1988) and although PCP binds preferentially to PCP receptors, it also binds, with a ten-fold lower affinity, to σ receptors (Zukin & Zukin 1979, Su 1982). It was found that those steroids that bind to σ receptors are also active in an anti-inflammatory test that assessed granuloma formation in rats (Siiteri et al 1977, Su et al 1988b); steroids which showed [^{3}H] d-SKF-10 047-displacing ability, such as progesterone, deoxycorticosterone and corticosterone, were effective in preventing granuloma formation whereas many other steroids, such as all oestrogens, hydrocortisone, 17α-hydroxyprogesterone and pregnenolone, were inactive at σ receptors and in the anti-inflammatory test (see footnote to Table 1; Siiteri et al 1977, Su et al 1988b). These results suggest that σ receptors are involved in immune functions. However, testosterone shows a relatively high affinity for σ receptors but is inactive in the anti-inflammatory test. An antagonistic action of testosterone at the σ receptor might explain this apparent discrepancy. Further tests are required to confirm this speculation.

In summary, although much remains to be learned about σ receptors, the interaction of steroids with σ receptors may provide a link between the endocrine, nervous and immune systems.

Acknowledgement

We should like to thank Professor Etienne Baulieu for providing a sample of RU486.

References

Freinhar JP, Alvarez W 1985 Androgen-induced hypomania (letter). J Clin Psychiatry 46:354–355

Gorski J, Gannon F 1976 Current models of steroid hormone action: a critique. Annu Rev Physiol 38:425–451

Keats AS, Telford J 1964 Narcotic antagonists as analgesics: clinical aspects. In: Gould RF (ed) Advances in chemistry, Series 45: Molecular modification in drug design. American Chemical Society, Washington, DC, p 170–176

Khansari N, Whitten HD, Fudenberg HH 1984 Phencyclidine-induced immuno-depression. Science (Wash DC) 225:76–78

Ling MHM, Perry PJ, Tsuang MT 1981 Side effects of corticosterone therapy. Arch Gen Psychiatry 38:471–477

Luby ED, Cohen BD, Rosenbaum G, Gottlieb JS, Kelley R 1959 Study of a new schizophrenomimetic drug—Sernyl. Arch Neurol Psychiatry 81:363–369

Martin WR, Eades CG, Thompson JA, Huppler RE, Gilbert PE 1976 The effects of morphine and nalorphine-like drugs in the nondependent and morphine-dependent chronic spinal dog. J Pharmacol Exp Ther 197:517–532

Pope HG, Katz DL 1987 Bodybuilders' psychosis (letter). Lancet 1:863

Quirion R, Chicheportiche R, Contreras PC et al 1987 Classification and nomenclature of phencyclidine and sigma receptor sites. Trends Neurosci 10:444–446

Shannon HE 1982 Phencyclidine-like discriminative stimuli of (+)- and (−)-N-allylnormetazocine in rats. Eur J Pharmacol 84:225–228

Siiteri PK, Febres F, Clemens LE, Chang RJ, Gondos B, Stites D 1977 Progesterone and maintenance of pregnancy: is progesterone nature's immunosuppressant? Ann N Y Acad Sci 286:384–397

Snyder SH, Largent BL 1989 Receptor mechanisms in antipsychotic drug action: focus on sigma receptors. J Neuropsychiatry 1:7–15

Su T-P 1982 Evidence for sigma opioid receptor: binding of [^{3}H]SKF-10047 to etorphine-inaccessible sites in guinea-pig brain. J Pharmacol Exp Ther 223:284–290

Su T-P, Vaupel DB 1988 Further characterization of an endogenous ligand ('SIGMAPHIN') for sigma receptors in the brain. Soc Neurosci Abstr 14:545

Su T-P, Schell SE, Ford-Rice FY, London ED 1988a Correlation of inhibitory potencies of putative antagonists for σ receptors in brain and spleen. Eur J Pharmacol 148:467–470

Su T-P, London ED, Jaffe JH 1988b Steroid binding at σ receptors suggests a link between endocrine, nervous, and immune systems. Science (Wash DC) 240:219–221

Tam SW, Cook L 1984 Sigma opiates and certain antipsychotic drugs mutually inhibit (+)-[^{3}H]SKF 10,047 and [^{3}H]haloperidol binding in guinea pig brain membranes. Proc Natl Acad Sci USA 81:5618-5621

Taylor DP, Dekleva J 1987 Potential antipsychotic BMY 14802 selectively binds to sigma sites. Drug Dev Res 11:65–70

Vaupel BD, Jasinski DR 1979 Acute single dose effects of phencyclidine (PCP) in the dog. Fed Proc 38:435

Vincent JP, Kartalovski B, Geneste P, Kamenka JM, Lazdunski M 1979 Interaction of phencyclidine ('angel dust') with a specific receptor in rat brain membranes. Proc Natl Acad Sci USA 76:4678–4682

Wilson IC, Prange AJ, Lara PP 1974 Methyltestosterone and imipramine in men: conversion of depression to paranoid reaction. Am J Psychiatry 131:21–24

Wolfe SA Jr, Kulsakdinun C, Battaglia G, Jaffe JH, De Souza EB 1988 Initial identification and characterization of sigma receptors on human peripheral blood leukocytes. J Pharmacol Exp Ther 247:1114–1119

Zukin SR, Zukin RS 1979 Specific [^{3}H]phencyclidine binding in rat central nervous system. Proc Natl Acad Sci USA 76:5372–5376

DISCUSSION

Ramirez: Have you done experiments to resolve the issue of whether the sigma receptor is a protein, or is a carbohydrate or lipid?

Su: Phospholipase C destroys σ receptor ligand binding activity by 100%; trypsin destroys it by 60%. Boiling in water destroys binding activity totally, so most likely the receptor contains protein.

Martini: Have you tested steroids such as the active derivatives of vitamin D$_3$, for example 1,25-(OH)$_2$ vitamin D$_3$, in your binding assays?

Su: No.

Martini: Or the digitalis-like compounds present in blood?

Su: No.

Glowinski: Sigma receptors have been shown to be located on mesencephalic dopaminergic cells, either in the ventral tegmental area or in the substantia nigra. It would be interesting to see whether the σ receptors on these dopaminergic cells are affected or not by treatment with hormones such as progesterone.

Su: The A10 mesocorticolimbic dopamine neurons, when activated by a σ ligand (*d*-SKF-10 047, *d*-*N*-allylnormetazocine), can be antagonized by the prototypic σ receptor antagonists, haloperidol and BW 234U (*cis*-9-[3-(3,5-dimethyl-1-piperazinyl)propyl]carbazole hydrochloride) (Ceci et al 1988). Progesterone has not been tested.

Lambert: You are suggesting that some of the ligands for the σ receptor have major central actions in animals. Is it known whether the binding sites are on glia, or on blood vessels, or actually on neurons themselves? I gather that there is no electrophysiological correlate of that central activity.

Su: Our understanding of the σ receptor suffers from the drawback that it is poorly defined. We are now looking for an appropriate model in which to assay for the σ binding site. Dr Eckhart Weber has shown that σ ligands can act as antagonists at 5-HT$_3$ receptors in the guinea pig ileum preparation (Campbell et al 1989). This may be an interesting model, but he still has problems with it, especially in terms of the reverse activity of the + and − isomers of σ ligands. We think that the σ receptor is probably localized in plasma membranes (McCann & Su 1990), but we do not know whether σ receptors are confined to neurons or glia.

Lambert: 5-HT$_3$ antagonists such as ondansetron may have antipsychotic effects. I believe that ondansetron is currently in clinical trial for the treatment of schizophrenia (Abbott 1990).

Deliconstantinos: It has been reported (Cross 1987) that in mental disturbance there is a reduced production of oxygen free radicals by human T lymphocytes. It would be interesting if one were able to correlate the activity of σ receptors which are present in the brain with those that are present on T lymphocytes.

On the other hand, you have shown that in the σ ligands, the nitrogen atom plays an important role in σ receptor interactions. It would be interesting if there were an oxidation of the nitrogen atom to form nitric oxide (NO), which could explain the effect of this compound through cyclic GMP produced by the soluble guanylate cyclase.

Su: On the first point, σ receptors in the brain and lymphocytes have been shown to be very similar (Wolfe et al 1988). Related to this, I would be interested to know whether for instance there is any evidence that haloperidol treatment of schizophrenic patients will alter their immune responses.

Kordon: There are several known effects of haloperidol on the immune system. These have been recorded in animals rather than in schizophrenic patients; some of them are supposed to be mediated by prolactin, because they are no longer observed in hypophysectomized rats.

Makriyannis: Regarding the molecular superpositions that you described, Dr Su, the nitrogen-containing σ ligands seem to show a certain pattern, and one could make an argument in favour of some stereochemical compatibility between them and haloperidol. However, I have a problem in extending this to the steroids. Have you considered the possibility that steroids bind to a different site on the sigma receptor?

Su: We have measured the binding of radioactive *d*-SKF-10 047 and radioactive haloperidol to σ sites and have shown by Scatchard analysis that progesterone competitively displaces those two ligands from those sites (Su et al 1988). There appears to be a direct competitive interaction.

Makriyannis: The other molecular feature in which the ligands and steroids are dissimilar is their physical properties; progesterone is very insoluble in water, for example. I suspect that the nitrogens of the various ligands might all bind to the same site, as you suggest, but not the steroids.

Johnston: I would like to support Dr Su's comments on the importance of electrostatic potentials, because we have been doing similar molecular modelling studies on cortisol and cortisone and have found the electropotential models to be very revealing of major differences between stereochemically similar molecules. The superposition of the electrostatic potential maps is very interesting.

Su: There are two levels of ESP calculation, the semi-empirical and *ab initio* calculations. Our data so far are based on semi-empirical calculations but we are now going to a higher level of *ab initio* calculations. This work is being done by my collaborators, Drs Tamara Gund and Kenhiya Shukla, at the New Jersey Institute of Technology.

Johnston: You discussed the isolation of the brain material, and you used cation exchange resins, Dr Su. Did that hold on to your biological material?

Su: Actually, some of it went right through the cation exchange column, indicating that it was not positively charged at the elution pH.

Johnston: You use NMR in your studies and you identify a lot of methylene groups in the putative endogenous ligand. However, the most characteristic feature of the NMR spectrum of a steroid is the angular methyl groups, which stand out very strongly. Did you see those on the spectrum of the brain-extracted material?

Su: The methylene groups dominated the spectrum, but the methyl group was also present.

Karavolas: The steroid-like brain substance that you isolated has a relative molecular mass of about 480. I wonder if this might reflect the fact that it is a steroid with an ester group, a sulphate or other conjugate, which would increase the M_r to something above 400–450. Is there any evidence that when you hydrolyse you yield a 300–350 M_r compound, and is there any esterase activity in your σ receptor, which could generate some sort of steroid sulphate, or other ester?

Su: Unfortunately, we have not done the necessary hydrolysis experiments, but obviously that is a very interesting point. In fact, pregnenolone is inactive in the sigma receptor assay; only the sulphated form is active in that assay. We have not checked the esterase activity of the σ receptor yet.

McEwen: The condition in which effects of σ receptors on the immune system, and perhaps on the brain, might be most significant is pregnancy. The alterations in the immune system during pregnancy are not simply describable as immunosuppression, however; they are much more complicated than that. I suspect that you may be able to find out more about the ways in which progesterone alters immune function, which could then be very applicable to the whole pregnancy state.

Su: I agree that the possible involvement of σ receptors in immune responses certainly needs more investigation.

References

Abbott A 1990 5-HT$_3$ antagonists and ligands for dopamine D$_1$- and autoreceptors offer new leads for antipsychotic drugs. Trends Pharmacol Sci 11:49–51

Campbell BG, Scherz MW, Keana JFW, Weber E 1989 Sigma receptors regulate contractions of the guinea-pig ileum longitudinal muscle/myenteric plexus preparation elicited by both electrical stimulation and exogenous serotonin. J Neurosci 9:3380–3391

Ceci A, Smith M, French ED 1988 Activation of the A_{10} mesolimbic system by the σ-receptor agonist (+)SKF10,047 can be blocked by rimcazole, a novel putative antipsychotic. Eur J Pharmacol 154:53–57

Cross CE 1987 Oxygen radicals and human disease. Ann Int Med 107:526–545

McCann DJ, Su T-P 1990 Haloperidol-sensitive (+)[^{3}H]SKF-10047 binding sites (σ sites) exhibit a unique distribution in rat brain subcellular fractions. Eur J Pharmacol 188:211–218

Su T-P, London ED, Jaffe JH 1988 Steroid binding at σ receptors suggests a link between endocrine, nervous, and immune systems. Science (Wash DC) 240:219–221

Wolfe SA Jr, Kulsakdinun C, Battaglia G, Jaffe JH, De Souza EB 1988 Initial identification and characterization of sigma receptors on human peripheral blood leukocytes. J Pharmacol Exp Ther 247:1114–1119

General discussion I

Gene-mediated corticosteroid effects on neuronal excitability

de Kloet: The mineralocorticoid and glucocorticoid receptors have been cloned. Their primary structures indicate the presence of three domains, the steroid binding, DNA binding and N-terminal domains. The DNA binding domains of these two receptors are very similar, sequence homology being about 94%. The steroid binding domains show about 57% sequence homology (Evans 1988). In the rat brain (hippocampus), corticosterone and aldosterone show affinity for both types of receptor but the affinity differs by an order of magnitude; corticosterone and aldosterone show high affinity for the mineralocorticoid receptor (K_d 0.5×10^{-9} M) but a 10-fold lower affinity for the glucocorticoid receptor. Therefore, *in vivo* the mineralocorticoid receptor is 80–100% occupied by endogenous ligands, whereas the glucocorticoid receptor is 10–80% occupied during episodic changes in circulating steroid levels (Reul & de Kloet 1985, de Kloet & Reul 1987).

When an animal is stressed the corticosteroid level in the blood rises, so the glucocorticoid receptor may be considered to be a 'stress' receptor which mediates the stress-induced effects of corticosteroids in the brain. One approach by which to show an effect of corticosteroids is to remove the adrenals so that there are no endogenous adrenal steroids. Next one can investigate whether a disturbance in neural functioning develops that can be restored by steroid replacement.

Using *in situ* hybridization we have observed that the mineralocorticoid and glucocorticoid receptors seem to be expressed in the same neurons in the hippocampus of the rat (Van Eekelen et al 1988). So we faced the problem of the function of two corticosteroid receptors that are co-localized in the neurons of the hippocampus, that both bind corticosterone and, probably, bind to the same hormone-responsive element.

My colleague, Dr Marianne Joëls, incubated 300 µm hippocampal slices from adrenalectomized rats for 20 minutes with steroids, aldosterone or corticosterone. Then the perfusion was stopped and the incubation medium changed, so that no steroid remained. The slice will now only contain steroid that is bound to a receptor.

Intracellular recordings from pyramidal CA1 neurons were made and it was found that 1 nM aldosterone and 1 nM corticosterone increased the number of spikes, so these steroids increased neuronal excitability. After the 20 minute treatment with 1 nM aldosterone the level of excitability remained elevated during

117

the next 60 minutes. Interestingly, after the corticosterone treatment the number of spikes decreased slowly, returning to control level by 60 minutes. However, after a 20 minute incubation with 30 nM corticosterone there was no increase in excitability, and, after 60 minutes, excitability was suppressed and was below control levels. Thus, we have shown that aldosterone, a mineralocorticoid, increases neuronal excitability, whereas corticosterone, a glucocorticoid, first enhances excitability, then causes a suppression of excitability that remains for at least 4–5 hours (Joëls & de Kloet 1989). In experiments with RU28362, a potent glucocorticoid antagonist, we also found a long-lasting suppression of neuronal excitability after a brief initial exposure to the steroid.

Afterhyperpolarization (AHP) was also influenced by these steroids; 1 nM aldosterone and 1 nM corticosterone reduce the magnitude of afterhyperpolarization, but if the concentration of corticosterone is increased to over 30 nM and the time of incubation is increased, the size of the AHP also increases. AHP is the time during which the neuron shows reduced responsiveness to an excitatory stimulus. It is believed to be associated with a Ca^{2+}-dependent potassium conductance. The time dependency and the mode of action of aldosterone and corticosterone are consistent with the idea that these steroids might trigger a genomic event which may lead to alteration of a calcium flux (Joëls & de Kloet 1990, Nicoll 1988).

The effects of aldosterone and corticosterone that I have described are clearly genomically mediated; the effects have a slow onset and have long-lasting consequences. Binding of the steroids to mineralocorticoid and glucocorticoid receptors has opposite effects on neuronal excitability; the mineralocorticoid receptors maintain excitability, whereas glucocorticoid receptors suppress excitability, which is transiently raised by excitatory input. The two types of receptors probably interact with the same DNA sequence.

Glowinski: Do you think this can be due to a genomic effect, since the response is seen quickly?

de Kloet: I do not think the effects are rapid. Please note that the effects develop after removal of the steroid from the medium. The effect of aldosterone via the mineralocorticoid receptor develops slowly over 20–40 minutes and the effect of corticosterone via the glucocorticoid receptor was seen only after 60 minutes.

Hall: We have seen enhancement of excitability by methylprednisolone in cat spinal motor neurons. Using intracellular microelectrodes, we saw enhanced excitability within minutes of the intravenous injection of 30 mg/kg methylprednisolone. When we increased the dose to 60 mg/kg, we saw a biphasic dose–response curve where the enhancement of excitability seen at the lower dose was lost (Hall 1982). We have not measured ionic fluxes, but the modifications of the action potential are consistent with the idea that calcium conductance is greatly enhanced by a high dose of methylprednisolone.

de Kloet: I would like to see the detailed design of that experiment, because if you used concentrations much higher than those I used, you are probably dealing with a different phenomenon.

Hall: That is my point. I think that the effects that I described are non-genomic and in fact non-receptor-mediated membrane effects.

McEwen: If most of the type I receptors (the mineralocorticoid receptors) are occupied by steroid under normal conditions *in vivo*, how does the effect on neuronal excitability that Dr de Kloet described relate to the physiological situation? Could there be partial occupancy of the receptor, or are the neurons always maximally excited?

de Kloet: Using this approach we can distinguish between the response to the mineralocorticoid and the response to the glucocorticoid. In the intact animal I think the rate-limiting factor for the glucocorticoid receptor will be the level of circulating hormone, which will vary according to the time of the day and after stress. We found the mineralocorticoid receptor to be 80–90% occupied under all circumstances. In this case the receptor itself could be rate limiting. Perhaps activity of the receptor itself determines the degree of response to mineralocorticoids. Of course, at any given moment in the intact animal the two receptors will act in coordination to determine the state of excitability of these hippocampal CA1 neurons. When these results are extrapolated to physiological situations, I think the glucocorticoid receptor is involved in the response to stress, whereas the mineralocorticoid receptor determines the state of arousal that the animal is in at the moment it receives a stressful stimulus.

McEwen: Another possibility is that the mineralocorticoid type I receptor is largely, or at least partly, unoccupied at some times during the day (Chao et al 1989). We have found type I receptors to be largely unoccupied in the morning hours in the absence of stress, so there may be times of the day, and times in an animal's life, when it is like an adrenalectomized animal.

Feldman: It has been suggested that a membrane effect of a steroid might be the initial trigger for a genomic effect. What mechanism might this involve?

McEwen: We know that there are *trans*-acting factors, DNA-binding proteins, whose state of phosphorylation is regulated by second messenger systems such as those involving Ca^{2+} calmodulin kinase, protein kinase C or adenylate cyclase. These proteins bind to DNA and work like steroid receptors, so they might provide a connection between cell surface events, intracellular second messengers and genes.

Feldman: Do you think the negative feedback of glucocorticoids on the release system, and their early membrane effect and subsequent genomic effects, could be exerted through such a mechanism?

McEwen: Yes, I think so.

de Kloet: Before one can decide on this one needs first to show that the rapid effects seen in response to glucocorticoids are really due to an effect at the membrane. Jacques Glowinski said that for adenylate cyclase activity to be affected a continuous exposure to oestradiol is needed. Clearly, it is necessary to probe these steroid target cells at different levels (membrane, second messenger, gene) to establish whether the effects are membrane mediated and involve secondary genomic events. There is at present no reason to assume that the glucocorticoid-mediated phenomenon that I described is one which is secondary to a glucocorticoid membrane-evoked response, because the steroid specificity and the time and dose dependencies are all in favour of a long-term, gene-mediated response involving intracellular steroid receptors.

Ramirez: In an *in vitro* rat hypothalamic preparation we have found that cyclic AMP releases LHRH, and Dr Kim has shown that it also increases messenger RNA specific for LHRH (Kim et al 1989). So an initial membrane mechanism seems plausible. Cyclic AMP could activate LHRH release mechanisms very quickly but later, through a genomic mechanism, cyclic AMP stimulates the synthesis of LHRH, to allow the system to respond again to an appropriate signal.

Baulieu: There is at least one example where the initial response to a steroid is followed later by other effects. For instance, in *Xenopus* oocytes, progesterone immediately alters adenylate cyclase activity, then meiosis follows two hours later. In between there is a complex series of events that might involve protein phosphorylation and protein synthesis.

Each of us is looking at the effects of particular hormones or mediators at different times after their application; if you look for a response immediately, then you may see one, but if you wait, you may see protein synthesis or cell division. Growth factors have an initial effect at the membrane level but, in fact, after a cascade of intracellular events, they ultimately exert their effects through the genome. When we see an immediate electrophysiological response to a steroid, mediated by a neuronal membrane effect, we should also look at other components of the response, which may take longer to be detected, since they are metabolic changes of the cell.

Kordon: The regulation of gene transcription and of exocytosis can be dissociated. For instance, gonadotropin releasing hormone (GnRH) binds to a membrane receptor coupled to phospholipase C. Hence, the hormone activates protein kinase C, production of inositol trisphosphate and Ca^{2+} mobilization. McArdle & Conn (1989) have been able to dissociate GnRH-induced gonadotropin secretion and LH gene transcription by inhibiting protein kinase C. After such blockade, the cell is still able to secrete LH in response to GnRH but the peptide no longer induces gene transcription. Although pleiotypic under most conditions, second messengers thus exhibit a certain degree of specialization.

Dubrovsky: I agree with Professor Baulieu's view that we need to specify in what cell region (membrane or cytoplasm) and for how long a particular hormone acts. In fact, early and late effects of a hormone may be different in a specific phenomenon. Thus, thyrotropin releasing hormone (TRH) produces an increase in population spike amplitude (PS) without affecting the excitatory postsynaptic potential (EPSP) of the evoked potential produced in the dentate gyrus by stimulation of the perforant path. This effect takes place after intracerebroventricular injection. In contrast, TRH significantly reduces the EPSP of the same response after the induction of long-term potentiation (LTP). These dissociated effects of TRH on EPSP can relate to different states of the cell or be mediated via different neuronal mechanisms (Morimoto & Goddard 1985).

Neuronal responses to steroids can be state dependent, and this in turn may depend on different neuronal mechanisms. Thus, while tonically firing neurons do not respond to iontophoretically released cortisol, cortisol release changes the nature and intensity of the response of the neuron to distant stimuli (Feldman 1981). Dr Hall demonstrated that the synthetic steroid methylprednisolone increased the excitability of the axon hillock but decreased excitability in somadendritic regions. Thus a hormone may have different effects on a neuron depending on when and where it acts (Hall 1982). As Danielli (1953) wrote: '. . . evolution is the history of changing uses of molecules, and not of changing synthetic abilities.' Studying the phylogenetic history of receptors might help us to understand what each receptor is doing at a specific site, and to avoid seeing apparent discrepancies when the receptors do not behave according to our preconceptions. Looking for antecedents can be more illuminating than looking for final causes of biological phenomena.

de Kloet: I object to the generalization of these phenomena, because there are sufficient arguments to maintain that intracellular receptors are involved. As I have pointed out previously, there is, in our experiments, after steroid exposure, no change in the electrical properties of the cell membrane until the neuron is subjected to an excitatory stimulus. In the experiments I described, the effects of steroids took time to develop, and the time differed between the mineralocorticoid and the glucocorticoid: it took 20 minutes for the mineralocorticoid response to aldosterone to develop and 60 minutes for the glucocorticoid response to corticosterone. This is a situation completely different from the one where a transmitter or peptide binds to a membrane receptor, triggering a sequence of events, one of which is genomic. Membrane-mediated and gene-mediated primary effects can be distinguished because they involve different signal transduction systems.

Kordon: Bruce McEwen was talking about the reversal of transmitter effects by steroids. This is particularly conspicuous in the hypothalamus. There are numerous examples of diverse neuroendocrine responses to neurotransmitters, such as dopamine or noradrenaline, depending upon whether or not the tissue has been exposed to steroids. This is true for instance of the dopamine-induced release of oxytocin, and the GnRH release induced by noradrenaline and dopamine, but also by peptides such as angiotensin II, neuropeptide Y and cholecystokinin (see reviews in Weiner et al 1988 and Kordon et al 1989).

As in Jacques Glowinski's model, a steroid-induced commutation of transduction mechanisms accounts for such response shifts. This is a very economical system by which a cell does not need to down-regulate or up-regulate its receptors: a simple change in the balance between G protein subunits within the membrane can completely reset the reading frame of the cell. This is an interesting and ultimately simple model for understanding the influence of steroids on membrane-dependent signal transduction processes.

Baulieu: In the *Xenopus* oocyte system, besides the reduction of adenylate cyclase activity, there were other changes in the membrane induced by progesterone. For example, the membrane became less permeable (leucine transport was decreased: Baulieu & Schorderet-Slatkine 1983, Pennequin et al 1975), although the molecular basis of this change is unknown. Also the IGF-I receptor system became more sensitive to its ligand (El Etr et al 1979, Wallace et al 1980). So, when a steroid hormone binds to a cell membrane, a variety of events may result within a short time.

In the *Xenopus* oocyte, progesterone triggers meiosis. If after two hours you wash out the hormone completely from the cell, meiosis continues because it has already been triggered at the membrane. Progesterone treatment alters the phosphorylation state of various factors that are involved in cell division and you can take these proteins from the progesterone-treated oocyte and transfer them to another oocyte, where they will reinitiate meiosis. Wash-out experiments are difficult to do in the CNS.

Simmonds: With the *Xenopus* oocyte system you presumably work at a reasonably low temperature?

Baulieu: At room temperature.

Simmonds: With mammalian tissue slices or fragments or cell cultures, many people work at room temperature for simplicity. How temperature dependent are these slower, probably genomic effects? Can you assume they will be absent if you are working at room temperature, or do you have to take them into account?

Ramirez: Pulses of progesterone in the rat hypothalamus elicited LHRH release at 37 °C but were ineffective at 30 °C. So the response of the LHRH neural apparatus is temperature dependent.

I would like to emphasize the fact that most circulating hormones are secreted in a pulsatile manner. So, receptors can be modulated by changes in the frequency of hormone signals in addition to changes in hormone concentration; both frequency modulation and amplitude modulation are important. We have evidence (see my paper in this volume and Ramirez et al 1985) that a change in the frequency of progesterone or P-3-BSA infusion to corpus striatum superfused *in vitro* (that is, a continuous infusion) blocks amphetamine-evoked dopamine release.

McEwen: Thinking about issues of pulsatility of hormone application leading to transient responsiveness, I wonder if we can distinguish between receptor desensitization that results from continuous infusion and the possibility that the hormone induces effects which oppose one another. Such opposing effects might have different time courses and would result in a net biphasic response. The two mechanisms are different, but they probably both operate at the same time in some systems.

Simmonds: That is a very important point. I think it would be very difficult to separate these.

References

Baulieu EE, Schorderet-Slatkine S 1983 Steroid and peptide control mechanisms in membrane of *Xenopus laevis* oocytes resuming meiotic division. In: Molecular biology of egg maturation. Pitman, London (Ciba Found Symp 98) p 137–158

Chao H, Choo P, McEwen BS 1989 Glucocorticoid and mineralocorticoid receptor mRNA expression in rat brain. Neuroendocrinology 50:365–371

Danielli JF 1953 Postscript. On some physical and chemical aspects of evolution. In: Evolution. Cambridge University Press, Cambridge (Symp Soc Exp Biol, vol 7) p 430–438

de Kloet ER, Reul JMHM 1987 Feedback action and tonic influence of corticosteroids on brain functions: a concept arising from the heterogeneity of brain receptor systems. Psychoneuroendocrinology 12:83–105

El Etr M, Schorderet-Slatkine S, Baulieu EE 1979 Meiotic maturation in *Xenopus laevis* oocytes initiated by insulin. Science (Wash DC) 205:1397–1399

Evans RM 1988 The steroid and thyroid hormone receptor superfamily. Science (Wash DC) 240:889–895

Feldman S 1981 Electrophysiological effects of adrenocortical hormones on the brain. In: Fuxe K et al (eds) Steroid hormone regulation of the brain. Pergamon Press, Elmsford, NY, p 175–190

Hall ED 1982 Glucocorticoid effects on central nervous system excitability and synaptic transmission. Int Rev Neurobiol 23:165–195

Joëls M, de Kloet ER 1989 Effects of glucocorticoids and norepinephrine on the excitability in the hippocampus. Science (Wash DC) 245:1502–1505

Joëls M, de Kloet ER 1990 Mineralocorticoid receptor-mediated changes in membrane properties of rat CA1 pyramidal neurons *in vitro*. Proc Natl Acad Sci USA 87:4495–4498

Kim K, Byung JL, Wan KC 1989 Effects of forskolin and phorbol ester on LHRH mRNA in the rat hypothalamus. Society for the Study of Reproduction 22nd Annual Meeting Abstract #153 (p 98)

Kordon C, Drouva SV, Enjalbert A, Gautron JP, Leblanc P 1989 The hypothalamic control of GnRH secretion. In: Delamarre–van de Waal H et al (eds) Control of the onset of puberty III. Elsevier, Amsterdam, p 79–88

McArdle CA, Conn PM 1989 Use of protein kinase C-depleted cells for investigation of the role of protein kinase C in stimulus–response coupling in the pituitary. Methods Enzymol 168:287–301

Morimoto K, Goddard GV 1985 Effects of thyrotropin-releasing hormone on evoked responses and long-term potentiation in dentate gyrus of rat. Exp Neurol 90:401–410

Nicoll RA 1988 The coupling of neurotransmitter receptors to ion channels in the brain. Science (Wash DC) 241:545–551

Pennequin P, Schorderet-Slatkine S, Drury KC, Baulieu EE 1975 Decreased uptake of ^{3}H-leucine during progesterone induced maturation of *Xenopus laevis* oocytes. FEBS (Fed Eur Biochem Soc) Lett 51:156–160

Ramirez VD, Kim K, Dluzen D 1985 Progesterone action on the LHRH and the nigrostriatal dopamine neuronal systems: *in vitro* and *in vivo* studies. Recent Prog Horm Res 41:421–472

Reul JMHM, de Kloet ER 1985 Two receptor systems for corticosterone in rat brain: microdistribution and differential occupation. Endocrinology 121:2505–2511

Wallace RA, Misulovin Z, El Etr M, Schorderet-Slatkine S, Baulieu EE 1980 The role of zinc and follicle cells in insulin-initiated meiotic maturation of *Xenopus laevis* oocytes. Science (Wash DC) 210:928–930

Weiner RI, Findell PR, Kordon C 1988 Role of classic and peptide neuromediators in the neuroendocrine regulation of LH and prolactin. In: Knobil E, Neill J (eds) The physiology of reproduction. Raven Press, New York, p 1235

Van Eekelen JAM, Jiang W, de Kloet ER, Bohn MC 1988 Mineralocorticoid and glucocorticoid receptor messenger RNA in the rat hippocampus. J Neurosci Res 21:88–94

Effects of progesterone and its metabolites on neuronal membranes

V. D. Ramirez, D. E. Dluzen and F. C. Ke

Department of Physiology and Biophysics, University of Illinois, 524 Burrill Hall, 407 South Goodwin Avenue, Urbana, IL 61801, USA

Abstract. Evidence supporting a membrane site of action for progesterone includes the rapidity of its effects when directly infused into tissue containing mainly nerve terminals, the absence of functional intracellular progesterone receptors *in vitro* and the fact that progesterone conjugated to bovine serum albumin (BSA) in the C-3 position (P-3-BSA) activates the release of hypothalamic luteinizing hormone releasing hormone (LHRH) or modulates amphetamine-evoked striatal dopamine release. In addition, P_2 membrane fractions from different areas of the CNS but not P_1 fractions or P_2 membranes from peripheral progesterone targets have specific binding sites for P-11-^{125}I-BSA. Among several BSA-conjugated steroids tested for competition displacement P-3-BSA had the highest affinity with an estimated inhibition constant of 28.5 ± 2.1 nM. This binding depends on the presence of cations such as Ca^{2+} and Mg^{2+} and after chemical depolarization of the P_2 membranes the binding curve of P-3-BSA shifts to the right. While progesterone is effective in releasing LHRH from the hypothalamus, 5β-pregnan-3β-ol-20-one (a 5β reduced metabolite) is at least 1000-fold more potent than the parent compound when tested *in vitro* and *in vivo*. This action is indirect because tetrodotoxin at 10^{-6} M blocks the LHRH releasing action, although 5β-prenan-3β-ol-20-one is still capable of releasing noradrenaline. Although 5β-pregnan-3β-ol-20-one can replace progesterone in activating the LHRH neural apparatus this is not true for the nigro-striatal dopamine system where only progesterone or P-3-BSA is effective, an action which is also indirect since tetrodotoxin blocks the effect of either compound. These results indicate that progesterone acts at membrane sites to modulate specific functions of the CNS and that site-specific mechanisms exist within the CNS which may differentially control its conversion to more active compounds.

1990 Steroids and neuronal activity. Wiley, Chichester (Ciba Foundation Symposium 153) p 125–144

Progesterone influences a number of important physiological functions in the CNS of mammals, particularly those affecting reproduction and mental functions. This steroid hormone is known to trigger neuronal activity by two mechanisms, one that activates the genomic pathway (McEwen et al 1987) and the other that involves a non-genomic transmembrane signalling mechanism

(Ramirez et al 1985, Majewska 1987). In this chapter we shall review evidence indicating an important role for progesterone and its reduced metabolites in neuronal membrane functions in relation to the control of LHRH (luteinizing hormone releasing hormone) and dopamine release from the hypothalamus and the nigro-striatal dopamine (NSDA) system, respectively. We shall also discuss some of the characteristics of progesterone binding to membrane fractions, as revealed using progesterone conjugated to ^{125}I-labelled bovine serum albumin (BSA) as a ligand.

Effects of progesterone and its metabolites on the activity of the LHRH neural apparatus

The LHRH neural apparatus can be considered as a network of neurons whose activation leads to either increases or decreases in the secretion of the decapeptide, LHRH. It is well established that inhibitory neurons, notably GABA and β-endorphin neurons, and excitatory neurons, such as noradrenaline (norepinephrine), neuropeptide Y and aspartate-glutamate neurons (Kalra & Kalra 1986, Bourguignon et al 1989, Masotto et al 1989), are key components of the LHRH neural apparatus. However, little is known about the exact connectivity of this neuronal network.

The interaction between neural and steroid signals in the hypothalamus which leads to the release of the LHRH decapeptide through activation of non-genomic mechanisms is one aspect that our laboratory has addressed. For example, pulses of progesterone were capable of releasing LHRH when administered directly into superfusion chambers containing a preparation from rat median eminence (Fig. 1A) known to contain mainly nerve terminals (Zamora & Ramirez 1983). A remarkable aspect of this effect of progesterone was that practically each pulse of the steroid triggered a peak response within 10–20 min after infusion. This action of progesterone resembled the effects of depolarizing pulses of K^+ (30 mM) in a comparable preparation (Fig. 1B). From this similarity of responsiveness, it is not unreasonable to postulate that progesterone pulses could somehow open Ca^{2+} channels of nerve terminals in the median eminence, leading to rapid activation of the LHRH pulse generator. Evidence indicating a role for Ca^{2+} in this phenomenon was obtained earlier by Drouva et al (1985), whose data revealed that removal of Ca^{2+} from, or addition of D-600 (a blocker of voltage-dependent calcium channels) to hypothalamic slices superfused *in vitro* blocked the stimulatory action of progesterone on LHRH release. In addition, the effect of progesterone on LHRH release involves the mediation of calmodulin and a calmodulin-dependent kinase system, because a calmodulin inhibitor (trifluoroperazine, 30 μM) or a calmodulin-dependent tubulin kinase inhibitor (phenytoin, 50 μM) antagonized the stimulatory action of progesterone. Moreover, recently Nikezic et al (1988) have found that *in vivo* administration of progesterone (2 mg) inhibited the potassium-depolarization

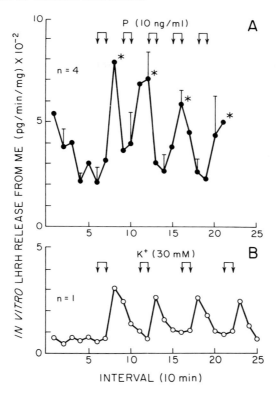

FIG. 1.   Effect of pulses of progesterone (P) (A: 10 min every 20 min) and K^+ (B: 10 min every 40 min) on the release of lutenizing hormone releasing hormone (LHRH) from the median eminence (ME) from ovariectomized oestrogen-primed (OVX + E) 30-day-old rats. Means ± SEM are shown in A. Notice in both cases relatively rapid release of LHRH from the nerve terminals. *, peak value significantly different ($P < 0.05$ by Student's t-test) from nadir value.

dependent $^{45}Ca^{2+}$ uptake by crude synaptosomal preparations (P_2 membrane fractions) from rat brain, notably from the striatum and hippocampus.

An alternative approach by which to examine a membrane site of action for progesterone is to use the steroid (P) linked to bovine serum albumin (BSA) to generate a large complex that does not diffuse across the axolemma (Ke & Ramirez 1987). Only one of these complexes, P-3-BSA, and not P-11-BSA or deoxycorticosterone-21-BSA (DOC-21-BSA), when administered at similar concentrations to that of progesterone, was effective in releasing LHRH from hypothalamic preparations derived from ovariectomized oestrogen-primed (OVX + E_2) 30-day-old rats (Kim & Ramirez 1985). This not only supports the hypothesis of a membrane site of action but indicates the necessity of a precise stereospecific orientation of the progesterone molecule in the complex for effective transmembrane activation. The progesterone-stimulated LHRH response is present only if the hypothalamus is physiologically primed with oestrogen, as it is during the rat oestrous cycle (Kim & Ramirez 1986), or when ovariectomized rats are pretreated with oestrogen (Kim & Ramirez 1985). Further, the progesterone-evoked LHRH release response is faster than that evoked by the P-3-BSA conjugate. Among several steroids tested in such hypothalamic preparations, including the synthetic progestin R5020, known to bind to progesterone receptors (Kato 1985), only progesterone itself and P-3-BSA elicited LHRH release, but with different latencies, probably due to different diffusion rates (Fig. 2). These results further confirm the assumption that progesterone acts through a non-genomic mechanism at a membrane site,

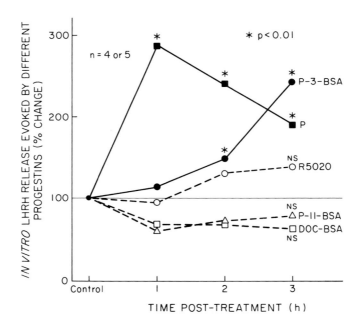

FIG. 2. *In vitro* LHRH release from hypothalamic preparations as a function of super-fusion time and evoked by different progestins administered in pulses; the first hour of basal LHRH release was considered control and expressed as 100%. Only free progesterone (P) and progesterone conjugated to BSA through C-3 were effective in augmenting the release of LHRH from hypothalamic preparations derived from OVX + E 30-day-old rats. Maximal effect was observed 1 h after the P pulses (10 min on, 20 min off), whereas with P-3-BSA the maximal effect was observed in the last hour of superfusion. Concentration values for P-3-BSA, progesterone, R5020, P-11-BSA and deoxycorticosterone-BSA (DOC-BSA) were approximately 1.7×10^{-7} M of P, 10^{-7} M, 10^{-7} M, 1.6×10^{-7} M of 11-hydroxyprogesterone (11-OH-P), and 1.8×10^{-7} M of DOC, respectively. *, values significantly different from controls ($P < 0.05$ by Student's t-test). NS, not significant.

because a rapid decline in the so-called cytoplasmic progesterone receptors (Kato 1985), without evidence of accumulation in the nuclear fraction, occurs in such preparations (Fig. 3).

Structure–functional studies of a variety of steroids similar in structure to the progesterone molecule, and also of several metabolites of progesterone (Park & Ramirez 1987, Ramirez & Dluzen 1987), revealed that only one of these steroids, 5β-pregnan-3β-ol-20-one, was active and, more importantly, that the apparent minimal effective dose was at least 1000-fold lower than that of the parent compound. The requirements for this potent action of 5β-pregnan-3β-ol-20-one mimic closely those of progesterone in at least two aspects: first, the

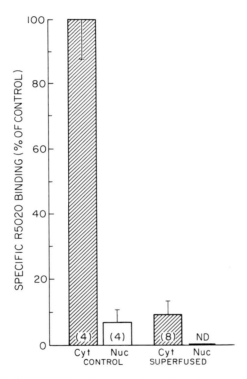

FIG. 3.   Binding of [³H] R5020 to the cytosolic and nuclear compartments of super-fused hypothalamic tissue. Hypothalamic-preoptic area fragments from ovariectomized, oestrogen-primed 30-day-old rats were kept in an ice bath (Control) or were superfused for 2 h in modified superfusion medium (Krebs-Ringer phosphate containing 0.1% BSA, 10 mM glucose, 0.1% [w/v] ascorbic acid, 3.5×10^{-4} M pargyline and 1×10^{-4} M bacitracin, pH 7.4). Progestin–receptor binding was determined in both the cytosol (Cyt) and the KCl-extractable nuclear fractions combined with the membrane (Nuc) fractions and are expressed (mean ± SEM) as a percentage of the binding measured in the Control cytosol fraction (15.4 fmol/mg of protein). The numbers in parentheses represent the numbers of superfusions in each group. ND, not detectable.

metabolite is effective only if hypothalamic preparations have been primed with oestrogen, and second, a pulsatile mode of administration is required, because a continued infusion of 5β-pregnan-3β-ol-20-one failed to activate the LHRH neural apparatus. In addition, this 5β-reduced progesterone metabolite was also effective and more potent when tested *in vivo*, since local infusion into the hypothalamus of freely moving rats by means of a push-pull cannula at concentrations of 10^{-11} M (Park & Ramirez 1987) and in rabbits at concentrations of 10^{-12} M (Lin & Ramirez 1990) was capable of stimulating LHRH release. Interestingly, the stimulatory effect of 5β-pregnan-3β-ol-20-one on the activity of the LHRH neural apparatus was blocked when the sodium channel blocker tetrodotoxin (TTX) $(10^{-6}$ M) was present in the perfusion medium, even though the metabolite still significantly released ($P < 0.01$ by Student's t-test) noradrenaline from the *in vitro* hypothalamic preparations (Fig. 4).

In short, the data reviewed in this section support the concept that progesterone activates the LHRH neural apparatus by a non-genomic mechanism through binding to stereospecific sites in the axolemma of neurons belonging to the neural circuit involved in the control of LHRH release. The fact that 5β-pregnan-3β-ol-20-one and not its epimer, 5α-pregnan-3α-ol-20-one, is active in releasing LHRH at doses at least 1000-fold lower than those of progesterone from *in vitro* and *in vivo* hypothalamic preparations in two species, the rat and the rabbit, suggests that it is this 5β-reduced metabolite of progesterone that may play an important physiological role in the control of LHRH release. Lastly, but not least, the effect of 5β-pregnan-3β-ol-20-one appears to be mediated by a direct action on noradrenaline terminals within the hypothalamus, because in the absence of axonal transmission, after blockade of Na^+ channels, 5β-pregnan-3β-ol-20-one is still capable of increasing the release of this neurotransmitter, which is known to play a paramount role in the control of LHRH release.

Effects of progesterone and its metabolites on the nigro-striatal dopamine system

Our laboratory for some time now has been studying the role of steroids and proteins in the activity of the NSDA system (Ramirez & Dluzen 1987). In the course of such studies we have clearly demonstrated that progesterone administered to female rats either systemically or directly into the corpus striatum has profound stimulatory or inhibitory modulatory effects on dopaminergic neurotransmission. As in the hypothalamus, the action of progesterone requires that the NSDA system be exposed to an oestrogen-priming regimen, either by exogenous replacement therapy (Dluzen & Ramirez 1984) or by an endogenous source, as in the intact cycling female rat (Dluzen & Ramirez 1985). An important finding was the demonstration that the mode and temporal characteristics of progesterone administration are crucial in eliciting either the stimulatory or the inhibitory component of progesterone. When this steroid is infused in pulses

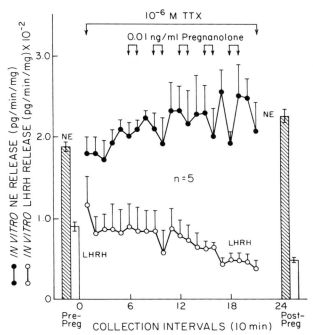

FIG. 4.   Changes in noradrenaline (norepinephrine, NE) and LHRH levels as determined in perfusates collected every 10 min from individual hypothalami from adult OVX + E rats. The superfusion medium (Krebs-Ringer phosphate buffer, 10 mM glucose, 0.1% BSA and 0.1 mM bacitracin, pH 7.3–7.4) contained 1 μM tetrodotoxin (TTX) and pulses of 5β-pregnan-3β-ol-20-one (pregnanolone) were applied for 150 min in a 10 min on, 20 min off cycle after 1 h of control basal release. The bars represent the mean values corresponding to the first hour (control release) and the last hour after treatment for NE and LHRH, respectively. Notice the divergence in the release of the two neurochemicals as a function of treatment. The increase in NE release and decrease in LHRH release were significantly different ($P < 0.05$ by Student's t-test) from the respective control values. Error bars indicate SEM values.

or at 2–12 h before the rat is killed, it exerts a stimulatory action, whereas when progesterone is infused continuously or at 24 h before death, the inhibitory component is observed (Dluzen & Ramirez 1987). Among several steroids tested in this system at identical doses, none was as effective as progesterone. Particularly relevant to this discussion was the lack of effect of 5β-pregnan-3β-ol-20-one and oestradiol (Dluzen & Ramirez 1987). The stimulatory effect of progesterone can be reproduced with a single pulse of the steroid but over a rather limited dose–response range, maximal stimulation occurring at 4 ng/ml and minimal at 2 ng/ml (Dluzen & Ramirez 1990a). It is also present in the corpus striatum from male rats, provided they are castrated and receive 17β-oestradiol benzoate priming (Dluzen & Ramirez 1990b). Interestingly, the latency required for 4 ng/ml progesterone to induce a significant modulatory action on amphetamine-evoked dopamine release was between 10 and 30 minutes.

Using a similar strategy to that described in the first section, we tested P-3-BSA in this system (Dluzen & Ramirez 1989a,b). Pulses of the complex at doses approximately equivalent to 2 ng/ml of free progesterone, which are known to be effective, were clearly stimulatory and led to an increase in the responsivity of the dopaminergic terminals to a subsequent 10^{-5} M amphetamine challenge (Fig. 5, panel A). In confirmation of our previous results with free progesterone (Dluzen & Ramirez 1984), a continuous infusion of the complex virtually shut off the responsiveness of the dopamine terminals to 10^{-5} M amphetamine (Fig. 5, panel B). More importantly, superfusion of striatal fragments with a medium containing 10^{-6} M TTX blocked the inhibitory effect of the continuous infusion of P-3-BSA on the responsiveness of the dopamine terminals to 10^{-5} M amphetamine, with dopaminergic responses recovering to levels detected in control preparations superfused with TTX alone (Fig. 5, panel C).

These data indicate that free progesterone, or progesterone immobilized through C-3 to BSA, but not 5β- nor 5α-reduced compounds, can modulate the NSDA system. Though progesterone and P-3-BSA are effective in both the LHRH and the NSDA systems, in the hypothalamus 5β-pregnan-3β-ol-20-one is exquisitely potent whereas in the corpus striatum it is completely inactive. In both systems, however, the effect of progesterone appears to be mediated by an interneuron, since TTX abolished the action of the steroid. We do not yet have firm evidence of which interneuron may be involved in the modulatory role of progesterone in the NSDA or LHRH system, although, in the latter, one of such neurons appears to be noradrenergic. However, a reasonable candidate for the inhibitory activity of progesterone in the NSDA system would be the GABA output neurons from the corpus striatum, because progesterone and its metabolites can enhance the inhibitory effect of GABA in spontaneous and evoked unit activity of cerebellar Purkinje cells (Smith et al 1987), and alphaxalone, a steroid anaesthetic, and some reduced progesterone metabolites can modulate $GABA_A$ receptors (Callachan et al 1987, Majewska 1987) by increasing Cl^- conductance and thereby hyperpolarizing target cells (Vicini et al 1987). Indeed, the amphetamine-evoked peak dopamine response of corpus striatum preparations superfused with medium containing TTX was higher than, though not significantly different from, that of controls without the Na^+ channel blocker ($\bar{x} \pm SEM$, 20.4 ± 8.8 vs 11.7 ± 3.0, $n = 4$). If we accept the concept that amphetamine-evoked dopamine release is largely due to blockage of the reuptake mechanism for this neurotransmitter (Fisher & Cho 1979), it is tempting to speculate that hyperpolarization of dopaminergic terminals, caused by release of GABA after continuous infusion of P-3-BSA, can lead to alterations in the dopamine reuptake mechanism such that amphetamine is now a poor blocker, whereas in the presence of TTX dopamine reuptake is facilitated. Further experiments are necessary to test such a challenging hypothesis.

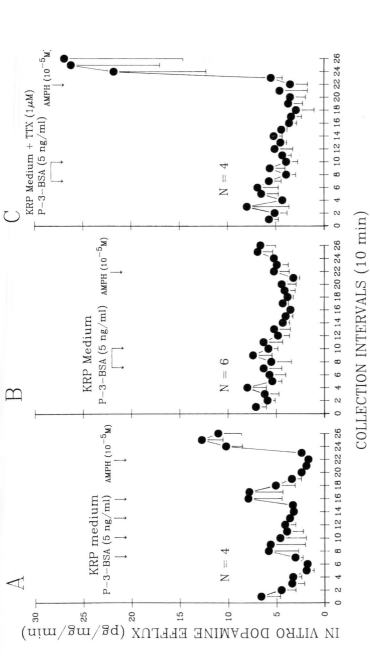

FIG. 5. The effect of P-3-BSA on basal and amphetamine (AMPH)-evoked dopamine (DA) efflux from *in vitro* striatal fragments derived from adult OVX + E rats. In A, pulses of the complex were effective in evoking increases in DA efflux and potentiated amphetamine (AMPH)-stimulated DA efflux. In B, a continuous infusion of the complex did not stimulate basal DA efflux and virtually shut off the AMPH-evoked DA response. In C, when the Krebs-Ringer phosphate (KRP) superfusion medium contained 1 μM tetrodotoxin (TTX), the continuous infusion of P-3-BSA was no longer effective in suppressing the AMPH-evoked DA response. Means ± SEM are shown.

Binding of progesterone-BSA conjugates to P_2 brain membranes and functional changes

Three main reasons led us to investigate the capacity of brain synaptosomal membranes (P_2 fractions) to bind progestins conjugated to radioiodinated bovine serum albumin. First was the inability of R5020 to modify the activity of either the LHRH neural apparatus or the NSDA system. Second was the failure to demonstrate specific binding sites for [^{3}H]progesterone in P_2 fractions (O. K. Park & V. D. Ramirez, unpublished work 1990). And, third, there was the fact that P-3-BSA could substitute for progesterone in its capacity to activate either of the two neuronal systems under study.

Though P-3-^{125}I-BSA binds specifically to P_2 fractions, the ligand of choice was P-11-^{125}I-BSA, because it binds less tightly to filters, thereby generating a lower non-specific binding (Ke & Ramirez 1990). Fig. 6 (left) illustrates the temporal binding characteristics of P-11-^{125}I-BSA to P_2 fractions prepared from rat cerebellum. The binding was specific for brain P_2 fractions, since similar fractions prepared from peripheral target tissue for progesterone (either

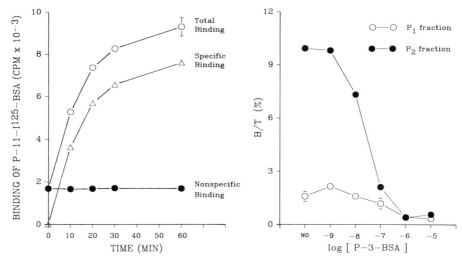

FIG. 6. *Left*: time course of the binding of P-11-^{125}I-BSA to rat cerebellum P_2 fractions. The concentration of total added P-11-^{125}I-BSA was about 4.9×10^{-11} M. The binding reactions were conducted in the absence (total binding) or presence (non-specific binding) of 10^{-5} M P-3-BSA. Bound and unbound ligand were separated by rapid filtration. Specific binding was determined by subtracting the non-specific binding from the total binding. *Right*: P-3-BSA displacement curves of the P-11-^{125}I-BSA binding to P_1 and P_2 fractions from rat cerebellum. The control tubes (without P-3-BSA) are designated as NO. The percentage binding is presented as B (bound)/T (total added P-11-^{125}I-BSA). The data represent means $\pm$ SEM of triplicates. Absence of an SEM bar indicates that the variation falls within the size of the symbols.

ovary or uterus) did not show binding. Moreover, the binding is site specific within the neural tissue, as only the P_2 but not the P_1 (pellets obtained from centrifugation of homogenates at $1000\,g$ for ten minutes) fractions bound the ligand (Fig. 6 right), and within the P_2 fraction only the axolemma subfraction showed a high affinity constant, estimated as $47\,nM$ (Ke & Ramirez 1990). Structure–binding competition studies revealed that P-3-BSA competes with the highest affinity for the P-11-^{125}I-BSA sites in the P_2 fractions, by comparison with any of the other structurally related complexes. Importantly, neither albumin nor oestrogen conjugated to albumin was able to compete for the binding sites, over a large range of doses (Ke & Ramirez 1990).

Table 1 presents the calculated K_i values from these studies as determined according to the Cheng and Prusoff equation. The binding of P-11-^{125}I-BSA to brainstem P_2 fractions depends on the presence of specific bivalent cations in the incubation medium such as Ca^{2+}, Mg^{2+}, Ba^{2+}, Mn^{2+} and Sr^{2+} but is absent in presence of Ni^{2+}, Cd^{2+}, Co^{2+}, Fe^{2+}, Zn^{2+} and Cu^{2+} (Fig. 7). Interestingly, the binding to brainstem P_2 fractions can be modulated by different concentrations of Mg^{2+} in the incubation medium ($50\,mM$ Tris-HCl, $120\,mM$ NaCl, $5\,mM$ KCl, 0.5, 2 or $5\,mM$ MgSO$_4$, pH 7.4 at $4\,°C$). Fig. 8 shows that at low concentrations of Mg^{2+}, little or no binding is detectable, whereas at the high concentration of $5\,mM$ a shift to the right of the P-3-BSA displacement curve was detected compared to the normal competition curve obtained at the $2\,mM$ concentration.

Lastly, a chemical depolarization of the brainstem P_2 fractions achieved by increasing K^+ and decreasing Na^+ concentrations iso-osmotically led to a drastic shift to the right of the P-3-BSA displacement curve, indicating a change from a high to a lower affinity of the cold ligand for the binding sites. The specificity of this phenomenon is further attested by the fact that depolarization of the membranes in the absence of Ca^{2+} (by addition of EDTA) markedly reduced the binding to the lower affinity binding sites (Fig. 9).

Concluding remarks

The data discussed here indicate that progesterone binds stereospecifically to neuronal membranes prepared from different brain regions all known to be target sites of progesterone, including the hypothalamus (Ramirez et al 1985), striatum (Ramirez & Dluzen 1987), cerebellum (Smith et al 1987) and brainstem (Sakuma & Pfaff 1981), although the specific functions of this steroid in these brain areas are only partially established. In two of the brain regions, the striatum and the hypothalamus, extensively investigated for the functional effects of progesterone, the complex P-3-BSA, which has the highest dissociation constant for the membrane sites of the BSA complexes tested (about $28\,nM$), can clearly substitute for free progesterone, since this complex is capable of mimicking all the functional effects of the free hormone at similar equivalent concentrations.

TABLE 1 Chemical structure of different steroid conjugates and their K_i values estimated from curves of their displacement of P-11-^{125}I-BSA binding to rat cerebellar P_2 fractions

Chemical structure	Steroid conjugate	K_i (nM)
CH₃ / CO ... CMO:BSA	Progesterone 3-(o-carboxymethyl) oxime BSA (P-3-BSA)	28.2
CH₃ / CO ... O HemiS:BSA	6β-Hydroxyprogesterone-6-hemisuccinate BSA (P-6-BSA)	69.2
OH ... BSA:CMO	Testosterone 3-(o-carboxymethyl) oxime BSA (T-3-BSA)	302.0
H₂CO HemiS:BSA / CO	Deoxycorticosterone-21-hemisuccinate BSA (DOC-21-BSA)	607.2
H₂COAc / CO HO... CMO:BSA	Corticosterone 21-acetate 3-(o-carboxymethyl) oxime BSA (11 OH, 21 Ac P-3-BSA)	1258.9
CH₃ / CO BSA:HemiSO	11α-Hydroxyprogesterone 11-hemisuccinate BSA (P-11-BSA)	1737.6
OH ... HO CMO:BSA	17β-Oestradiol 6-(−o-carboxymethyl) oxime BSA (E-6-BSA)	No displacement

It is not unreasonable to propose that the binding sites of progestins to neuronal membranes in the P_2 brain fractions represent real receptors, coupled to and capable of regulating channel functions. There is ample circumstantial evidence to indicate that progesterone and/or its metabolites can modify Ca^{2+} channels (Wasserman et al 1980, Drouva et al 1985, Kubli-Garfias et al 1985, Nikezic et al 1988) in addition to Cl^- channels (Majewska 1987). The fact that the binding of P-3-BSA to brain P_2 membranes can be modified by bivalent cations, particularly by high doses of Mg^{2+}, known to block Ca^{2+} channels (Miller 1988), and that depolarization of the membranes by high doses of K^+,

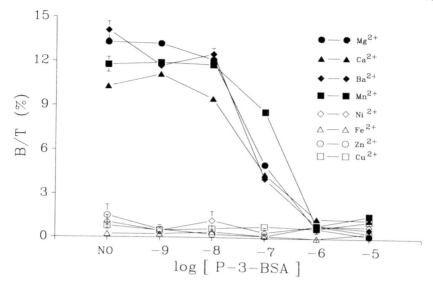

FIG. 7. The effect of different species of divalent cations (2 mM) on the curve of P-3-BSA displacement of the P-11-^{125}I-BSA binding to rat brainstem P_2 fractions. The incubation media contained 50 mM Tris-HCl, 120 mM NaCl, 5 mM KCl, 0.1% BSA and 2 mM of the divalent cation as indicated. The designations NO and B/T and the data presentation are as described for Fig. 6.

which opens voltage-sensitive Ca^{2+} channels (Capponi et al 1986), led to significant changes in the binding parameters of the progestin, strongly suggests that progesterone affects the gating and permeability of Ca^{2+} channels in neuronal tissue.

Since progesterone has two opposite actions on neuronal membranes, depending on its mode of administration, we should like to propose the following hypothesis, schematically depicted in Fig. 10, which can be tested experimentally. The *pulsatile* mode of P-3-BSA administration leads to the opening of Ca^{2+} channels in a specific interneuron linked to the chain of neuronal events resulting in LHRH and dopamine release from the hypothalamus and the striatum, respectively. The *continuous* mode of P-3-BSA administration leads to release of GABA, which then hyperpolarizes dopaminergic terminals in the striatum or LHRH nerve terminals in the hypothalamus. In addition and conversely, the continuous binding of the progestins to the dopaminergic or LHRH terminals may facilitate the so-called open state of the Cl^- channels or maintain the so-called inactive state of the Ca^{2+} channels (Triggle 1989), ultimately resulting in decreases in the secretion of these neurochemicals.

Lastly but not least, the fact that the 3β,5β-reduced metabolite of progesterone, 5β-pregnan-3β-ol-20-one, is at least three orders of magnitude

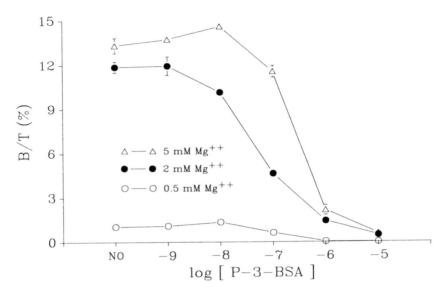

FIG. 8. The effect of different concentrations of Mg^{2+} on the curve of P-3-BSA displacement of P-11-^{125}I-BSA binding to rat brainstem P_2 fractions. The incubation media contained 50 mM Tris-HCl, 120 mM NaCl, 5 mM KCl, 0.1% BSA and Mg^{2+} (concentrations of Mg^{2+} as indicated). The designations NO and B/T and the data presentation are as described for Fig. 6.

more potent than progesterone itself, and can effectively substitute for the parent compound in its effect in the LHRH neural apparatus but not in the striatum, indicates a possible site-specific physiological role for this elusive metabolite. Proof that progesterone can be converted to 5β-pregnan-3β-ol-20-one in the hypothalamus of the rat will require sensitive methods, because the effect of this metabolite requires very low concentrations, of the order of picomoles.

It is concluded that progesterone acts at membrane receptors, possibly through coupling to Ca^{2+} and/or Cl^- channels in specific neurons, to modulate specific functions of the CNS. Moreover, it is likely that site-specific mechanisms exist within the CNS which may differentially control its conversion to more potent compounds.

Acknowledgements

We thank Ms E. Wilks for her assistance in preparing this manuscript and the National Science Foundation for partially supporting this work through a grant, # 85-09064, to V.D.R.

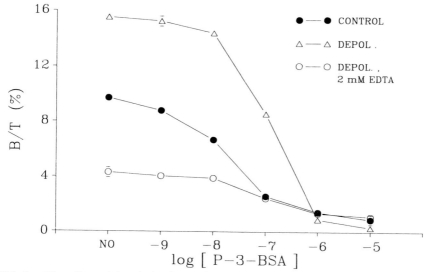

FIG. 9. The effect of depolarization and EDTA on the P-3-BSA displacement curve of the P-11-^{125}I-BSA binding to rat brainstem P_2 fractions. The depolarization (DEPOL.) was produced by increasing the K^+ concentration in the medium from 5 mM to 80 mM and iso-osmotically decreasing the Na^+ concentration from 120 mM to 45 mM. Divalent cations were replaced by EDTA in the other group as indicated. The designations NO and B/T and the data presentation are as described for Fig. 6.

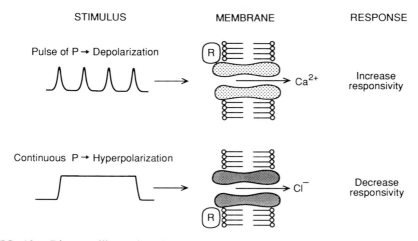

FIG. 10. Diagram illustrating the hypothesis that pulses of progesterone or P-3-BSA evoke secretion of neurochemicals by binding to membrane receptors coupled to Ca^{2+} channels, whereas continuously infused progesterone or P-3-BSA complex binds to membrane receptors coupled to Cl^- channels. In the former case, depolarization ensues and thereby the responsivity of the terminals is increased. In the latter case, hyperpolarization ensues and responsivity of the terminals is decreased.

References

Bourguignon JP, Gerard A, Franchimont P 1989 Direct activation of gonadotropin-releasing hormone secretion through different receptors to neuroexcitatory amino acids. Neuroendocrinology 49:402–408

Callachan H, Cottrell GA, Hather NY, Lambert JJ, Nooney JM, Peters JA 1987 Modulation of GABA$_A$ receptors by progesterone metabolites. Proc R Soc Lond B Biol Sci 231:359–369

Capponi AM, Lew PD, Schlegel W, Pozzan T 1986 Use of intracellular calcium and membrane potential fluorescent indicators in neuroendocrine cells. Methods Enzymol 124:116–135

Dluzen DE, Ramirez VD 1984 Bimodal effect of progesterone on *in vivo* dopamine function of the rat corpus striatum. Neuroendocrinology 39:149–155

Dluzen DE, Ramirez VD 1985 *In vitro* dopamine release from the rat striatum: diurnal rhythm and its modification by the estrous cycle. Neuroendocrinology 41:97–100

Dluzen DE, Ramirez VD 1987 Intermittent infusion of progesterone potentiates whereas continuous infusion reduces amphetamine-stimulated dopamine release from ovariectomized estrogen-primed rat striatal fragments superfused *in vitro*. Brain Res 406:1–9

Dluzen DE, Ramirez VD 1989a Progesterone effects upon dopamine release from the corpus striatum of female rats. I. Evidence for interneuronal control. Brain Res 476:332–337

Dluzen DE, Ramirez VD 1989b Progesterone effects upon dopamine release from the corpus striatum of female rats. II. Evidence for a membrane site of action and the role of albumin. Brain Res 476:338–344

Dluzen DE, Ramirez VD 1990a *In vitro* progesterone modulation of amphetamine-stimulated dopamine release from the corpus striatum of ovariectomized estrogen-treated female rats: response characteristics. Brain Res 517:117–122

Dluzen DE, Ramirez VD 1990b *In vitro* progesterone modulates amphetamine stimulated dopamine release from the corpus striatum of castrated male rats treated with estrogen. Neuroendocrinology, in press

Drouva SV, Laplante E, Kordon C 1985 Progesterone-Induced LHRH release *in vitro* is an estrogen—as well as Ca^{++}—and calmodulin-dependent secretory process. Neuroendocrinology 40:325–331

Fisher JF, Cho AK 1979 Chemical release of dopamine from striatal homogenates: evidence for an exchange diffusion model. J Pharmacol Exp Ther 208:203–209

Kalra PS, Kalra SP 1986 Steroidal modulation of the regulatory neuropeptides: luteinizing hormone releasing hormone, neuropeptide Y and endogenous opioid peptides. J Steroid Biochem 25:733–740

Kato J 1985 Progesterone receptors in brain and hypophysis. Curr Top Neuroendocrinol 5:31–81

Ke FC, Ramirez VD 1987 Membrane mechanism mediates progesterone stimulatory effect on LHRH release from superfused rat hypothalami *in vitro*. Neuroendocrinology 45:514–517

Ke FC, Ramirez VD 1990 Binding of progesterone to nerve cell membrane of rat brain using progesterone conjugated to ^{125}I-bovine serum albumin as a ligand. J Neurochemistry 54:467–472

Kim K, Ramirez VD 1985 *In vitro* luteinizing hormone-releasing hormone release from superfused rat hypothalami: site of action of progesterone and effect of estrogen priming. Endocrinology 116:252–258

Kim K, Ramirez VD 1986 *In vitro* LHRH release from superfused hypothalamus as a function of the rat estrous cycle: effect of progesterone. Neuroendocrinology 42:392–398

Kubli-Garfias C, Ortega-Suarez P, Hoyo-Vadillo C, Ponce-Monter H 1985 Evidence that 5β-progestins produce uterine relaxation by diminishing cellular calcium permeability. Drug Dev Res 6:103–107

Lin W, Ramirez VD 1990 Infusion of progestins into the hypothalamus of female New Zealand white rabbits: effect on *in vivo* luteinizing hormone-releasing hormone release as determined with push-pull perfusion. Endocrinology 126:261-272

Majewska MD 1987 Steroids and brain activity. Essential dialogue between body and mind. Biochem Pharmacol 36:3781–3788

Masotto C, Wisniewski G, Negro-Vilar A 1989 Different γ-aminobutyric acid receptor subtypes are involved in the regulation of opiate-dependent and independent luteinizing hormone-releasing hormone secretion. Endocrinology 125:548–553

McEwen BS, Jones KK, Pfaff DW 1987 Hormonal control of female behavior in the female rat: molecular, cellular and neurochemical studies. Biol Reprod 36:37–45

Miller JR 1988 Calcium signalling in neurons. Trends Neurosci 11:415–419

Nikezic G, Horvat A, Milenkovic LJ, Martinovic JC 1988 Ca^{++} uptake by brain region synaptosomes following *in vivo* administration of ovarian steroids. Mol Cell Endocrinol 57:77–80

Park OK, Ramirez VD 1987 Pregnanolone, a metabolite of progesterone, stimulates LHRH release: *in vitro* and *in vivo* studies. Brain Res 437:237–252

Ramirez VD, Dluzen D 1987 Is progesterone a pre-hormone in the CNS? J Steroid Biochem 27:589–598

Ramirez VD, Kim K, Dluzen D 1985 Progesterone action on the LHRH and the nigrostriatal dopamine neuronal systems: *in vitro* and *in vivo* studies. Recent Prog Horm Res 41:421–472

Sakuma Y, Pfaff DC 1981 Mesencephalic mechanism for integration of female reproductive behavior in the rat. Am J Physiol 237:285–290

Smith SS, Waterhouse BD, Woodward DJ 1987 Locally applied progesterone metabolites alter neuronal responsiveness in the cerebellum. Brain Res Bull 48:739–747

Triggle DJ 1989 Drugs active at voltage-dependent calcium channels. In: Neurotransmission (Research Biochemicals Inc) V(2):1–4

Vicini S, Mienville JM, Costa E 1987 Actions of benzodiazepine and β-carboline derivatives on γ-aminobutyric acid activated Cl^- channels recorded from membrane patches of neonatal rat cortical neurons in culture. J Pharmacol Exp Ther 243:1195–1201

Wasserman WJ, Pinto LH, O'Conner CM, Smith LD 1980 Progesterone induces a rapid increase in $[Ca^{2+}]$ in *Xenopus laevis* oocytes. Proc Natl Acad Sci USA 77:1534–1536

Zamora AJ, Ramirez VD 1983 Vesicular and plasmalemmal changes in nerve endings of rat median eminence from mediobasal hypothalami superfused with media containing high potassium concentrations. Neurosciences (Kobe) 10:463–473

DISCUSSION

Simmonds: You used 5β-pregnan-3β-ol-20-one. Did you look at the effects of the 3α-hydroxy metabolite on the release of LHRH and on amphetamine-induced dopamine release? I ask this because the 3α-hydroxy metabolite is the one that is most potent at the GABA receptor. 5β-Pregnan-3β-ol-20-one failed to affect the amphetamine-induced release of dopamine in your studies, so I wonder whether the 3α-hydroxy form might have been active.

Ramirez: We have not yet tested the effect of the 3α-hydroxy metabolite on amphetamine-induced dopamine release.

Glowinski: There is something I do not understand about the effect of progesterone on the amphetamine-evoked release of dopamine. As you know, amphetamine acts on dopamine release through two mechanisms; by inhibiting the reuptake of dopamine and and by facilitating its release, this latter process being for a large part independent of nerve activity. It is therefore difficult for me to understand how progesterone acts directly on dopaminergic nerve terminals and modulates these two processes. In addition, your experiments with tetrodotoxin suggest that the effect of progesterone is indirect, mediated by other type(s) of neurons which connect with or synapse on dopaminergic nerve terminals (axo-axonic contacts). Therefore, progesterone must abolish or facilitate the release of a neurotransmitter originating from these neurons which in turn will modify the amphetamine-evoked release of dopamine. To my knowledge, however, it has not been described yet that the release of a neurotransmitter from a neuron in the striatum can significantly modify the amphetamine-evoked dopamine release. This is conceivable, but remains to be demonstrated.

Ramirez: We too were surprised by our results. We think that continuous application of progesterone might activate GABAergic terminals acting on GABA neurons or on recurrent fibres. The released GABA could hyperpolarize the dopaminergic neuron. We are now doing experiments to see if continuous infusion of progesterone does cause GABA release. Another possibility is that in addition to releasing GABA, or perhaps instead of releasing GABA, the continuous infusion of progesterone potentiates the effect of GABA.

Glowinski: I agree with your interpretation, but this would be more demonstrable if you were interested for instance in the effect of progesterone on the acetylcholine-evoked release of dopamine (a process which is mediated by muscarinic and nicotinic receptors). Again, amphetamine acts directly on dopaminergic nerve terminals and its effect is for a large part independent of the state of polarization of the membrane. I have some difficulty in understanding the molecular basis by which progesterone could influence the amphetamine-evoked release of dopamine.

Ramirez: We should perhaps look at the effect of progesterone with different doses of amphetamine.

Glowinski: Or look for the effects of compounds that affect the influx of calcium in nerve terminals, such as acetylcholine or substance P, rather than amphetamine, which does not act through a receptor located on dopaminergic nerve terminals.

McEwen: Do you iodinate the BSA and then conjugate it to progesterone through the C-11 position of the steroid?

Ramirez: No; we make the conjugated complex before we do the iodination.

McEwen: You showed that BSA conjugated to the steroid in the C-11 position is not an effective agonist, but you use this complex as a radioligand. The binding of the radioligand can be displaced by other conjugated complexes with the specificity that would be expected from their effects. But the LHRH and dopamine release experiments suggest that the conjugate which is the same as the radioligand is inactive. Isn't there a contradiction?

Ramirez: We have shown that iodinated P-3-BSA binds to P_2 membranes, but it shows high non-specific binding to the filter. So we can use P-11-BSA to look at binding (because it has lower non-specific binding), even though it is not active in the LHRH release assay, just as antagonists are used for binding studies in other systems. Using this heterologous binding assay we found K_i values for P-3-BSA that correlate well with the effects observed in the biological LHRH release assay.

Recently we have done some experiments in the striatum using P-11-BSA at a concentration higher than that used previously and we saw a stimulatory effect on amphetamine-evoked dopamine release, so we should try a wider range of doses before we can definitely say whether these ligands are active or not.

Martini: Is the binding of P-11-BSA to membranes prepared from ovariectomized, non-oestrogenized rats the same as it is from ovariectomized, oestrogenized animals?

Ramirez: This is a question that we hope to answer in the future, now that we are satisfied that the assay is specific. We are now doing experiments on ovariectomized animals, and also investigating whether P-11-^{125}I-BSA binds to brain membranes from male rats. I would like to emphasize that for progesterone to affect amphetamine-evoked release of dopamine or the release of LHRH, the animal must be oestrogen primed (Ramirez et al 1985). There is an absolute requirement for oestrogen, and this finding agrees well with the work of Dr Kordon and others.

Baulieu: Progesterone and P-3-BSA both evoked LHRH release, but had different latencies. Have you an explanation for this difference?

Ramirez: Under our conditions of *in vitro* superfusion, progesterone probably diffuses to the membrane more rapidly than P-3-BSA, which is a much larger molecule than progesterone. I think this difference in timing can be explained by the molecules having different diffusion rates, although we have not actually measured those rates.

Baulieu: Have you used a range of concentrations of P-3-BSA?

Ramirez: Progesterone concentrations from 2 ng/ml to 50 ng/ml will induce LHRH release, with maximal activity at 20 ng/ml. We have not tried different concentrations of P-3-BSA.

Baulieu: Did you ensure that your conjugate was stable, and thus did not release progesterone during your experiments?

Ramirez: Levels of free progesterone detected in the perfusate were below the sensitivity of our radioimmunoassay (less than 20 pg/tube), so we never detected free progesterone (Ke & Ramirez 1987). By extrapolation from the threshold value of the assay we estimated a possible contamination of free progesterone in the conjugate of about 100 pg/ml, a dose at least 100-fold less than the effective stimulating dose of progesterone for LHRH release.

References

Ke FC, Ramirez VD 1987 Membrane mechanism mediates progesterone stimulatory effect on LHRH release from superfused rat hypothalami *in vitro*. Neuroendocrinology 45:514–517
Ramirez VD, Kim K, Dluzen D 1985 Progesterone action on the LHRH and the nigrostriatal dopamine neuronal systems: *in vitro* and *in vivo* studies. Recent Prog Horm Res 41:421–472

In vitro effects of 17β-oestradiol on the sensitivity of receptors coupled to adenylate cyclase on striatal neurons in primary culture

Marion Maus, Joel Prémont and Jacques Glowinski

Laboratoire de Neuropharmacologie, INSERM U 114, Collège de France, 11 place Marcelin Berthelot, 75231 Paris Cedex 05, France

Abstract. Pretreatment of intact striatal neurons from the mouse embryo in primary culture with 17β-oestradiol (10^{-9} M, 24 hours) enhanced the stimulation of adenylate cyclase activity induced by either dopamine (D_1 receptors), isoproterenol, serotonin or 2-chloroadenosine (maximal effective concentrations) but suppressed inhibitory responses evoked by agonists of D_2-dopaminergic or enkephalin (μ and δ) receptors. Binding studies indicated that some of these effects are (β_1) or are not (D_1 and D_2) associated with changes in the number of receptors. Similar effects were partially seen with testosterone but not with 17α-oestradiol, progesterone or dexamethasone and those induced by 17β-oestradiol were abolished when cells were exposed to inhibitors of mRNA transcription (α-amanitin) or protein synthesis (cycloheximide). Modifications in the properties of G_s or $G_{o,i}$ proteins were postulated because the number of adenylate cyclase catalytic subunits was not affected by 17β-oestradiol pretreatment. Results of ADP-ribosylation experiments with cholera toxin or pertussis toxin and of immunoblot experiments with anti-Gα$_o$ and anti-Gβ sera led us to suggest that 17β-oestradiol induces qualitative modifications in $G_{o,i}$ proteins leading to a stabilization of the associated form of the heterotrimer Gα$_{o,i}$βγ. In fact, pretreatment with pertussis toxin (which impairs Gα$_{o,i}$βγ dissociation) mimics the effects of 17β-oestradiol on responses of adenylate cyclase to stimulatory and inhibitory agonists.

1990 Steroids and neuronal activity. Wiley, Chichester (Ciba Foundation Symposium 153) p 145–155

Several studies have indicated that oestrogens can modify dopaminergic transmission in the striatum, a part of the basal ganglia involved in sensory-motor and cognitive processes (for review see McEwen & Parsons 1982, Van Hartesveldt & Joyce 1986). Indeed, oestrogen treatment seems to aggravate some symptoms of Parkinson's disease, which is linked in part to the progressive degeneration of nigro-striatal dopaminergic neurons (Bedard et al 1977). This steroid hormone has also been shown to affect the intensity of abnormal movements and stereotyped behaviour induced by dopamine agonists in rats with unilateral lesions of nigro-striatal dopaminergic neurons (Hruska & Silbergeld 1980, Euvrard et al 1980, Van Hartesveldt & Joyce 1986). In addition, modifications in the firing rate of nigral dopaminergic cells (Chiodo & Caggiula 1980), in the turnover of dopamine in the striatum (McEwen & Parsons 1982) and in the density or sensitivity of dopamine receptors have all been shown in ovariectomized rats after acute injection of 17β-oestradiol (McEwen & Parsons 1982, Hruska & Silbergeld 1980, Euvrard et al 1980, Hruska & Nowak 1988). However, these studies do not allow us to determine the precise sites of action of the steroid hormone, which could act either directly on striatal target cells of dopaminergic neurons or indirectly through a primary effect on nigral dopaminergic cells. This led us to perform *in vitro* studies on striatal neurons from the mouse embryo (16-day-old) in primary culture. These cells possess dopamine receptors and other types of receptors coupled either positively or negatively to adenylate cyclase or to other transduction systems (Prémont et al 1983, Chneiweiss et al 1988). Although embryonic neurons in primary culture could differ from adult cells in their *in vivo* environment, they are not influenced by dopaminergic neurons or by endocrine factors, such as prolactin, which could intervene in the *in vivo* effects of 17β-oestradiol (McEwen & Parsons 1982, Euvrard et al 1980).

Effects of 17β-oestradiol on striatal D_1- and D_2-dopaminergic receptors

It is well established that D_1- and D_2-dopaminergic receptors are respectively coupled positively and negatively to adenylate cyclase in the striatum (Stoof & Kebabian 1981). By acting on D_1 receptors, dopamine stimulates the activity of adenylate cyclase in membranes from striatal neurons cultured for five days *in vitro*. Its inhibitory effect, mediated by D_2 receptors, can also be demonstrated in particular assay conditions: high concentration of GTP, presence of chloride ions and of an antagonist of D_1 receptors, and activation of adenylate cyclase by a strong agonist such as VIP (vasoactive intestinal peptide).

In a first series of experiments the stimulatory effect of dopamine (3×10^{-5} M, maximal effective concentration) on adenylate cyclase activity in membranes (D_1 receptors) was enhanced markedly when intact striatal neurons in culture were exposed for 24 hours to a physiological concentration of 17β-oestradiol (10^{-9} M). Conversely, this 17β-oestradiol pretreatment completely suppressed the D_2-induced inhibition of cyclic AMP formation (Table 1). Similar results were obtained using cultures of anterior pituitary cells which possess only D_2 receptors (Maus et al 1989a). These findings are in agreement with the anti-D_2 dopaminergic inhibitory effect of oestrogens on acetylcholine (ACh) release from striatal interneurons and on prolactin release from pituitary cells (Euvrard et al 1980, Raymond et al 1978). Binding studies with [^{125}I] SCH 23982

TABLE 1 Effects of 17β-oestradiol (E2) on neuronal striatal receptor-associated adenylate cyclase coupling systems

Agonist	Adenylate cyclase responses to stimulatory agonists[a]			Receptor densities[c]		Associated G proteins (G protein and subunits)	Effects of E2
	Control	E2	PTX	Control	E2		
D1-Dopaminergic	100	190*	135*	18	15	G_s ($\alpha_s\beta\gamma$)	No modification in the level of α_s after E2 pretreatment (estimated by ADP-ribosylation with cholera toxin)
β1-Adrenergic	125	210*	217*	15	30*		
A2-Purinergic	40	100*	140*	ND	ND		No modification in the level of $\beta\gamma$ subunits by E2
5-HT-Serotonergic	30	80*	ND	ND	ND		

Agonist	Adenylate cyclase responses to inhibitory agonists[b]			Receptor densities[c]		G protein and subunits	Effects of E2
	Control	E2	PTX	Control	E2		
D2-Dopaminergic	−19	−3*	−3*	29	23	$G_{o,i}$ ($\alpha_{o,i}\beta\gamma$)	E2 enhances (by 28%) the PTX-catalysed ADP-ribosylation of $\alpha_{o,i}$
μ and δ opiate	−21	−4*	−4*	ND	ND		

Values correspond to the variations (increase [a] or decrease [b]) in adenylate cyclase activity expressed as a percentage of that estimated in the absence of stimulatory or inhibitory agonists. Dopamine (D1-dopaminergic agonist) was used at 3×10^{-5} M; isoproterenol (β1-adrenergic agonist), 2-chloroadenosine (A2-purinergic agonist) and serotonin (5-HT-serotonergic agonist) were all used at 10^{-5} M.

[a]Basal adenylate cyclase activities (in the absence of agonists) were (in pmol cyclic AMP/mg protein) 32 ± 3, 39 ± 4 and 15 ± 2 in control culture conditions, in E2- and in pertussis toxin (PTX)-treated neurons respectively.

[b]Inhibition of adenylate cyclase activity was observed in the presence of vasoactive intestinal polypeptide (VIP, 10^{-6} M). Dopamine (D2-dopaminergic agonist) was used at 3×10^{-5} M in the presence of SCH 23390 (2×10^{-7} M), a D1-dopaminergic antagonist. Morphine (μ and δ opiate agonist) was used at 10^{-5} M. Adenylate cyclase activities in the absence of inhibitory agonists were (in pmol cyclic AMP/mg protein) 75 ± 6, 64 ± 6 and 53 ± 5 in control culture conditions, in E2- and in PTX-treated neurons respectively.

[c]D1-dopaminergic, D2-dopaminergic and β1-adrenergic binding sites were estimated using [125I]SCH 23982, [125I]iodosulpride and [125I]iodocyanopindolol respectively. Receptor densities (B_{max}) were expressed in fmol/mg protein.

*, $P < 0.05$, Student's t-test.
ND, not done.

and $[^{125}I]$iodosulpride, two antagonists which bind respectively to D_1 and D_2 receptors, indicated that the modifications of D_1- and D_2-dopamine-mediated effects on adenylate cyclase activity induced by 17β-oestradiol were not linked to changes in the density of D_1 and D_2 receptors (Table 1) (Maus et al 1989a).

Effects of 17β-oestradiol on other receptors coupled to adenylate cyclase in striatal neurons in primary culture

In previous studies we have shown that striatal neurons in primary culture possess noradrenergic (β_1), purinergic (adenosine) (A_2) and serotonergic (5-HT) receptors coupled positively to adenylate cyclase as well as opiate receptors (μ and δ) coupled negatively to the enzyme (Prémont et al 1983, Chneiweiss et al 1988). Responses induced by agonists of these receptors were modified in a way similar to that found for D_1 and D_2 receptors when striatal neurons were pretreated for 24 hours with 17β-oestradiol (10^{-9} M). Indeed, the increase in adenylate cyclase activity evoked by isoproterenol, 2-chloroadenosine or 5-HT (used at their maximal effective concentrations) was markedly potentiated by the 17β-oestradiol pretreatment (Maus et al 1989b), whereas the inhibitory effect induced by agonists of μ and δ opiate receptors was no longer seen (Table 1).

Binding studies with $[^{125}I]$iodocyanopindolol, an antagonist of β-adrenergic receptors, revealed that 17β-oestradiol enhances not only the isoproterenol-evoked effect on adenylate cyclase activity but also the density of β_1-noradrenergic binding sites (Table 1) (Maus et al 1989b). In fact, similar modifications in the number of β-noradrenergic and 5-HT (serotonin) binding sites have been seen in the brain after the *in vivo* administration of oestrogens (for review see McEwen & Parsons 1982). Therefore, depending on the receptors examined, 17β-oestradiol pretreatment of striatal neurons may (β_1-noradrenergic) or may not (D_1- and D_2-dopaminergic) modify the density of receptor sites. No explanation can be provided yet for this difference.

Nuclear site of action of 17β-oestradiol

It is well known that steroid hormones mediate most of their effects through nuclear receptors (King & Greene 1984). The pharmacological specificity and the kinetic characteristics of the effects of 17β-oestradiol on responses evoked by agonists of receptors coupled to adenylate cyclase suggest that this steroid hormone indeed acts through a nuclear receptor ($K_d = 10^{-10}$–10^{-9} M). In fact, in contrast to 17β-oestradiol, 17α-oestradiol (an inactive isomer of 17β-oestradiol) and progesterone or dexamethasone did not modify the responses mediated by receptors coupled to adenylate cyclase. Testosterone, however, reproduced partially the effects of 17β-oestradiol on the sensitivity of receptors to biogenic amines. In addition, the effects of 17β-oestradiol were seen only after a long exposure (eight hours at least) of striatal neurons to the steroid hormone, and dose–response curves indicated that its EC_{50} (concentration for half-maximal effect) was in the range of 10^{-10} M. Finally, the 17β-oestradiol-induced potentiation of responses mediated through receptors coupled positively to adenylate cyclase was prevented by inhibitors of mRNA transcription (α-amanitin) or protein synthesis (cycloheximide). Altogether, these observations are in favour of a genomic action of 17β-oestradiol (Maus et al 1989a,b).

Mechanism of action of 17β-oestradiol on the adenylate cyclase complex

Results obtained on D_1- or D_2-dopaminergic receptors indicate that changes in the sensitivity of receptors coupled to adenylate cyclase induced by 17β-oestradiol are not necessarily linked to changes in the number of receptor sites. Through its genomic action and by a cascade of events which have still to be elucidated, 17β-oestradiol must affect the adenylate cyclase complex indirectly. The steroid pretreatment (24 hours, 10^{-9} M) of striatal neurons does not seem to modify the levels of adenylate cyclase catalytic units. In fact, $MnCl_2$ or forskolin, two powerful direct activators of the enzyme, increased cyclic AMP formation in a similar way in membranes from either control or 17β-oestradiol-treated striatal neurons. Therefore, modifications at the level of transduction proteins (G_s and/or $G_{o,i}$) must occur in order to explain the 17β-oestradiol-induced amplification or inhibition of responses mediated by receptors coupled positively or negatively to adenylate cyclase (Maus et al 1989b).

G_s and $G_{o,i}$ proteins, which have a heterotrimeric structure ($\alpha_s\beta\gamma$ and $\alpha_{o,i}\beta\gamma$), can be dissociated respectively into α_s and $\alpha_{o,i}$ and their common $\beta\gamma$ subunits. Once dissociated, α_s subunits stimulate adenylate cyclase activity, whereas inhibition of the enzyme activity results mainly from the reassociation of α_s with $\beta\gamma$ subunits (Gilman 1987) (Fig. 1). The α_o and $\alpha_{i(1,2,3)}$ subunits can also be coupled to some K^+ and Ca^{2+} ionic channel subtypes (Hescheler et al 1988, Yatani et al 1988). The 17β-oestradiol pretreatment of striatal neurons could induce covalent modifications and/or changes in the levels of the G_s and $G_{o,i}$ subunits. This was investigated in ADP-ribosylation experiments with cholera toxin or pertussis toxin and by immunoblot experiments using specific polyclonal antibodies against β and against α_o, the main substrate of pertussis toxin in the brain (Gierschik et al 1986). These studies were performed in collaboration with V. Homburger and J. Bockaert.

In appropriate conditions, using [32P]-labelled NAD, cholera toxin can be shown to ADP-ribosylate the dissociated α_s subunits (Cassel & Pfeuffer 1978). Quantitative information can be obtained on the level of α_s using [32P]NAD. Actually, our experiments with cholera toxin and [32P]NAD indicated that the 17β-oestradiol pretreatment of striatal neurons (24 hours, 10^{-9} M) did not modify the levels of α_s (see Table 1, p 147).

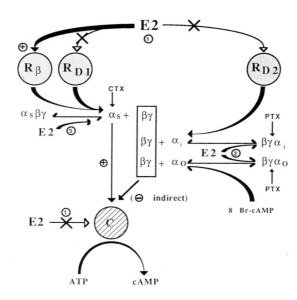

FIG. 1.   Model of action of 17β-oestradiol (E2) on the different components of the striatal adenylate cyclase system.

⊸✕⊳   No effect of E2 on D_1- and D_2-dopaminergic binding sites (R_{D1} and R_{D2}) and on catalytic units (C) of adenylate cyclase.

①→   E2 increases β_1-adrenergic binding sites (R_β).

②→   E2 increases pertussis toxin (PTX) substrates $\beta\gamma\alpha_i$ and $\beta\gamma\alpha_o$ without affecting levels of α_o and β, thus blocking adenylate cyclase responses to inhibitory agonists.

③→   E2 potentiates agonist responses mediated by α_s.

Pertussis toxin ADP-ribosylates $\alpha_{o,i}$ only when these subunits are associated with $\beta\gamma$ (Ui 1986). In ADP-ribosylation experiments with pertussis toxin and $[^{32}P]$NAD we demonstrated a higher labelling of $\alpha_{o,i}$ subunits from membranes of striatal neurons exposed to 17β-oestradiol (Table 1). The immunoblot experiments showed that 17β-oestradiol pretreatment did not modify the levels of α_o and β. The ADP-ribosylation experiments with pertussis toxin therefore suggest that this steroid treatment stabilizes the heterotrimeric associated form $\alpha_{o,i}\beta\gamma$. This process could explain the suppressive effect of 17β-oestradiol on responses mediated by receptors coupled negatively to adenylate cyclase, the lack of dissociation, or reduced dissociation, of $\alpha_{o,i}\beta\gamma$ preventing inhibitory responses mediated by free $\beta\gamma$ subunits. By the law of mass action, G_s could be dissociated more easily into α_s and $\beta\gamma$ subunits in 17β-oestradiol-treated neurons to compensate for the reduced level of free $\beta\gamma$ subunits. The potentiating effect of 17β-oestradiol on responses mediated through receptors coupled positively to adenylate cyclase (D_1-dopaminergic, 5-HT and A_2-adenosine receptors) could therefore be explained (Fig. 1).

The enhanced pertussis toxin-induced ADP-ribosylation of $\alpha_{o,i}$ observed after 17β-oestradiol pretreatment of striatal neurons was specific. Steroids which did not affect responses mediated through receptors coupled either positively or negatively to adenylate cyclase did not modify the pertussis toxin-induced ADP-ribosylation of $\alpha_{o,i}$. Finally, by uncoupling receptors inhibiting adenylate cyclase activity from their $G_{o,i}$ proteins, and thus stabilizing the associated heterotrimeric form $\alpha_{o,i}\beta\gamma$ (Ui 1986), the pertussis toxin pretreatment of intact striatal neurons (1 µg/ml, 24 hours) reproduced most of the effects observed with 17β-oestradiol. In fact, it almost completely suppressed inhibitory responses mediated through D_2-dopaminergic and enkephalin/opiate (µ and δ) receptors, while it potentiated responses induced by dopamine D_1 receptors, isoproterenol or 2-chloroadenosine.

Conclusion

Several processes could be responsible for the covalent modifications of $G_{o,i}$ proteins induced by the 17β-oestradiol pretreatment of striatal neurons. These include a phosphorylation, alkylation, myristoylation or even an endogenous ADP-ribosylation of their subunits, $\alpha_{o,i}$ particularly (Watanabe et al 1988, Buss et al 1987, Tanuma et al 1988). Experiments are in progress that are designed to elucidate the mechanism involved in the enhanced pertussis toxin-induced ADP-ribosylation of $\alpha_{o,i}$ seen in membranes from 17β-oestradiol-pretreated neurons. In fact, in contrast to the results with 17β-oestradiol, we have recently observed that the pretreatment of these striatal cells with either 8-bromo-cyclic AMP or phorbol 12-myristate 13-acetate (12-O-tetradecanoylphorbol 13-acetate) decreases the pertussis toxin-induced ADP-ribosylation of $\alpha_{o,i}$ subunits. In addition, the effect of 8-bromo-cyclic AMP was prevented by the isoquinolinesulphonamide H_7, a non-specific inhibitor of protein kinases. These results favour the intervention of phosphorylation processes mediated by protein kinases A and C respectively. We have still to demonstrate whether or not $\alpha_{o,i}$ or β proteins are the substrates of protein kinases A or C. In any case, these observations suggest that 17β-oestradiol could modify the levels of intracellular second messengers regulating protein kinases A or C. We already have evidence indicating that a decrease in cyclic AMP levels occurs in 17β-oestradiol-pretreated neurons. This suggests that the enhanced pertussis toxin-induced ADP-ribosylation of $\alpha_{o,i}$ evoked by the steroid hormone involves a dephosphorylation linked to a reduced activity of protein kinase A. Interestingly enough, Liu & Greengard (1976) had already shown that 17β-oestradiol regulates the extent of the cyclic AMP-dependent phosphorylation of proteins.

We have shown here that 17β-oestradiol acts in a uniform way on all pertussis toxin-sensitive G proteins of striatal neurons. Other transduction systems involving G proteins could also be affected by the steroid treatment. In support of this statement, other authors have shown a desensitization of the angiotensin-induced activation of phospholipase C in the pituitary of ovariectomized female rats after prolonged treatment with 17β-oestradiol (Schoepp & Bailly 1987). Hypersensitivity of L-type calcium channels of pituitary cells exposed to 17β-oestradiol has also been reported (Drouva et al 1988). In fact, in preliminary experiments, we could show that pretreatment of striatal neurons with 17β-oestradiol (24 hours, 10^{-9} M) increases the sensitivity of phospholipase C to carbachol (a muscarinic agonist), a transduction process involving a G protein insensitive to both cholera and pertussis toxins.

Since several receptors of neurotransmitters have been recently described on astrocytes from various brain structures in primary culture, it remains to be established whether or not oestrogens exert pleiotropic effects on the sensitivity of these receptors, as shown for that of neuronal receptors. If this is the case, this will also have to be taken into account in the variety of mechanisms by which oestrogens could affect astrocyte–neuron interactions during development and in adult mammals.

Acknowledgements

This study was supported by INSERM, Rhône Poulenc Santé and DRET (87/201).

References

Bedard P, Langelier P, Villeneuve A 1977 Oestrogens and extrapyramidal system. Lancet 2:1367–1368
Buss JE, Mumby SM, Casey PJ, Gilman AG, Sefton BM 1987 Myristoylated α subunits of guanine nucleotide-binding regulatory proteins. Proc Natl Acad Sci USA 84:7493–7497
Cassel D, Pfeuffer T 1978 Mechanism of cholera-toxin action : covalent modification of the guanyl nucleotide-binding protein of the adenylate cyclase system. Proc Natl Acad Sci USA 75:2669–2673
Chiodo LA, Caggiula AR 1980 Alterations in basal firing rate and autoreceptor sensitivity of dopamine neurons in the substantia nigra following acute and extended exposure to estrogen. Eur J Pharmacol 67:165–166
Chneiweiss H, Glowinski J, Prémont J 1988 Mu and delta opiate receptors coupled negatively to adenylate cyclase on embryonic neurons from the mouse striatum in primary cultures. J Neurosci 8:3376–3382
Drouva SV, Rérat E, Bihoreau C et al 1988 Dihydropyridine-sensitive calcium channel activity related to prolactin, growth hormone, and luteinizing hormone release from anterior pituitary cells in culture : interactions with somatostatin, dopamine, and estrogens. Endocrinology 123:2762–2773
Euvrard C, Oberlander C, Boissier JR 1980 Antidopaminergic effect of estrogens at the striatal level. J Pharmacol Exp Ther 214:179–185
Gierschik P, Milligan G, Pines M et al 1986 Use of specific antibodies to quantitate the guanine nucleotide-binding protein G_o in brain. Proc Natl Acad Sci USA 83:2258–2262
Gilman AG 1987 G proteins : transducers of receptor-generated signals. Annu Rev Biochem 56:615–649

Hescheler J, Rosenthal W, Wulfern M et al 1988 Involvement of the guanine nucleotide binding protein, N_o, in the inhibitory regulation of neuronal calcium channels. Adv Second Messenger & Phosphoprotein Res 21:165–174

Hruska RE, Silbergeld EK 1980 Increased dopamine receptor sensitivity after estrogen treatment using the rat rotation model. Science (Wash DC) 208:1466–1468

Hruska RE, Nowak MW 1988 Estrogen treatment increases the density of D1 dopaminergic receptors in the rat striatum. Brain Res 442:349–350

King WG, Greene GL 1984 Monoclonal antibodies localize oestrogen receptor in the nuclei of target cells. Nature (Lond) 307:745–747

Liu AYC, Greengard P 1976 Regulation by steroid hormones of phosphorylation of specific proteins common to several target organs. Proc Natl Acad Sci USA 73:568–572

Maus M, Bertrand P, Drouva S et al 1989a Differential modulation of D1 and D2 dopamine-sensitive adenylate cyclases by 17-β oestradiol in cultured striatal neurons and anterior pituitary cells. J Neurochem 52:410–418

Maus M, Cordier J, Glowinski J, Prémont J 1989b 17-β oestradiol pretreatment of mouse striatal neurons in culture enhances the responses of adenylate cyclase sensitive to biogenic amines. Eur J Neurosci 1:154–161

McEwen BS, Parsons B 1982 Gonadal steroid action on the brain : neurochemistry and neuropharmacology. Annu Rev Pharmacol Toxicol 22:555–598

Prémont J, Daguet de Montety MC, Herbet A, Glowinski J, Bockaert J, Prochiantz A 1983 Biogenic amine- and adenosine-sensitive adenylate cyclases in primary cultures of striatal neurons. Dev Brain Res 9:53–61

Raymond V, Beaulieu M, Labrie F, Boissier J 1978 Potent antidopaminergic activity of estradiol at the pituitary level on prolactin release. Science (Wash DC) 200:1173–1175

Schoepp DD, Bailly DA 1987 Estrogen modulation of angiotensin-stimulated phosphoinositide hydrolysis in slices of rat anterior pituitary. Neurochem Int 11:149–154

Stoof JC, Kebabian JW 1981 Opposing roles for D1 and D2 dopamine receptors in efflux of cyclic AMP from rat neostriatum. Nature (Lond) 294:366–368

Tanuma S, Kawashima K, Endo H 1988 Eukaryotic mono(ADP-ribosyl)transferase that ADP-ribosylates GTP-binding regulatory Gi protein. J Biol Chem 263:5485–5489

Ui M 1986 Pertussis toxin as a probe of receptor coupling to inositol lipid metabolism. In: Putney JW (ed) Phosphoinositides and receptor mechanisms. Alan R Liss, New York, vol 7:163–195

Van Hartesveldt C, Joyce JN 1986 Effects of estrogens on basal ganglia. Neurosci Biobehav Rev 10:1–14

Watanabe Y, Imaizumi T, Misaki W, Iwakura K, Yoshida H 1988 Effects of phosphorylation of inhibitory GTP-binding protein by cyclic AMP-dependent protein kinase on its ADP-ribosylation by pertussis toxin, islet-activating protein. FEBS (Fed Eur Biochem Soc) Lett 236:372–374

Yatani A, Mattera R, Codina J et al 1988 The G protein-gated atrial K^+ channel is stimulated by three distinct $G_i\alpha$-subunits. Nature (Lond) 336:680–682

DISCUSSION

Karavolas: In the steroid-specificity studies, did you test the non-oestrogenic steroids at concentrations within their effective physiological concentrations? You tested them at a concentration of 10^{-9} M but many of these steroids exert their normal physiological effects at concentrations of 10^{-7} or 10^{-8} M, so you may have used subthreshold doses.

Glowinski: The dose–response curve for 17β-oestradiol covered a broad range of concentrations, including 10^{-7} M and 10^{-8} M. The effects of the non-oestrogenic steroids on the sensitivity of receptors coupled to adenylate cyclase were examined over a similar concentration range.

Karavolas: Have you investigated the effect of glucocorticoids?

Glowinski: We have not performed experiments to study the effects of glucocorticoids on neurons. However, we have shown that adenosine potentiates the noradrenaline-induced activation of phospholipase C in striatal astrocytes; this potentiation is abolished by glucocorticoids.

McEwen: Intracellular oestrogen receptors have not so far been detected in the striatum, although perhaps the new iodinated oestradiol with its high specific radioactivity will reveal such receptors. Do you think this effect of oestrogen might involve a genomic mechanism that is initially triggered by binding of oestrogen to a membrane receptor?

Glowinski: This cannot be excluded. It is correct to say that intracellular oestrogen receptors have not so far been demonstrated in the striatum. Such receptors could nevertheless be present in our cultures. However, our *in vitro* findings are in agreement with observations made *in vivo* in the adult rat showing similar changes in the sensitivity of dopaminergic receptors. These experiments have been done recently by J. D. Vincent's group in Bordeaux (unpublished). In fact, once again, our study was initiated to determine how oestrogen treatment *in vivo* was affecting dopaminergic transmission. Our results, which imply the existence of oestrogen receptors on striatal neurons (either nuclear or membrane), confirm data on (or are in agreement with) observations made *in vivo*. I therefore wonder whether the techniques which have been used to look for oestrogen receptors in the striatum of adult animals were sensitive enough. This has to be investigated further.

McEwen: Binding studies using tritiated oestradiol may not reveal intracellular oestrogen receptors where their numbers are small, but as I said, studies using iodinated oestradiol may clarify this problem. Lability of the receptors might be the reason they have not been found in binding studies, but autoradiography, in which lability should be less important, hasn't revealed any intracellular receptors either. This is why I think there might be a membrane receptor for oestrogen that no one has yet detected.

Glowinski: At the present stage I do not think that a membrane receptor could mediate the opposite effects on receptors coupled positively and negatively to adenylate cyclase seen in our study, taking also into account that a rather long time is required to see the appearance of the 17β-oestradiol-evoked responses. However, your suggestion is of particular interest and the relationship between membrane receptors (if they exist) and nuclear events undoubtedly deserves to be considered.

Baulieu: Using striatal slices from rat brain, Martine El Etr has observed a (probably) membrane-mediated effect of the steroid pregnenolone sulphate on the muscarinic acetylcholine receptor; the carbachol-induced production of inositol trisphosphate was decreased by pregnenolone sulphate (10^{-5} M). The effect was not reproduced in striatal neurons in culture, even in the presence of astrocytes. I agree with Bruce McEwen's suggestion. You might have a membrane effect that results, through the action of an enzyme such as protein kinase, in the activation, perhaps by phosphorylation, of protein(s) that ultimately affect the genome.

Bäckström: When we measured oestradiol levels in different areas of the female rat brain we found that the striatum has a very high concentration, the second highest of the regions we looked at (Bixo et al 1986).

Glowinski: This is interesting. However, unfortunately this does not necessarily indicate that there are oestrogen receptors in the striatum.

Bäckström: No, and also the intracellular concentration may not be as high as the concentration measured in the whole-brain extracts.

Kordon: Dr Glowinski's explanation of the multiplicity of oestrogen's effects on transduction parameters of cultivated neurons is quite interesting. It also fits with results from comparable experiments which we performed on pituitary cells. In that case, however, I do not understand why the response to vasoactive intestinal peptide is not amplified. There is no indication that VIP receptors are coupled to different coupling proteins from those mediating the effect of the D_1 receptors that you mentioned.

Glowinski: VIP was used at a concentration which induces a maximal activation of adenylate cyclase, and all adenylate cyclase subunit molecules seem to be activated, from the amplitude of the response (similar to that observed with forskolin). This is why 17β-oestradiol did not potentiate the response to VIP, in contrast to the response observed to other transmitters which act on receptors associated with part of the adenylate cyclase present in the cells.

Kordon: Maybe you could try smaller concentrations of VIP?

Glowinski: I agree with you; we should have done a dose–response curve with VIP in order to determine whether 17β-oestradiol potentiates responses evoked by a low concentration of VIP. In fact, the agonists in our study were in most cases used at their maximal effective concentration.

Kordon: I also appreciate your suggestion that calcium channels may be involved in the oestrogen modulation of transduction processes that you have described. In the rat pituitary, we found that treatment of cells with oestrogens for at least 8 h strikingly increased the opening frequency of voltage-dependent L-type calcium channels.

Reference

Bixo M, Bäckström T, Winblad B, Selstam G, Andersson A 1986 Comparison between pre- and postovulatory distributions of oestradiol and progesterone in the brain of the PMSG-treated rat. Acta Physiol Scand 128:241–246

Effect of oestradiol on dopamine receptors and protein kinase C activity in the rat pituitary: binding of oestradiol to pituitary membranes

D. Joubert-Bression, A. M. Brandi, P. Birman and F. Peillon

INSERM U 223, Faculté de Médecine Pitié-Salpêtrière, 105 Boulevard de l'Hôpital, 75634 Paris Cedex 13, France

Abstract. Oestradiol exerts an important modulatory influence on the release of prolactin which is accomplished partly through disruption of the inhibitory influence of dopamine. We have focused on the status of the anterior pituitary D_2 dopamine receptor in female rats treated chronically with oestradiol or progesterone. A direct membrane effect of these steroids on the dopamine system was also investigated *in vitro*. Both steroids affected the status of the D_2 receptor, oestradiol decreasing the number of sites *in vitro* and progesterone increasing it both *in vitro* and *in vivo*. The *in vitro* studies demonstrated that these steroids exert a direct membrane effect on the D_2 receptor. These results correlated with an *in vitro* short-term physiological effect of oestradiol and progesterone on the dopaminergic inhibition of prolactin release, oestradiol decreasing it while progesterone had the opposite effect. Binding studies with [^{3}H]oestradiol on pituitary membranes revealed a site for oestradiol of high affinity and low capacity, indicating that oestradiol's membrane effects could be mediated by a specific receptor. *In vivo* treatment with oestradiol also induces proliferation of prolactin-secreting cells (lactotrophs). We focused on the effect of oestradiol on protein kinase C activity, which is involved in both secretion and proliferation. In female rats treated with oestradiol total protein kinase C activity was increased by 74% (particulate 90%, soluble 71%) in comparison with controls. This effect was reversed by concomitant treatment with a dopamine agonist. Thus in the pituitary oestradiol and progesterone affect the characteristics of membrane components that are implicated in the physiological control of the cell. Whether these effects are post-transcriptional only or are also mediated through direct membrane mechanisms needs further investigation.

1990 Steroids and neuronal activity. Wiley, Chichester (Ciba Foundation Symposium 153) p 156–171

The anterior pituitary gland is a target organ for steroids such as oestradiol, which has a major role in the control of lactotrophs. These cells, which secrete the lactogenic hormone prolactin, possess specific nuclear receptor sites for oestradiol. It is largely accepted that this steroid exerts its effect on transcription of the prolactin gene after it has bound to its nuclear sites. Oestradiol increases prolactin synthesis and mRNA accumulation *in vitro* and increases the transcription rate of the prolactin gene in the intact animal. Beside this well-known physiological action, 17β-oestradiol also affects the growth of the cells that produce prolactin (Lloyd et al 1975); it also modulates the release of this hormone, primarily through disrupting the dopaminergic control of the lactotrophs. The mechanisms underlying the effects on both proliferation and dopaminergic control are still not completely understood.

Oestradiol and the pituitary dopamine receptor

Specific receptor sites for dopamine have been identified in the anterior pituitary gland. They have been defined pharmacologically as belonging to the D_2 subcategory of dopamine receptors (Sibley et al 1982) and are predominantly localized to the cells that synthesize and secrete prolactin. Dopamine inhibits prolactin release through biochemical mechanisms that include reduction in the level of intracellular cyclic AMP, inhibition of phosphatidylinositol turnover and reduction of calcium influx. Although the sites of oestrogen action on dopamine inhibition may be multiple, oestradiol appears capable of exerting a direct effect at the level of the anterior pituitary gland; treatment of primary cultures of rat pituitary cells with oestrogens has been demonstrated to reverse the ability of dopaminergic agonists to inhibit prolactin release (Giguère et al 1982).

In vivo, oestradiol and progesterone influence the inhibitory control exerted on prolactin by dopamine. Chronic treatment with oestradiol decreases hypothalamic dopamine turnover and lowers dopamine levels in the portal blood and in the anterior pituitary gland. It also affects the number of dopamine receptor sites in the anterior pituitary. Several studies have been conducted on this particular point, using intact male or female rats, or ovariectomized females. In our experimental model we used intact and ovariectomized female rats (Bression et al 1983). We detected dopamine sites using [^{3}H]domperidone, a highly specific dopamine antagonist. This ligand, under the conditions used in our study, detects two dopamine sites which differ in both their K_d and B_{max} (high affinity site: $K_d = 0.30 \pm 0.08$ nM [$\bar{x} \pm$ SEM], $B_{max} = 74 \pm 9$ fmol/mg protein; low affinity site: $K_d = 17.4 \pm 3.2$ nM, $B_{max} = 214 \pm 22$ fmol/mg protein). Oestradiol treatment of intact female rats induced an increase in the K_d and B_{max} of the low affinity sites (Fig. 1). In contrast, the same oestradiol treatment had no effect in ovariectomized rats. The difference between the two results was in fact due to the difference in the plasma progesterone level, which was high in oestrogenized intact females and low in oestrogenized ovariectomized animals. Thus, the oestrogen-induced increase observed in the number of

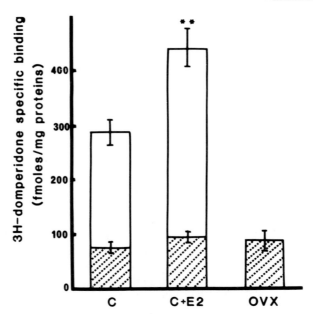

FIG. 1. Total number of specific [^{3}H]domperidone binding sites in the anterior pituitary of control (C, $n = 11$), oestrogenized (E$_2$, $n = 11$) and ovariectomized (OVX, $n = 4$) rats after *in vivo* treatment. The amounts of high and low affinity sites are illustrated by the hatched and open parts of each bar respectively (mean $\pm$ SEM). n, = number of experiments. **, $P < 0.01$ (by Student's t-test) for low affinity sites vs control.

dopamine receptor sites in intact females was a consequence of high plasma progesterone levels: after treatment of ovariectomized rats with both oestradiol and progesterone an increase in [^{3}H]domperidone binding sites was seen (Fig. 2A). The importance of progesterone in the *in vivo* modulation of dopamine sites in the anterior pituitary gland was well documented recently by Pilotte et al (1989). The authors concluded that treatment of ovariectomized rats with oestradiol followed by treatment with both oestradiol and progesterone increases the density of dopamine receptor sites. Other studies have demonstrated a reduction in the number of dopamine receptors when ovariectomized rats were treated with oestradiol. In contrast, treatment of male rats with oestradiol does not seem to affect the number of dopamine sites, but rather to affect the coupling mechanisms of the receptors (Munemura et al 1989). These authors suggest that in male rats, oestrogen is capable of attenuating the functional coupling of the D$_2$ receptor with its biochemical effector system (the adenylate cyclase system) in the anterior pituitary gland. Using the MtTF$_4$ pituitary tumour, Albaladejo et al (1984) have also demonstrated a reduction in the number of dopamine sites after treatment with oestradiol. Taken together, these results argue in favour

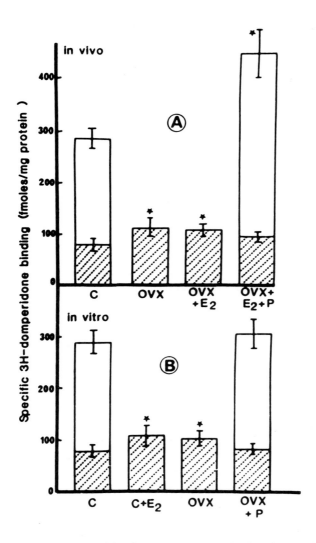

FIG. 2. Total number of specific [^{3}H]domperidone binding sites (A) in the anterior pituitary of control (C), ovariectomized (OVX), oestrogenized ovariectomized rats (OVX + E2) and ovariectomized rats treated *in vivo* with oestradiol and progesterone (OVX + E2 + P) and (B) in pituitary membranes from control (C) and ovariectomized (OVX) rats incubated *in vitro* with oestradiol for controls (C + E2) and with progesterone for ovariectomized rats (OVX + P). For details, see legend of Fig. 1. *, $P < 0.01$ (by Student's *t*-test) for total binding vs control.

of an *in vivo* effect of oestradiol and progesterone on the D_2 receptor in the anterior pituitary. Such an effect could form part of the mechanism through which these steroids affect the dopaminergic control of lactotrophs and thus prolactin secretion.

During the rat oestrus cycle, in which oestradiol and progesterone plasma levels vary, the amount of dopamine secreted from the hypothalamus and reaching the pituitary gland and the number of dopamine receptors change in parallel to changes in prolactin levels. In particular, Pasqualini et al (1984) have demonstrated a rapid decrease in the number of dopamine receptors that occurs at the same time as the onset of the preovulatory prolactin surge; this decrease might be a decisive component in the initiation or maintenance of this surge in the rat. More recently, Brandi et al (1990) have shown that in parallel to the variation in dopamine receptor number, the sensitivity of the anterior pituitary gland to dopamine also varies during the oestrous cycle; minimum sensitivity is found at the moment of the prolactin surge, which occurs after the oestradiol peak and concomitantly with the pro-oestrus progesterone increase (Fig. 3). Thus, gonadal steroids might play a physiological role in the dopaminergic control of lactotrophs.

The action of steroids on the *in vivo* dopaminergic inhibition of prolactin release may therefore involve several mechanisms, including regulation of dopamine receptor number and of receptor–effector coupling mechanisms. The fact that oestradiol exhibits antidopaminergic properties *in vitro* has led several investigators to look for a direct *in vitro* regulation of the number of dopamine sites. In our study, we demonstrated an antagonistic regulation by oestradiol and progesterone of the rat pituitary dopamine receptor sites, oestradiol decreasing the number of binding sites (the low affinity ones) whereas progesterone increased it (Figs. 2B and 4) (Bression et al 1985). This effect of oestradiol was a short-term one, contrasting with previous work showing a long-term effect, detected only after several days of treatment in culture (Giguère et al 1982). We observed a correlation between the modulation of the number of dopamine sites and ovarian steroid regulation of the dopaminergic inhibition of prolactin secretion from pituitary explants *in vitro*. Oestradiol decreased the sensitivity of the lactotrophs to dopamine, whereas progesterone was necessary for a normal response of these cells. These results were partially confirmed by Pasqualini et al (1986) who also found that *in vitro* oestradiol treatment of pituitary explants led to a decrease in the number of dopamine sites (using [3H]spiperone as the ligand) that occurred in parallel to increased prolactin secretion. This effect was detectable after a seven minute incubation with oestradiol, ruling out the possibility of a genomic action of oestradiol. Thus, these studies demonstrate that, in addition to a modulatory effect of oestradiol on hypothalamic dopamine turnover, the antidopaminergic properties of oestradiol may be explained partly by a direct effect on pituitary dopamine receptors.

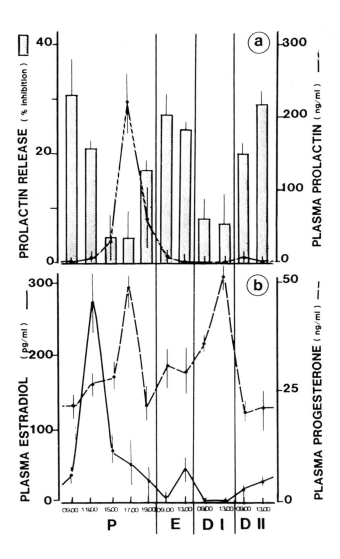

FIG. 3.   (a) Relationship between changes in inhibition of prolactin release by 10 nM dopamine and plasma prolactin levels and (b) changes in oestradiol and progesterone levels during the four-day oestrous cycle of the rat (P, pro-oestrus; E, oestrus; D I, dioestrus 1; D II, dioestrus 2). Each value of plasma prolactin, oestradiol and progesterone is the mean ± SEM of nine determinations.

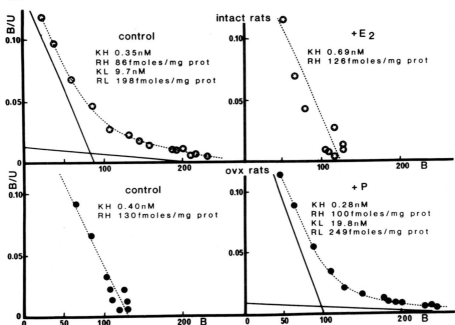

FIG. 4. Computer analysis of $[^3H]$domperidone binding to crude membrane preparations from the pituitaries of intact or ovariectomized (OVX) rats. Membranes from intact rats were incubated in the presence or absence of 10^{-8} M oestradiol (E2) and those from ovariectomized rats were incubated in the presence or absence of 10^{-8} M progesterone (P). KH and KL (nM), dissociation constants of the high and low affinity sites; RH and RL (fmol/mg protein), maximum number of binding sites of the high and low affinity sites. B, concentration of bound; U, concentration of unbound ligand (both fmol/mg protein).

Oestradiol binding to pituitary membranes

The direct short-term effects of oestradiol and progesterone on dopamine receptor status in the anterior pituitary gland raise questions about the mechanism leading to such effects. It is generally assumed that steroid hormones passively diffuse to nuclear receptors that determine the cellular specificity of the response. However, several experiments indicate that these hormones interact with components of biological membranes and that they may bind to the plasma membrane. Electrophysiological studies on neurons in the CNS have demonstrated rapid changes in firing patterns after treatment with steroids. Such alterations suggest the presence of specific steroid receptors that mediate changes in membrane responsiveness in less than 100 milliseconds (Kelly et al 1977). Synaptosomes from the rat brain have been shown to respond to the presence of glucocorticoids by either increasing their uptake of tryptophan or reducing their release of corticotropin releasing factor. Baulieu and coworkers have demonstrated that progesterone and other steroid molecules are able to promote the maturation of *Xenopus laevis* oocytes, although these cells do not contain cytoplasmic steroid receptors (Godeau et al 1978). They therefore suggested that progesterone may exert its effects by first interacting with the cell membrane.

Given the wide spectrum of membrane functions and the multiplicity of the recognized effects of steroids in cell biology, it is not surprising that these molecules are able to modify several membrane functions. However, even if most of the effects steroids have on membrane properties do not represent direct effects of the drugs, several of them argue in favour of the presence of specific steroid binding sites on membranes. Such sites have already been identified. Pietras and Szego made a major contribution when they characterized oestrogen binding sites in uterine plasma membranes (Pietras & Szego 1979); a partial purification and characterization of oestrogen receptors was obtained from subfractions of hepatocyte plasma membranes (Pietras & Szego 1980). Towle & Sze (1983) have shown glucocorticoid and gonadal steroid binding to synaptic plasma membranes. In a study using a fluorescent oestradiol conjugate,

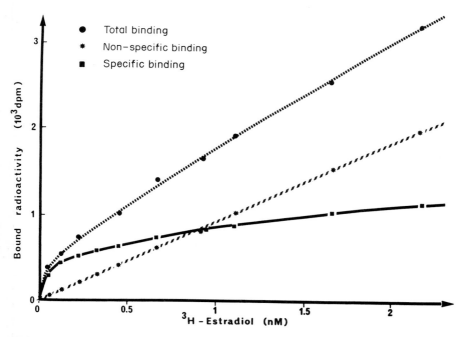

FIG. 5. Saturation binding experiment. Rat pituitary membranes were incubated at 0 °C overnight in the presence of increasing concentrations of [^{3}H]oestradiol (0.02–2.0 nM) with or without diethylstilboestrol (10^{-6} M). Bound ligand was separated from unbound ligand by filtration.

Berthois et al (1986) have shown the existence of membrane binding sites for oestradiol in human breast cancer tissue. In the rat anterior pituitary gland, a specific interaction of corticosteroids with binding sites in the plasma membrane has been suggested by the work of Koch et al (1978).

In our study (Fig. 5), we have shown that in pituitary membranes oestradiol binds to one homogeneous population of sites with high affinity ($K_d = 0.041$ nM) and low capacity (14 fmol/mg protein) (Bression et al 1986). The binding is thermolabile. Extensive washing of the membranes did not decrease the number of sites. This fact indicates that the binding activity was not loosely associated with the membranes, which were devoid of the cytosolic enzyme marker, lactate dehydrogenase. Binding was specific for oestrogenic compounds. The presence of pituitary membrane oestrogen binding sites was also proposed by Sokolovsky et al (1981). In addition, these authors demonstrated a direct effect of oestradiol on muscarinic acetylcholine receptor sites in rat pituitary membranes.

All these findings indicate that our understanding of the cellular mechanism of steroid hormone action is not complete. Our results suggest that oestradiol affects dopamine's inhibition of prolactin secretion by modulating the number of dopamine receptors. Thus oestradiol might act not only by a regulation of gene expression but also by a direct regulation of membrane function. Furthermore, our results do not restrict such mechanisms to oestradiol but suggest that progesterone may also operate in this way.

In vivo oestradiol treatment and pituitary protein kinase C activity

In the pituitary gland a close relationship exists between the effects of hormones (steroids or neurohormones) on mitotic activity and on pituitary hormone release. Indeed, neurohormones such as somatostatin and dopamine inhibit both processes, whereas other hormones—thyroliberin (TRH), somatocrinin (GHRH) or vasoactive intestinal peptide (VIP)—in addition to oestradiol stimulate both release and mitotic activity. In the pituitary the proliferative effects of oestrogens are especially pronounced on lactotrophs. These effects can be blocked by *in vivo* treatment with dopamine receptor agonists (Kalberman et al 1980). The mechanisms by which mitotic activity is induced are still unresolved. Because of the fundamental role of protein kinase C in signal transduction, growth control and tumour promotion, we have been interested in the *in vivo* effect of oestradiol treatment on anterior pituitary gland protein kinase C activity and in the influence of concomitant treatment with a dopamine agonist, CV 205-502. Protein kinase C is activated by diacylglycerol which is generated during phosphoinositide turnover by hydrolysis of membrane phospholipids by a specific phospholipase C. The introduction of diacylglycerol into the cell is sufficient to stimulate DNA synthesis. Oestrogens have been reported to stimulate lipid synthesis in the rat uterus (Spooner & Gorski 1972) and phosphatidylinositol metabolism in mouse uterine tissue (Grove & Korach 1987). Tamoxifen, *in vitro*, inhibits protein kinase C activity in the rat brain; an increase in phospholipid concentration overcomes this inhibition (O'Brien et al 1985). It therefore seems likely that oestradiol may also affect the activity of protein kinase C. In our study we looked at the long-term effects of oestradiol treatment on protein kinase C activity in female rats, to investigate whether this enzyme is implicated in the pathogenesis of human pituitary adenomas (Birman et al 1989). In humans, a worsening of pituitary tumours during pregnancy has been described (Peillon et al 1970). A possible role for oestrogens in the pathogenesis of prolactin-secreting adenomas has been proposed (Peillon et al 1984) and oestrogen-induced prolactinoma has recently been described in a man. In our experimental animal model both lactotroph proliferation and prolactin release are greatly stimulated by oestradiol; this mimics the situation which exists in patients with prolactin-secreting adenomas. After eight days of *in vivo* treatment in our model, oestradiol stimulates both the protein kinase C activity associated with plasma membranes and that found in the cytosol; stimulations were of 90% and 71% respectively. After fifteen days of treatment, stimulation of only the cytosolic protein kinase C activity was found. Cytosolic protein kinase C activity increased dramatically to 188% of control activity. Treatment with the dopamine agonist CV 205-502, which exerts effects opposite to those of oestradiol on both cell proliferation and prolactin release, decreased protein kinase C activity when it was administered alone and prevented the increase in activity that was induced by 15 days of oestradiol treatment (Fig. 6).

This study, conducted *in vivo*, did not help us to determine whether the mechanism by which oestradiol or dopamine treatment modulates protein kinase C activity involves a direct or an indirect action. Oestradiol-induced translocation of protein kinase C from the cytosol into the cell membrane and activation of the enzyme by oestradiol were recently demonstrated in cells from oestradiol-dependent rat mammary gland tumours (Sidorkina et al 1988). These effects were observed 10–15 minutes after the administration of oestradiol (10 µg intraperitoneally) to ovariectomized rats. Oestradiol had a similar effect on protein kinase C in uterine tissue. In contrast, oestradiol did not induce any redistribution of protein kinase C between the cytosol and the cell membrane in hormone-independent rat mammary gland tumour cells. The authors suggested that oestradiol might, like the peptide growth factors, exert its stimulatory effect on cell division via a coupling of its membrane receptors with the system for activation of protein kinase C. The effects detected in our study may represent a modulation of the amount of enzyme and/or a modulation of its activity. These results are of interest in view of those already obtained from studies of human pituitary adenomas; in these tumours, protein kinase C activity is increased considerably by comparison to that of normal human pituitaries. Thus, in pituitary adenomas as in other tumours, protein kinase C seems to play a critical role in cellular growth. Furthermore, results concerning

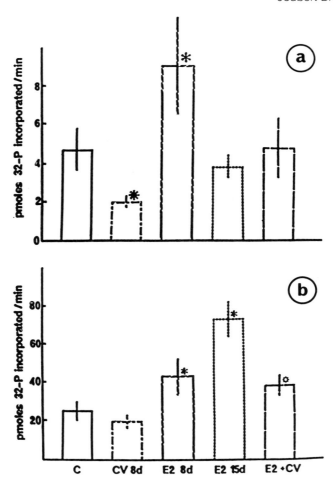

FIG. 6.   Protein kinase C activity in pituitary particulate (a) and soluble (b) fractions from controls (C) or from rats treated with CV 205-502 for eight days (CV 8d) or oestradiol for eight (E_2 8d) or 15 days (E_2 15d), or with oestradiol alone for seven days, then in combination with CV 205-502 for the last eight days (E2 + CV). Results are expressed in pmol ^{32}P incorporated per min per 10 mg protein of particulate or soluble fractions applied to the DE-52 column. *$P < 0.05$ vs control; ✻$P < 0.02$ vs control; ✿, $P < 0.02$ vs E2 15d.

protein kinase C activity obtained after oestradiol treatment suggest that this hormone may, like peptide growth factors, affect cell proliferation by interacting with membrane components.

The two examples described here—the interaction between oestradiol and the dopaminergic inhibition of prolactin release, and the effect of oestradiol treatment on protein kinase C—raise an important question: what are the primary recognition sites for oestradiol and other steroid hormones? Despite progress in the analysis of molecular events, this question remains unresolved, largely because the binding of steroid hormones to sites detected on plasma membranes has not been clearly coupled to physiological events.

The presence of recognition sites for neurotransmitters, neuropeptides and steroids on the outer plasma membrane of the cell could explain, at least in part, some of their common biological activities, such as the regulation of hormone release and the regulation of cell proliferation at the level of the pituitary gland.

Acknowledgement

We thank Mrs M. Le Guennec for her helpful secretarial assistance.

References

Albaladejo V, Collu R, André J 1984 Down regulation by 17β-estradiol of D2 dopamine receptors in the MtTF4 pituitary tumor. Endocrinology 114:2344–2348

Berthois Y, Pourreau-Schneider N, Gandilhon Ph, Mittre H, Tubiana N, Martin PM 1986 Estradiol membrane binding sites on human breast cancer cell lines. Use of a fluorescent estradiol conjugate to demonstrate plasma membrane binding systems. J Steroid Biochem 25:963–972

Birman P, Touraine Ph, Bai-Grenier F et al 1989 The stimulated C-kinase activity in estradiol-treated rat pituitaries is reduced by chronic treatment with the dopamine agonist CV 205-502. Acta Endocrinol 121:489–494

Brandi AM, Joannidis S, Peillon F, Joubert D 1990 Changes of prolactin response to dopamine during the rat estrous cycle. Neuroendocrinology 51:449–454

Bression D, Brandi AM, Le Dafniet M et al 1983 Modifications of the high and low affinity pituitary domperidone-binding sites in chronic estrogenized rats. Endocrinology 113:1799–1805

Bression D, Brandi AM, Pagesy P et al 1985 In vitro and in vivo antagonistic regulation by estradiol and progesterone of the rat pituitary domperidone binding sites: correlation with ovarian steroid regulation of the dopaminergic inhibition of prolactin secretion in vitro. Endocrinology 116:1905–1911

Bression D, Michard M, Le Dafniet M, Pagesy P, Peillon F 1986 Evidence for a specific estradiol binding site on rat pituitary membranes. Endocrinology 119:1048–1051

Giguère V, Meunier H, Veilleux R, Labrie F 1982 Direct effects of sex steroids on prolactin release at the anterior pituitary level: interactions with dopamine, thyrotropin-releasing hormone, and isobutylmethylxanthine. Endocrinology 111:857–862

Godeau JF, Schorderet-Slatkine S, Hubert P, Baulieu EE 1978 Induction of maturation in Xenopus laevis oocytes by a steroid linked to a polymer. Proc Natl Acad Sci USA 75:2353–2357

Grove RI, Korach K 1987 Estrogen stimulation of phosphatidylinositol metabolism in mouse uterine tissue. Endocrinology 121:1083–1088

Kalberman LE, Machiavelli GA, De Nicola AF, Weissenberg LS, Burdman JA 1980 Synthesis of DNA in oestrogen-induced pituitary tumours in rats: effect of bromocriptine. J Endocrinol 87:221–224

Kelly MJ, Moss RL, Dudley CA 1977 The effects of microelectrophoretically applied estrogen, cortisol and acetylcholine on medial preoptic-septal unit activity throughout the estrous cycle of the female rat. Exp Brain Res 30:53–64

Koch B, Lutz-Bucher B, Briaud B, Mialhe C 1978 Specific interaction of corticosteroids with binding sites in the plasma membranes of the rat anterior pituitary gland. J Endocrinol 79:215–222

Lloyd HM, Meares JD, Jacobi J 1975 Effects of oestrogen and bromocriptine on in vivo secretion and mitosis in prolactin cells. Nature (Lond) 255:497–498

Munemura M, Agui T, Sibley D 1989 Chronic estrogen treatment promotes a functional uncoupling of the D2 dopamine receptor in rat anterior pituitary gland. Endocrinology 124:346–355

O'Brien CA, Liskamp RM, Solomon DH, Weinstein IB 1985 Inhibition of protein kinase C by tamoxifen. Cancer Res 45:2462–2465

Pasqualini C, Lenoir V, El Abed A, Kerdélhué B 1984 Anterior pituitary dopamine receptors during the rat estrous cycle. Neuroendocrinology 38:39–44

Pasqualini C, Bojda F, Kerdélhué B 1986 Direct effect of estradiol on the number of dopamine receptors in the anterior pituitary of ovariectomized rats. Endocrinology 119:2484–2489

Peillon F, Vila-Porcile E, Olivier L, Racadot J 1970 L'action des oestrogènes sur les adénomes hypophysaires chez l'homme. Documents histologiques en microscopie optique et électronique et apport de l'expérimentation. Ann Endocrinol 31:259–270

Peillon F, Bression D, Brandi AM, Racadot J 1984 Pathogenesis of prolactinomas. The role of estrogens and dopamine receptors. In: Lamberts SWJ et al (eds) Trends in diagnosis of pituitary adenomas. Free University Press, Amsterdam, p 103–113

Pietras R, Szego C 1979 Estrogen receptors in uterine plasma membrane. J Steroid Biochem 14:1471–1483

Pietras R, Szego C 1980 Partial purification of oestrogen receptors in subfractions of hepatocyte plasma membranes. Biochem J 191:743–760

Pilotte N, Burt DR, Barraclough ChA 1989 Ovariectomy permits progesterone to increase the binding of ^{3}H-spiperone to the anterior pituitary gland in estrogen-primed rats. Endocrinology 124:805–811

Sibley DR, De Léan A, Creese I 1982 Anterior pituitary dopamine receptors. Demonstration of interconvertible high and low affinity states of the D2 dopamine receptor. J Biol Chem 257:6351–6361

Sidorkina OM, Morozova TM, Rau VA 1988 Translocation of protein kinase C under the action of estradiol from the cytosol into the cell membranes and activation of the enzyme in the target cells. Biokhimiya 53:406–412

Sokolovsky M, Egozi Y, Avissar S 1981 Molecular regulation of receptors: interaction of β-estradiol and progesterone with the muscarinic system. Proc Natl Acad Sci USA 78:5554–5558

Spooner PM, Gorski J 1972 Early estrogen effects on lipid metabolism in the rat uterus. Endocrinology 91:1273–1279

Towle A, Sze PY 1983 Steroid binding to synaptic plasma membrane: differential binding of glucocorticoids and gonadal steroids. J Steroid Biochem 18:135–143

DISCUSSION

Su: We are searching for a physiological function for the σ receptor, and I am wondering if it might be involved here. Haloperidol has an effect on prolactin release, usually thought to be exerted through a direct effect on the dopamine

D_2 receptor system. You have shown that progesterone can affect prolactin release, so perhaps you should experiment with σ receptor-specific ligands such as *d*-pentazocine or *d*-SKF-10 047 (*d*-*N*-allylnormetazocine), in your assay. It would be interesting to see if they have any effects.

Joubert-Bression: Yes, we could try that.

Simmonds: In pituitary membranes from ovariectomized rats the number of dopamine binding sites was decreased compared to that in intact animals. I gather that you could restore the number of sites to control levels by adding progesterone *in vitro* to the membranes.

Joubert-Bression: Yes; we added progesterone to the incubation medium.

Simmonds: You were using broken cell membranes?

Joubert-Bression: Yes.

Baulieu: Do you need oestradiol in the medium to see the effect of progesterone?

Joubert-Bression: No. We incubated the membranes with either progesterone or oestradiol, not both together.

Baulieu: Do you need pretreatment with oestradiol *in vivo* to see the effect of progesterone?

Joubert-Bression: No.

Simmonds: Where do these additional dopamine receptors come from in the membrane fragments? Presumably they must be present in the membranes from ovariectomized rats but do not bind ligand until progesterone makes them active in some way.

Joubert-Bression: This is a good question, but I do not know the answer.

Majewska: Perhaps some of them are 'cryptic' receptors, hidden within the membrane, and progesterone exposes them. The physical properties of the membrane can alter the availability of some receptors—for example, the serotonin receptor (Heron et al 1980). When you alter membrane fluidity you may hide or expose certain ligand binding sites.

Joubert-Bression: Similarly, binding of epidermal growth factor to pituitary membranes is increased if you first treat the membranes with a buffer of high ionic strength.

Ramirez: Have you investigated the time course of this effect, or looked at the phenomenon in more detail? It is a rather puzzling result. What concentration of progesterone did you use?

Joubert-Bression: We used 10^{-8} M progesterone. We haven't looked at the time dependency.

Baulieu: Does the steroid antagonist RU486 prevent the progesterone-induced increase in dopamine receptor number?

Joubert-Bression: We have not tried using this antagonist. The rat pituitary is very small, which limits the number of binding assays we can do.

Ramirez: Were the membranes prepared from pituitary cells in culture or directly from animals, and what sort of membrane preparation was it?

Joubert-Bression: We prepared the membranes from animals and used the P_2 fraction.

Ramirez: So you probably have some contamination with cytosolic proteins.

Joubert-Bression: I do not think so, because we tested for the activity of the cytosolic marker lactate dehydrogenase and found contamination to be only 0.0001% of the cytosolic activity.

Kordon: When you treat animals with oestrogen *in vivo*, a number of factors could affect pituitary protein kinase C activity also in an indirect manner; for instance, there could be oestrogen-dependent changes in dopamine or neuropeptide fluxes to the pituitary. Under *in vitro* conditions, we never observed any rapid effect of the steroid on protein kinase C. All data were compatible with the hypothesis of a genomic mechanism; moreover, the effects were completely blocked by protein synthesis inhibitors (Drouva et al 1990). Unlike you, we did not see spontaneous translocation of the kinase after oestrogen treatment. Don't you think the translocation you have seen may reflect indirect effects of oestrogen—effects on GnRH release, for instance?

On the other hand, I think you should not correlate protein kinase C activation with cell proliferation only. Many other parameters, such as phosphorylation of K^+ or Ca^{2+} channels, or changes in the sensitivity of adenylate cyclase receptor coupling, are also affected by protein kinase C (Drouva et al 1988, 1990).

Joubert-Bression: Yes, I agree. We did not however relate the changes in protein kinase C activity only to proliferation, but also to hormone secretion. In addition, in our experimental model, activation of proliferation and hormone secretion are never dissociated. Both are either stimulated or inhibited.

Su: Specific binding in your oestrogen binding assay was about 50% or more of total binding, which is quite high for this type of assay. There are σ receptors in the pituitary, so one would like to be able to measure progesterone binding. Have you assayed binding of radioactive progesterone?

Joubert-Bression: No.

McEwen: Did 4-hydroxytamoxifen interfere with the membrane binding of [^{3}H]oestradiol?

Joubert-Bression: It had no effect on the binding.

McEwen: This gives you the opportunity to discriminate between the genomic and non-genomic effects of oestrogen, because tamoxifen would certainly interfere with intracellularly mediated effects, so you should make use of this compound.

Joubert-Bression: Yes, this is a good suggestion.

Baulieu: RU486, an antagonist at the intracellular progesterone receptor, could be used in the same way, to distinguish genomic and non-genomic effects.

Joubert-Bression: Yes.

Ramirez: Have you investigated the effect of temperature or pH on [^{3}H]oestradiol binding?

Joubert-Bression: The binding was thermolabile. We had to do the binding assay at 0 °C, because at 20 °C or 37 °C binding was not stable.

Kordon: Did you see any effect of progesterone on the membrane binding of dopamine at 0 °C?

Joubert-Bression: We didn't do the experiment at that temperature; we did it at 30 °C.

References

Drouva SV, Rérat E, Bihoreau C et al 1988 Dihydropyridine-sensitive calcium channel activity related to prolactin, growth hormone, and luteinizing hormone release from anterior pituitary cells in culture: interactions with somatostatin, dopamine, and estrogens. Endocrinology 123:2762–2773

Drouva SV, Gorenne I, Laplante E, Rérat E, Enjalbert A, Kordon C 1990 Estradiol modulates protein kinase C activity in the rat pituitary *in vivo* and *in vitro*. Endocrinology 126:536–544

Heron DS, Shinitzky M, Herskovitz M, Samuel D 1980 Lipid fluidity markedly modulates the binding of serotonin to mouse brain membranes. Proc Natl Acad Sci USA 77:7463–7467

The molecular features of membrane perturbation by anaesthetic steroids: a study using differential scanning calorimetry, small angle X-ray diffraction and solid state ^{2}H NMR

Alexandros Makriyannis, De-Ping Yang and Thomas Mavromoustakos

Section of Medicinal Chemistry & Pharmacognosy, School of Pharmacy, and Institute of Materials Science, University of Connecticut, Storrs, CT 06269, USA; Francis Bitter National Magnet Laboratory, Massachusetts Institute of Technology, Cambridge, MA 02139, USA

Abstract. We have studied the interactions of the anaesthetic steroid alphaxalone and its inactive isomer Δ^{16}-alphaxalone with model membrane bilayers using differential scanning calorimetry, small angle X-ray diffraction and solid state NMR. Our data show that the anaesthetic steroid broadens the membrane phase transition and increases the ratio of *gauche* to *trans* conformers in the membrane. Δ^{16}-Alphaxalone has only small effects on membrane and incorporates to a limited degree in the bilayer. The amphipathic anaesthetic steroid alphaxalone is located near the membrane interface (the junction of the polar and hydrophobic regions of the phospholipids forming the bilayer). It orients with its long axis parallel to the chains of the lipid membranes and its 3α-hydroxyl group near the *sn*-2 carbonyl. Anchoring of the steroid at the membrane interface and imperfect packing with the bilayer chains may be involved in membrane perturbation and eventually lead to anaesthesia.

1990 Steroids and neuronal activity. Wiley, Chichester (Ciba Foundation Symposium 153) p 172–189

In many classes of anaesthetics there is a good correlation between anaesthetic potency and oil/water partition coefficients, suggesting that anaesthetic activity results from non-specific interactions of the drug with membrane lipids (Seeman 1972). This generalization, however, does not hold true for the anaesthetic steroids, where small structural changes having no significant effect on partitioning properties can lead to large differences in anaesthetic activity (Atkinson et al 1965, Phillips 1975). To account for this structural specificity some investigators have suggested that anaesthetic steroids act after binding to a specific site on a target membrane protein (Richards et al 1978). Others have proposed that the sites of action are membrane lipids that are capable of a high degree of structural discrimination, evidence for which was obtained from electron spin resonance (ESR) experiments using spin-labelled lipid bilayers containing cholesterol (Lawrence & Gill 1975). These experiments showed that steroids with anaesthetic activity caused an increase in the fluidity of the model membrane whereas structurally related inactive analogues produced much less disorder.

In our initial studies, we focused on two structurally related pregnane steroids that had widely different physiological properties. Of these, alphaxalone (5α-pregnan-3α-ol-11,20-dione) has potent anaesthetic properties and was used clinically as the main active component in the commercially available anaesthetic, Althesin. The other steroid studied, Δ^{16}-alphaxalone (5α-pregn-16-en-3α-ol-11,20-dione), which differs from alphaxalone only by having a double bond in the C-16 position (see structures in Fig. 1, p 175), lacks anaesthetic activity (Atkinson et al 1965). First, we tested these two molecules for their effects on a membrane preparation not involved in the anaesthetic response, namely, the anion transport system in human erythrocytes (Makriyannis & Fesik 1980). We found that the steroid with anaesthetic activity inhibited anion transport more effectively than its inactive analogue; this indicated that the differences in activity between the two molecules were not restricted to their actions on neuronal membranes. We have also investigated the interactions of alphaxalone and Δ^{16}-alphaxalone using phosphatidylcholine bilayer vesicles as model membranes (Makriyannis & Fesik 1983). The steroids were incorporated into the bilayer and the preparations were studied by means of high resolution ^{1}H, ^{13}C and ^{2}H NMR spectroscopy. Our results showed that the two steroids had very different motional properties in the lipid bilayer, alphaxalone being considerably more mobile than Δ^{16}-alphaxalone in such preparations. This was interpreted as evidence that the biologically active steroid perturbs the phospholipid bilayer more effectively than its biologically inactive analogue.

In a later study we used a multilamellar bilayer dispersion of dimyristoylphosphatidylcholine with perdeuterated acyl chains (DMPC-d_{54}) as a model membrane (Fesik & Makriyannis 1985). We showed that alphaxalone consistently decreased the quadrupolar splittings in the solid state ^{2}H NMR spectra of DMPC-d_{54} in the liquid-crystalline phase. An increase in the number of *gauche* segments of the acyl chains of DMPC could explain this observation. The inactive steroid Δ^{16}-alphaxalone did not produce this effect. The ability of alphaxalone to perturb membrane lipids more effectively than Δ^{16}-alphaxalone can be related to the differences that exist in molecular geometry between the two molecules. Because of these differences, the active steroid requires more space in order to be accommodated between the phospholipid chains.

In another study, we used aqueous multilamellar dispersions of dipalmitoylphosphatidylcholine (DPPC) with specific ^{13}C and ^{2}H labels as endogenous probes to study the conformational and dynamic properties of the lipid bilayer as a function of temperature (Makriyannis et al 1986). The results showed no significant changes between the solid state ^{13}C and ^{2}H NMR spectra of the DPPC containing the inactive steroid and those of DPPC alone. However, the physiologically active steroid produced significant changes, including a lowering of the phase transition temperature, broadening of the transition and reduction of the ^{2}H quadrupolar splittings. These changes indicate that alphaxalone increases the relative number of *gauche* chain conformers when the DPPC chains are in the liquid-crystalline phase and increases the rate of axial diffusion in both the gel and liquid-crystalline phases.

We also studied the interactions of a series of structurally related pregnane analogues that have a wide range of anaesthetic potencies, using high resolution ^{1}H and ^{2}H NMR (Fesik 1981). The results of these studies, which used unilamellar membranes, showed a good correlation between the motional properties and anaesthetic potencies of the steroids.

In the studies described here we have probed further into the interactions of alphaxalone and Δ^{16}-alphaxalone with membranes and have sought to examine the role played by cholesterol during this interaction. Also, we have obtained information on the topography of the anaesthetic steroid in the bilayer at the molecular level. We have then attempted to correlate the steroid's orientation and site of incorporation in the bilayer with its ability to perturb membranes.

For our studies we used differential scanning calorimetry (DSC), small angle X-ray diffraction and solid state ^{2}H NMR. DSC is used to study the effects of drugs on the phase properties of membranes (Melchior & Steim 1976), whereas small angle X-ray diffraction can give information on the structural changes of the bilayer that are induced by the drug molecule and also help us to identify the exact location of the drug in the bilayer (Franks & Levine 1981, Herbette et al 1986). Solid state NMR gives the most detailed molecular information (Griffin 1981, Davis 1983, Smith & Oldfield 1984) and can identify changes in membrane conformation and dynamics produced by the drug (Makriyannis et al 1986). NMR can also be used to determine the orientation and conformation of the drug in the membrane (Makriyannis et al 1989).

Differential scanning calorimetry

We have studied the effects of the two pregnane analogues on the thermotropic behaviour of two model membranes, as shown in Fig. 1. The first preparation (left) is with fully hydrated DPPC and has a characteristic thermogram consisting of a broad low enthalpy transition ($T_c' = 35.3\ °C$) and a sharp high enthalpy main transition ($T_c = 41.3\ °C$). When incorporated into the membrane, the inactive steroid Δ^{16}-alphaxalone (20 molar per cent, or $x = 0.20$) broadens the

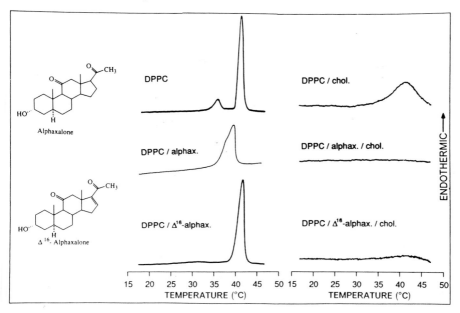

FIG. 1. Differential scanning calorimetric thermograms obtained from bilayer preparations of DPPC (dipalmitoylphosphatidylcholine), DPPC + alphaxalone (molar fraction, $x = 0.20$), DPPC + Δ^{16}-alphaxalone ($x = 0.20$), DPPC + cholesterol ($x = 0.20$), DPPC + alphaxalone ($x = 0.20$) + cholesterol ($x = 0.20$), and DPPC + Δ^{16}-alphaxalone ($x = 0.20$) + cholesterol ($x = 0.20$). Ordinate, rate of heat absorption (relative units). The thermograms on the right have been magnified 3.3 times relative to those on the left.

pretransition but does not alter T_c', while the main transition maintains the same half-width and T_c. In contrast, the anaesthetic steroid alphaxalone produces a significant broadening of the main transition, which now seems to be composed of two overlapping components. The pretransition is no longer discernible. The broadening of the main transition is an indication of decreased cooperativity at the phase transition. The second preparation (right) consists of fully hydrated DPPC containing $x = 0.20$ cholesterol. Cholesterol broadens the phase transition and significantly reduces its enthalpy. The thermogram consists of a broad two-component asymmetrical peak centred on 40 °C. Addition of alphaxalone ($x = 0.20$) to this preparation virtually eliminates the endotherm whereas its inactive analogue broadens it without significantly affecting T_c. The results with the cholesterol-containing preparation confirm those from hydrated DPPC and show that the anaesthetic molecule, in the presence and absence of cholesterol, greatly reduces the cooperativity of the chains at the phase transition. The inactive steroid produces a much smaller effect.

Small angle X-ray diffraction

In order to study the location of alphaxalone in the membrane we have carried out small angle X-ray diffraction experiments using bilayer preparations of DMPC and DMPC with cholesterol equilibrated at relative humidity 98% in the temperature range of 10 °C to 55 °C. The preparations were studied in the presence of each of the two steroids and the respective diffraction data were compared. Patterns of lamellar diffraction orders were observed and analysed to provide information on total period repeat distance (d-spacing) and the electron density profile across the bilayer, as described by Franks & Levine (1981).

Phase changes

As is characteristic for such systems, d-spacing decreases when the bilayer undergoes the gel to liquid-crystalline phase transition and continues to decrease gradually at temperatures above the transition. This is due to conformational changes in the bilayer at the phase transition temperature, which produce an increase in the *gauche : trans* conformer ratio in the lipid chains. We observed that for the DMPC preparations containing Δ^{16}-alphaxalone the d-spacing in the liquid-crystalline phase is identical to that of the control DMPC preparation, whereas the d-spacing of DMPC containing the anaesthetic steroid alphaxalone is always 1.5 Å smaller. Addition of cholesterol ($x = 0.15$) to each of the three preparations caused the transition to broaden. Again, the inactive steroid did not change the d-spacing whereas the active analogue reduced it slightly. The data provide evidence that alphaxalone increases the *gauche* conformer contribution in the lipid chains and thus has a fluidizing effect on the membrane.

Site of alphaxalone in the bilayer

Representative comparisons of electron density profiles of DMPC and DMPC + alphaxalone (with and without cholesterol) are shown in Fig. 2, where z is the distance across the bilayer, perpendicular to its plane, measured from the bilayer centre. As can be seen, the d-spacing above the phase transition is 48 Å for the DMPC preparations and becomes 50 Å when cholesterol is present. In each electron density profile, the middle trough corresponds to the centre of the bilayer, i.e., the terminal methyl group region, and the two maxima occurring at about 18 Å from the centre correspond to the phosphates of the head groups. We have superimposed the electron density profiles of the DMPC and DMPC + alphaxalone preparations and assumed identical electron densities at the highest and lowest points of the profiles. Furthermore, we have compared two preparations with identical d-spacings. This could be achieved only if the two preparations were at different temperatures, because the drug-containing

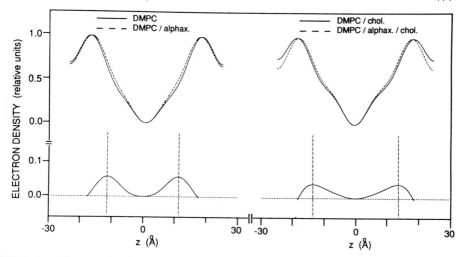

FIG. 2. Electron density profiles obtained from X-ray diffraction experiments using DMPC bilayers equilibrated at relative humidity 98%. *Left*: comparison between DMPC at 49 °C and DMPC + alphaxalone ($x = 0.10$) at 40 °C. *Right*: comparison between DMPC + cholesterol ($x = 0.15$) at 54 °C and DMPC + alphaxalone ($x = 0.10$) + cholesterol ($x = 0.15$) at 54 °C. Below each superposition is the difference between the two profiles with an expanded scale. z, distance across the bilayer, perpendicular to its plane, measured from the bilayer centre.

and pure lipid preparations generally have different d-spacings at the same temperature. We have described the rationale and validity of our approach elsewhere (Mavromoustakos et al 1990). The comparison revealed an electron density difference near the bilayer interface in the region centred at $z = 11.2$ Å. This can clearly be seen in the magnified vertical difference scale below the superposition. This increase in electron density should be due to the presence of alphaxalone; the peak position corresponds to the location of the centre of mass of alphaxalone in the DMPC bilayer. The width of the difference peak is of the order of 14 Å, which is approximately the length of the long axis of the alphaxalone molecule, indicating that in all likelihood the molecule orients with its long axis parallel to the lipid chains. The location of alphaxalone in the bilayer, as revealed by the X-ray diffraction data, positions the molecule in a manner that allows its 3α-hydroxyl group to be in the proximity of the *sn*-2 carbonyl group of DMPC. The inclusion of cholesterol in the DMPC preparations produces changes in the electron density profile. However, when we carried out a superposition of two DMPC/cholesterol preparations with and without alphaxalone using criteria similar to those described above, we obtained analogous results. The cholesterol-containing preparations give a difference plot from the electron density profiles with a peak centred at $z = 13.2$ Å, approximately 2 Å closer to the interface when compared to the preparation without cholesterol. Also, the width of the difference peak is now 16 Å, larger by 2 Å. The data from our second set of preparations indicate that cholesterol causes a slight shift in the time-averaged location of the steroid closer to the interface between the polar and hydrophobic regions of the phospholipid bilayer, although the steroid still maintains its proximity to the sn-2 carbonyl.

Solid state ^{2}H NMR spectroscopy

Solid state NMR has become the method of choice for obtaining information on membrane conformation and dynamics and can be extended to the study of the effects of drugs on model and biological membranes. In previous work (Makriyannis et al 1986) we used both ^{2}H and ^{13}C solid state NMR to obtain detailed molecular information on the interactions of alphaxalone and Δ^{16}-alphaxalone with the phospholipid bilayer. We associated the perturbing effects of the anaesthetic steroid with its ability to induce fast axial diffusion accompanied by an increase of *gauche* contributions in the phospholipid chains. In order to study the effect of cholesterol on these interactions, we have now done further studies and have obtained solid state ^{2}H NMR spectra due to the 2[7',7'-^{2}H$_2$]-methylene segment of the sn-2 chain from the following six preparations: DPPC, DPPC/alphaxalone, DPPC/ Δ^{16}-alphaxalone, DPPC/cholesterol, DPPC/alphaxalone/cholesterol and DPPC/Δ^{16}-alphaxalone/cholesterol (see Fig. 3 for molar ratios). Solid state ^{2}H NMR spectra were also obtained from DPPC preparations containing alphaxalone deuterated at the 9, 12, 17 and 21 positions, so that we could determine the orientation of alphaxalone in the bilayer.

Effects on the DPPC chains

Figure 3 shows the temperature dependence of representative solid state ^{2}H NMR spectra for each of the six preparations. Above the phase transition temperature all the ^{2}H spectra are axially symmetric powder patterns with sharp parallel and perpendicular edges. At 40 °C the DPPC preparation is very near its phase transition temperature and has a composite ^{2}H spectrum from gel (L$_{\beta'}$) and liquid-crystalline (L$_\alpha$) components. The L$_\alpha$ part of the spectrum has a residual quadrupolar splitting $\Delta\nu_Q = 29.5$ kHz. At the same temperature, the spectra from the preparations of both steroids are in the L$_\alpha$ phase. However, alphaxalone produces a small, but reproducible, reduction in the splitting ($\Delta\nu_Q = 29.0$ kHz) while Δ^{16}-alphaxalone slightly increases this splitting ($\Delta\nu_Q = 30.0$ kHz). In the cholesterol-containing preparations, the splittings for the alphaxalone and Δ^{16}-alphaxalone preparations are 40.4 and 43.2 kHz, respectively. In this more ordered membrane preparation, differences in the $\Delta\nu_Q$ values due to the presence of the two steroids are magnified. The smaller $\Delta\nu_Q$ value from the alphaxalone-containing preparation indicates that the

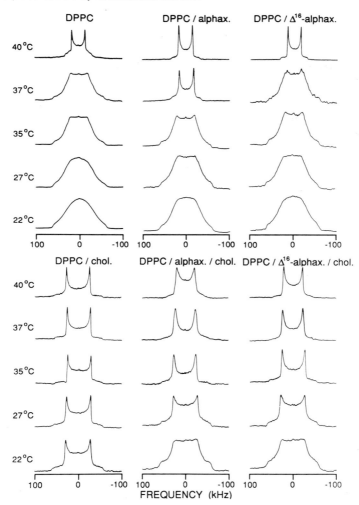

FIG. 3. Solid state ^{2}H NMR spectra due to the $2[7',7'-^2H_2]$-methylene segment of DPPC obtained from bilayer preparations of DPPC, DPPC + alphaxalone ($x = 0.30$), and DPPC + Δ^{16}-alphaxalone ($x = 0.30$), DPPC + cholesterol ($x = 0.30$), DPPC + alphaxalone ($x = 0.15$) + cholesterol ($x = 0.15$), and DPPC + Δ^{16}-alphaxalone ($x = 0.15$) + cholesterol ($x = 0.15$).

anaesthetic produces a more disordered membrane system that has a large *gauche* conformer contribution in the chains. In contrast, the preparation with higher cholesterol content has a much larger quadrupolar splitting (53.0 kHz), owing to the ordering effect of the excess cholesterol and a concomitant large increase in the *trans* conformer chain segment population.

The temperature variation of hydrated DPPC spectra (Fig. 3, *top*) shows that incorporation of Δ^{16}-alphaxalone produces only marginal changes. However, alphaxalone produced significant changes in the ^{2}H spectra: (a) a purely liquid crystalline-type spectrum appears at 39 °C (not shown in figure), approximately 2 °C below the corresponding temperature for pure DPPC; and (b) at 37 °C the spectra show a considerably more liquid-crystalline character than that of either pure DPPC or DPPC/Δ^{16}-alphaxalone at the same temperature.

Examination of the ^{2}H spectra from the cholesterol-containing preparations (Fig. 3, bottom) shows that in all these preparations the phase transition is broadened, as already observed by differential scanning calorimetry. A comparison of the ^{2}H spectra from the two steroid preparations shows that spectra from preparations containing the anaesthetic steroid have consistently lower $\Delta\nu_Q$ values. There are also qualitative differences between the two sets of spectra. For example, at 37 °C the spectrum from the alphaxalone preparation shows shoulders in the 90° edges, a characteristic of a two-component system. At 40 °C the spectrum is still not of the L_α type. It has sloping 90° edges and is two-thirds filled in the centre, spectral features which may indicate two components exchanging at an intermediate rate. The corresponding spectra after Δ^{16}-alphaxalone incorporation are closer to L_α in character. We are currently undertaking a more quantitative analysis of these spectra.

Incorporation in the bilayer

In Figure 4 we present typical solid state ^{2}H NMR spectra of DPPC bilayer preparations containing deuterium-labelled alphaxalone and Δ^{16}-alphaxalone at 42 °C, each in two different molar ratios (0.95/0.05 and 0.90/0.10). These four preparations have identical amounts of DPPC and the spectra were obtained using identical experimental parameters. This allowed us to correlate the spectral intensities with the amount of drug incorporated in the bilayer. In Fig. 4 (left) the spectra are represented on an absolute intensity scale while on the right the same spectra are shown on an arbitrary scale. In the alphaxalone-containing preparations, NMR spectral intensity increases with increasing drug concentration, whereas the two spectra from the inactive analogue are of equal intensity and approximately ten-fold less intense than the spectra from the alphaxalone-containing preparations. This experiment provides direct evidence that two steroids closely related in structure become incorporated very differently in the membrane. The observation may also explain, in part, the lack of anaesthetic activity of Δ^{16}-alphaxalone.

Orientation in the bilayer

^{2}H spectra from specifically ^{2}H-labelled molecules can be used to determine their orientation in an anisotropic membrane system. This method was initially

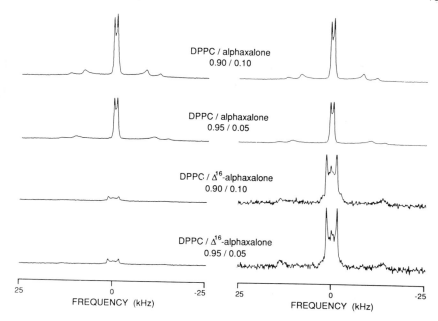

FIG. 4.   Solid state ^{2}H NMR spectra from fully hydrated DPPC bilayer preparations containing $(9,12\alpha,12\beta,17,21,21,21\text{-}d_7)$-alphaxalone or $(9,12\alpha,12\beta,21,21,21\text{-}d_6)$-$\Delta^{16}$-alphaxalone $(x = 0.05$ and $0.10)$. *Left*: spectra with absolute intensities. *Right*: same spectra with arbitrary intensities.

applied to the study of the orientation of cholesterol in a bilayer (Taylor et al 1981) and we have since expanded and broadened its applicability (Makriyannis et al 1989). We report here on a preliminary determination of the axis of orientation of alphaxalone in the DPPC bilayer. The ^{2}H spectrum (Fig. 4) from the alphaxalone-containing preparation $(x = 0.10)$ shows an intense powder pattern of $\Delta\nu_Q = 0.84$ kHz in the centre that is due to the three deuterons at the C-21 methyl group. In addition, there are two pairs of weaker peaks. One, having a $\Delta\nu_Q$ value of 16.5 kHz, is attributed to one label at the 12β position, and another at $\Delta\nu_Q = 23.6$ kHz originates from three labels at the 9, 12α and 17 positions. Our calculation is based on a model according to which the steroid undergoes fast axial diffusion about a director which is parallel to the lipid chains of the bilayer. The angle (θ) between a C—^{2}H bond and the director is related to the corresponding quadrupolar splitting through a molecular order parameter (S_{mol}) according to the equation (Taylor et al 1981):

$$\Delta\nu_Q = \frac{3}{4} A_Q \left(\frac{3 \cos^2\theta - 1}{2} \right) S_{\text{mol}}$$

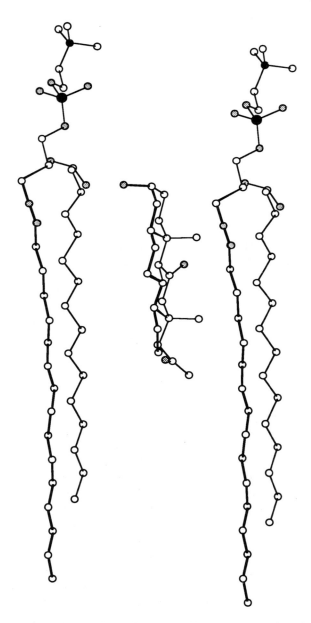

FIG. 5. Representation of a model showing the position and orientation of alphaxalone with respect to the DPPC bilayer. Alphaxalone anchors at the membrane interface and may form a hydrogen bond between its 3α-hydroxyl group and the *sn*-2 carbonyl group of DPPC.

where A_Q is the deuterium quadrupolar coupling constant ($\approx 170\,\text{kHz}$). When experimental data are available from a few labels on a rigid part of the molecule, S_{mol} is expected to be identical for all the labels. This allows us to compare the ratios of the predicted splitting values and of the experimentally observed ones. Using an iterative algorithm, the orientation of the director in the molecular frame can be determined. Our calculations showed that the director goes through H at C-3 and C-16 of alphaxalone and almost exactly coincides with the long axis of the steroid ring system. This permits alphaxalone in the bilayer to orient in such a manner that it is able to fit between the chains of two adjacent lipid molecules with its 3α-hydroxyl group presumably directed towards the interface region in the bilayer and near the *sn*-2 carbonyl. The result is consistent with the topographic information obtained from our small angle X-ray diffraction data. The position and orientation of alphaxalone in a DPPC bilayer is depicted graphically in Fig. 5. The model represents our experimentally determined results.

Conclusions

Our studies show that the anaesthetic steroid alphaxalone perturbs model membrane bilayers, whereas its inactive analogue, Δ^{16}-alphaxalone, does not. This perturbation involves an increase in the ratio of *gauche* to *trans* conformers in the bilayer chains. Also, work with other amphipathic molecules in our laboratory shows that the critical interaction occurs at the interface region of the membrane and may involve a conformational change in the glycerol backbone of the phospholipid bilayer. The ability of a steroid to induce such perturbations is related to its stereochemical characteristics, which are responsible for an imperfect steroid–bilayer packing. The anaesthetic steroid undergoes amphipathic interactions with the membrane and anchors itself at the interface with its 3α-hydroxyl group near the *sn*-2 carbonyl with which it may form a hydrogen bond. It acquires an orientation which places its long axis parallel to the bilayer chains.

Conversely, the inactivity of Δ^{16}-alphaxalone can be attributed to a combination of its favourable packing, which leads to insufficient lipid perturbation, and its inability to incorporate substantially in the membrane.

Thus, the perturbation of membrane lipids by anaesthetic steroids may affect the functions of important membrane-associated proteins and eventually lead to anaesthesia.

Acknowledgements

This work was supported by a grant from the National Institute on Drug Abuse (DA-3801). We should like to thank Professor R. G. Griffin for making the solid state NMR spectrometer available for the ^{2}H NMR experiments and Dr K. Beshah for timely help and stimulating discussions over the acquisition and analysis of the ^{2}H NMR spectra. We thank Professor L. G. Herbette for providing us with the X-ray diffraction facilities at the Biomolecular Structure Analysis Center of the University of Connecticut Health Center.

References

Atkinson RM, Davis B, Pratt MA, Sharpe HM, Tomich EG 1965 Action of some steroids on the central nervous system of the mouse. II. Pharmacology. J Med Chem 8: 426–432

Davis JH 1983 The description of membrane lipid conformation, order and dynamics by ^{2}H-NMR. Biochim Biophys Acta 737:117–171

Fesik SW 1981 A study of the mechanism of anesthetic action. The interaction of steroids with model membranes. PhD dissertation, University of Connecticut

Fesik SW, Makriyannis A 1985 Geometric requirements for membrane perturbation and anesthetic activity. Conformational analysis of alphaxalone and Δ^{16}-alphaxalone and ^{2}H NMR studies on their interactions with model membranes. Mol Pharmacol 27:624–629

Franks NP, Levine YK 1981 Low angle X-ray diffraction. In: Grell E (ed) Membrane spectroscopy. Springer-Verlag, New York, p 437–487

Griffin RG 1981 Solid state nuclear magnetic resonance of lipid bilayers. Methods Enzymol 72:108–174

Herbette LG, Chester DW, Rhodes DG 1986 Structural analysis of drug molecules in biological membranes. Biophys J 49:91–94

Lawrence DK, Gill EW 1975 Structurally specific effects of some steroid anesthetics on spin-labeled liposomes. Mol Pharmacol 11:280–286

Makriyannis A, Fesik SW 1980 Effects of anesthetics on sulfate transport in the red cell. J Neurosci Res 5:25–33

Makriyannis A, Fesik SW 1983 Mechanism of steroid anesthetic action: interaction of alphaxalone and Δ^{16}-alphaxalone with bilayer vesicles. J Med Chem 26:463–465

Makriyannis A, Siminovitch DJ, Das Gupta SK, Griffin RG 1986 Studies on the interaction of anesthetic steroids with phosphatidylcholine using ^{2}H and ^{13}C solid state NMR. Biochim Biophys Acta 859:49–55

Makriyannis A, Banijamali A, Jarrell HC, Yang D-P 1989 The orientation of (−)-Δ^9-THC in DPPC bilayers as determined from solid state ^{2}H-NMR. Biochim Biophys Acta 986:141–145

Mavromoustakos T, Yang D-P, Charalambous A, Herbette LG, Makriyannis A 1990 Study of the topography of cannabinoids in model membranes using X-ray diffraction. Biochim Biophys Acta 1024:336–344

Melchior DL, Steim JM 1976 Thermotropic transitions in biomembranes. Annu Rev Biophys Bioeng 5:205–237

Phillips GH 1975 Structure-activity relationships in steroidal anesthetics. J Steroid Biochem 6:607–613

Richards CD, Martin K, Gregory S et al 1978 Degenerate perturbations of protein structure as the mechanism of anaesthetic action. Nature (Lond) 276:775–779

Seeman P 1972 The membrane action of anesthetics and tranquilizers. Pharmacol Rev 24:583–655

Smith LR, Oldfield E 1984 Dynamic structure of membranes by deuterium NMR. Science (Wash DC) 225:280–288

Taylor MG, Akiyama T, Smith ICP 1981 The molecular dynamics of cholesterol in bilayer membranes: a deuterium NMR study. Chem Phys Lipids 29:327–339

DISCUSSION

Majewska: Can you predict the interaction of a molecule such as pregnenolone sulphate with the phospholipid membrane? This molecule has a sulphate group, so with what would the sulphate interact?

Makriyannis: Because of the sulphate in the 3β position, I don't think the steroid will sink into the membrane; I expect it to stay at the interface or perhaps a little higher and to interact with the positively charged lipid head groups. However, it is difficult to predict exactly how it will fit in the bilayer. Regarding the ability of pregnenolone sulphate to perturb the membrane, we have shown that 3β-hydroxy pregnanes, unlike their 3α isomers, do not perturb. However, the sulphate group is much larger than the hydroxyl and, in spite of its 3β stereochemistry, may induce membrane perturbation.

Baulieu: I feel that pregnenolone sulphate will not enter the membrane, but that's just my opinion. Pregnenolone itself has the same structure as cholesterol but without the C-22–C-27 side-chain. You said that cholesterol packs perfectly, so how important to the packing is the side-chain and how would pregnenolone, which I like to think of as a 'mini cholesterol', pack?

Makriyannis: Cholesterol has very drastic effects on the dynamics of the phospholipid chains and I think pregnenolone would work like a 'little cholesterol', with qualitatively similar but less drastic effects on the membrane bilayer.

Baulieu: Where would the C-20 carbonyl group of pregnenolone be positioned in the membrane?

Makriyannis: This carbonyl is probably buried in the membrane bilayer, as we have observed with alphaxalone.

Baulieu: Dehydroepiandrosterone is a C_{19} steroid with a carbonyl group at C-17, but no C-21–C-20 side-chain. Would this molecule cause more perturbation than pregnenolone?

Makriyannis: It might very well do that, but one needs to test it.

Baulieu: It would be excellent if you did the experiments!

Lambert: What sort of aqueous concentrations of the anaesthetic steroids would be required to produce the perturbation of membranes that you described? In the type of experiments that we do, we put a known concentration of steroid into the bath, but we don't know how much enters the membrane. I wonder what sort of aqueous concentration would result in a steroid concentration in the membrane that is sufficient to perturb its structure.

Makriyannis: I don't know the answer to that particular question, but let me try to answer it in a different way. If you perturb membrane lipids you can alter the functioning of a membrane protein. However, the quantitative aspects of this effect are not well understood. I suspect that even small lipid perturbations—considerably smaller than those I described with model membranes—can have major effects on membrane proteins. Packing of lipids around membrane proteins is very tight and one may be able to affect the functioning of such proteins with small amounts of lipid-perturbing drugs. For example, we found that you need only very small amounts of an ether lipid analogue (one to four molecules per protein) to produce 30% inhibition of the activity of the glucose-transporting protein in human erythrocytes (D. L. Melchior & A. Makriyannis, unpublished). However, quantifying the biophysical data or trying to quantitatively compare the biophysical data with changes in protein functioning is difficult.

Simmonds: Richards & White (1981) measured the partitioning of [^{14}C] alphaxalone from artificial cerebrospinal fluid into liposomes of phosphatidylcholine, phosphatidylserine and cholesterol. They obtained a coefficient of about 1000, so a 1 μM aqueous concentration of alphaxalone would give a concentration of 1 mM in the lipid.

Lambert: We showed that anaesthetic steroids applied intracellularly via the patch electrode had no effect on the GABA$_A$ receptor (see Fig. 4, p 66). Do you think the steroid should be able to perturb the membrane equally well from either side?

Makriyannis: It should be able to perturb from either side. We have shown that the steroids interact with many different lipids. Presumably, then, membrane asymmetry should not prevent drug interaction with either side. I would like to point out that people tend to report steroid concentrations in a membrane preparation in terms of molar concentrations, but sometimes they don't report the amount of membrane that they used. The amount of membrane present, however, will determine the steroid concentration in the membrane, because these molecules segregate almost entirely into the membrane. One should therefore provide this kind of information.

Lambert: So the membrane acts like a sink for steroids?

Makriyannis: They partition almost entirely into the membrane, so if you do an experiment with the same concentration of steroid in the preparations but different amounts of membrane, you will have different steroid concentrations in the membrane.

Su: Have you tested the effects of local anaesthetics in your model and tried to correlate their effects with their clinical potencies? Some local anaesthetics are known to exert their effects when they actually enter the cell (Narahashi & Frazier 1971).

Makriyannis: The pregnane steroids I have discussed are used as general anaesthetics, not local anaesthetics. We have looked at a number of anaesthetic steroids and found a good correlation between their membrane effects and anaesthetic potencies. We used high resolution and solid state NMR and found good correlations between the structures of anaesthetic steroids and their abilities to perturb membranes. I don't think it is known where general anaesthetics act, or whether they act inside or outside the cell.

Majewska: Would you expect barbiturates to perturb the membrane in the same way as steroids, such as tetrahydroprogesterone or alphaxalone? Their modulatory effects on $GABA_A$ receptors are very similar.

Makriyannis: I would expect membrane perturbation, but that does not necessarily explain their mechanism of action. I don't know whether the perturbation of the membrane lipids by barbiturates accounts for their pharmacological properties. This lipid perturbation model does not exclude the possibility of a direct interaction of the steroid with the protein. Such an interaction may be at a non-catalytic site and thus may have some features in common with the interactions of steroids with lipids. We tend to think of drug interactions as being unique for each molecule. However, in my opinion, the interactions of different drug molecules with membrane components may have many common features. Lipids are amphipathic, but so are membrane proteins, with polar and hydrophobic components and an interface. There may thus be some common features in the interactions of amphipathic drugs with either membrane lipids or proteins.

Baulieu: When thinking about whether steroids can enter the membrane from either side, we should remember that membranes are not symmetrical; there are choline-rich phospholipids in the extracellular side of the membrane and ethanolamine-rich lipids in the intracellular side. Is there any difference in steroid accessibility or perturbation between membranes with different lipid compositions? Have you tested different types of lipid to see if there is a side of the membrane that is more easily penetrated by steroids?

Makriyannis: We tested our steroids on different lipid preparations and found some variations between the different lipids. However, there is a commonality in these interactions; for example, the steroids anchor at the bilayer interface in all of the lipid membrane preparations. We are now using small angle X-ray diffraction to find out whether the drugs have a preference for the inner or outer leaflet of the bilayer.

Simmonds: One might expect a number of different proteins in the membrane to be affected by this sort of perturbation. Would the structure–activity profile of a series of steroids be similar for each of those proteins, or would that profile depend on the nature of the protein?

Makriyannis: The structure–activity profile should depend on the structure of the protein and on its microenvironment. In fact, the effects of the same drug on different proteins are not always in the same direction. The same drug may increase the function of one protein and reduce that of another protein. The commonly held view is that if you increase the fluidity of the membrane you will increase the function of all membrane proteins, and that if the membrane lipids are in the gel phase, then the protein's function will be totally inhibited. Melchior (Carruthers & Melchior 1988) has shown that this is not always the case and that the effects of membrane phospholipid dynamics and phase properties on protein function can be different from those expected.

I think that such a model allows for a great degree of variability and diversity in the effects of drug molecules on the function of different membrane proteins.

Johnston: You proposed that there is hydrogen bonding between the 3α-hydroxyl group of the steroid and the carbonyl group of DPPC. Do you see any changes in phosphorus NMR?

Makriyannis: The phosphorus is quite far from the hydrogen-bonding site, so ^{31}P NMR may not provide this information. However, we looked for hydrogen bonding using high pressure infrared spectroscopy. In this method you pack the membrane very tightly and thus you accentuate the differences between drug molecules vis-à-vis the bilayer. You begin with a non-hydrated preparation and then gradually hydrate it and observe the changes. Generally, it is difficult to detect hydrogen bonding in the presence of water, and Fourier transform infrared spectroscopy is probably the best method for this purpose.

Johnston: Your choice of Δ^{16}-alphaxalone as a control strikes me as a bit odd, because the acidity of the C-20 carbonyl of alphaxalone and Δ^{16}-alphaxalone will be different, so the electronic properties of the C-20 regions of these molecules will also be different.

Makriyannis: What would the implication of that be?

Johnston: This part of the molecule will be more acidic in Δ^{16}-alphaxalone than it is in alphaxalone because Δ^{16}-alphaxalone has an α–β unsaturated ketone group, so you wouldn't expect it to penetrate as far in the membrane as alphaxalone, and that's in fact what you saw.

Makriyannis: I don't think the acidity has anything to do with the extent of penetration; I think penetration depends on the shape of the molecule.

Johnston: But the acidity is dictating the interaction. The acidity results from the delocalization over the flat unsaturated ketone system.

Makriyannis: We can argue about this. We don't know why Δ^{16}-alphaxalone doesn't incorporate as well as alphaxalone in the bilayer, but I don't think acidity is important. I think incorporation depends more on the degree of self-association of these molecules, and whether they would pack better with each other than with the lipids of the membrane.

Deliconstantinos: Is it possible to use fluidizing agents to cause a change from a *trans* conformation to a 'kink' (*cis*) conformation of the phospholipid?

Makriyannis: That is what happens when the anaesthetic steroids interact with the bilayer. What you call *cis* are generally referred to as *gauche* conformers in the bilayer chains. When the lipid is in the gel phase, all the methylene segments are in the *trans* conformation. In the liquid-crystalline phase some methylene segments acquire the *gauche* conformation and the chain shortens. Anaesthetic steroids increase the number of *gauche* segments in the chain and we think that this is one of the features of membrane perturbation. We can measure how many *trans*-to-*gauche* transformations occur using solid state NMR.

Deliconstantinos: Where does the energy for this conformational change come from? I can see such a change when I estimate membrane fluidity at different temperatures, but when you use anaesthetics or other compounds that increase fluidity, there must be an energy source for the conformational change. I don't myself believe that these conformational changes take place. The techniques available are not sufficiently sensitive to detect these changes. I believe changes in packing occur, however. Changes in the packing of the acyl chains of the phospholipid are sufficient to explain the membrane fluidity changes.

Makriyannis: To pack the steroid in the bilayer, you need to change some methylene segments to the *gauche* conformation. Phospholipids in the all-*trans* conformation will not pack tightly with the drug. You need to alter the chain conformations to optimize packing of the drug in the bilayer.

Deliconstantinos: Packing also refers to the lattice structure of the membrane. It is possible that steroids alter membrane fluidity by changing the lattice structure, rather than by inducing a change in conformation, which is energetically difficult to achieve.

Makriyannis: You are talking about the lateral expansion of the membrane. You can gain information about lateral expansion from small angle X-ray diffraction, and alphaxalone does not cause any observable lateral expansion.

References

Carruthers A, Melchior DL 1988 Effects of lipid environment on membrane transport: the human erythrocyte sugar transport protein/lipid bilayer system. Annu Rev Physiol 50:257–271

Narahashi T, Frazier DT 1971 Site of action and active form of local anesthetics. Neurosci Res 4:65–99

Richards CD, White AE 1981 Additive and non-additive effects of mixtures of short-acting intravenous anaesthetic agents and their significance for theories of anaesthesia. Br J Pharmacol 74:161–170

Effects of prostaglandin E_2 and progesterone on rat brain synaptosomal plasma membranes

George Deliconstantinos

Department of Experimental Physiology, University of Athens, Medical School, GR-115 27 Athens, Greece

Abstract. The lipid fluidity of rat brain synaptosomal plasma membranes (SPM) labelled with 1,6-diphenyl-1,3,5-hexatriene (DPH) was increased by prostaglandin E_2 (PGE$_2$) and decreased by progesterone, as indicated by steady-state fluorescence anisotropy $[(r_0/r)-1]^{-1}$. Arrhenius-type plots of $[(r_0/r)-1]^{-1}$ indicated a lipid phase separation of SPM at $\approx 23.5\,°C$ which was reduced to $\approx 18.1\,°C$ by PGE$_2$ and increased to $\approx 34.6\,°C$ by progesterone. Treatment of SPM by PGE$_2$ and progesterone caused an increase of the lipid phase separation to $\approx 32.4\,°C$. Arrhenius plots of Na$^+$/K$^+$-ATPase activity in control SPM exhibited a break point at $\approx 23.1\,°C$ which was reduced to $\approx 17.8\,°C$ by PGE$_2$ and increased to $\approx 32.6\,°C$ by progesterone. SPM treated with PGE$_2$ plus progesterone showed an increased break point at $\approx 29.3\,°C$. Na$^+$/K$^+$-ATPase activity was increased at a PGE$_2$ concentration range between 0.1 and 3 µM; higher concentrations (up to 10 µM) led to a gradual inhibition of enzyme activity. Progesterone (0.1–10 µM) and PGE$_2$ plus progesterone both produced a gradual decrease in enzyme activity. The allosteric inhibition of Na$^+$/K$^+$-ATPase by fluoride (F$^-$) (as reflected by changes in the Hill coefficient) was modulated by PGE$_2$ and progesterone. The perturbations of membrane lipid structure and changes in membrane fluidity provide a basis for suggesting an independent non-genomic mechanism for the progesterone-induced alterations in the effects of PGE$_2$ on brain function.

1990 Steroids and neuronal activity. Wiley, Chichester (Ciba Foundation Symposium 153) p 190–205

Major prostaglandins (PGs) that are synthesized by brain tissue include PGE$_2$, PGF$_{2\alpha}$, PGD$_2$ and PGI$_2$ (Brown et al 1984). PGs have been reported to be involved in the modulation of neurotransmitter release (Hedqvist 1976), thermo-regulation (Bernheim et al 1980), convulsive threshold (Kontos 1981) and cerebro-vascular tone (Wolfe & Mamer 1975). The microinjection of PGs into the hypothalamus can modulate the release of peptides from the hypothalamus, such as luteinizing hormone releasing hormone (LHRH) (Ojeda et al 1979). An inter-action of progesterone and β-oestradiol with the muscarinic cholinergic system in rat hypothalamus and adenohypophysis has been reported (Sokolovsky et al 1981). The existence of specific binding sites for sex steroids in well-characterized synaptic plasma membranes isolated from rat brain has also been described (Towle & Sze 1983, Kopeikina-Tsiboukidou & Deliconstantinos 1986). Progesterone is structurally similar to cholesterol; it has a planar configuration which permits its insertion into membranes. Progesterone can intercalate into a phospholipid bilayer containing cholesterol, modulating the phase properties of the membrane phospholipid bilayer (Carlson et al 1983), as well as leading to an alteration in the three-dimensional structure of membrane proteins; this disorganization evokes functional changes of membrane-bound enzymes (Alivisatos et al 1981, Deliconstantinos 1988).

Recently we described studies on the interaction between steroids (oestradiol, oestrone, progesterone) and PGs (PGE$_2$, PGF$_{2\alpha}$) in rat myometrial plasma membranes where we showed that both PGF$_{2\alpha}$ and PGE$_2$ caused an increase in membrane fluidity (Deliconstantinos & Fotiou 1986). The present studies were undertaken to explore the mechanisms responsible for the modulation of lipid dynamics and lipid–protein interactions in rat brain synaptosomal plasma membranes, induced by PGE$_2$ and progesterone, using as a functional parameter the activity of the integral membrane enzyme Na$^+$/K$^+$-ATPase. An attempt was made to determine whether progesterone and PGE$_2$ alter membrane fluidity, which would account for the functional changes evoked in the Na$^+$/K$^+$-ATPase.

Materials and methods

Synaptosomal plasma membranes (SPM) from rat brain were prepared as previously described (Papaphilis & Deliconstantinos 1980). Compared with the original homogenate from which they were prepared, they showed a 7–10-fold increase in Na$^+$/K$^+$-ATPase (EC 3.6.1.3) activity.

The Na$^+$/K$^+$-ATPase activity of SPM was assayed in an incubation medium consisting of Tris.HCl 30 mM, pH 7.4; MgCl$_2$ 5 mM; disodium ATP 3 mM; NaCl 80 mM; KCl 20 mM; ouabain 1 mM; and indomethacin 50 µM, with traces of [γ-^{32}P]ATP and 0.1 mg of SPM protein, in a final volume of 1.0 ml. Incubations were carried out at 37 °C for 15 min. The reaction was started by the addition of ATP and stopped by adding to the mixture an acidified suspension of activated charcoal (British Drug Houses Co.). The untreated [γ-^{32}P]ATP (which adsorbs to charcoal) was then removed by centrifugation in the presence of glycerol. Na$^+$/K$^+$-ATPase activity was defined as the difference in the ^{32}P$_i$ released from [γ-^{32}P]ATP during incubation in the presence and absence of ouabain. The ouabain-inhibitable component of ATPase activity is the activity that is lost when Na$^+$ or K$^+$ is omitted from the reaction mixture.

Arrhenius plots of the enzyme activity at temperatures of 5–40 °C at 3–4 °C intervals were analysed using a least-squares minimalization process to determine the break points. In every case, initial rates were determined under maximal velocity conditions and constant pH to preclude artifactual breaks in the slope. For the assay of the inhibition by F^- of the Na^+/K^+-ATPase, the reaction mixture contained increasing amounts of NaF, as indicated in Fig. 4 (p 197).

Steady-state fluorescence polarization of 1,6-diphenyl-1,3,5-hexatriene (DPH) was studied in an AMINCO SPF-500 spectrofluorometer as described by Shinitzky & Barenholz (1978). The polarization of fluorescence was expressed as the fluorescence anisotropy, r, and the anisotropy parameter $[(r_0/r)-1]^{-1}$ was calculated using a value of $r_0 = 0.365$ for DPH, as previously described (Deliconstantinos et al 1987). The fluorescence anisotropy was calculated according to the equation

$$r = I_{VV} - I_{VH}/I_{VV} + 2I_{VH}$$

where I_{VV} and I_{VH} are the intensities of the emitted light oriented, respectively, parallel and perpendicular to the plane of the exciting beam. Light-scattering corrections, estimated as previously described (Deliconstantinos et al 1989a), were always $<5\%$ of the total signal and did not differ significantly between various preparations. The anisotropy parameter varies directly with the apparent rotational relaxation time of the probe and thus inversely with the fluidity. The temperature dependence of $[(r_0/r)-1]^{-1}$ was determined over the range 5–40 °C. Membranes (approx. 50 μg) were warmed initially to 40 °C and the fluorescence polarization was estimated every 1–2 °C as the suspension cooled slowly to 5 °C. Plots of log $[(r_0/r)-1]^{-1}$ versus $1/T$ were constructed to detect membrane lipid phase separation temperatures, as previously described (Kopeikina-Tsiboukidou & Deliconstantinos 1989).

SPM were preincubated with various concentrations of PGE_2 and progesterone for 1 h at 25 °C in an incubation mixture of 20 mM Tris.HCl/20 mM KCl, pH 7.4 containing 50 μM indomethacin and 0.2 mg of SPM protein in a final volume of 1.5 ml under continuous magnetic stirring. Na^+/K^+-ATPase activity and steady-state fluorescence polarization were estimated in portions of the membranous suspension as described above.

Results and discussion

Studies of the mechanisms of action of PGE_2 and progesterone have given impetus to the investigation of PG and sex steroid interactions in the brain (Chiu & Richardson 1985). The major targets of their actions have been thought to be specific membrane receptors coupled to adenylate cyclase for PGE_2 (Malet et al 1982), and intracellular receptors which bind to specific regions of chromatin or DNA (or both) to effect changes in the rate of transcription of specific genes, for progesterone (Chan & O'Malley 1976). However, recent studies have suggested that the actions of PGs and steroids may be the result of their interactions with cell plasma membranes (Duval et al 1983, Manevich et al 1985, Deliconstantinos et al 1988).

The ability of PGE$_2$ and progesterone to interact with SPM isolated from rat brain, and to cause significant changes in Na$^+$/K$^+$-ATPase activity by altering the membrane fluidity, was investigated in the present study. Curves representing changes in Na$^+$/K$^+$-ATPase activity at different concentrations of PGE$_2$ and progesterone are illustrated in Fig. 1. A considerable increase in enzyme activity ($\approx 45\%$) appeared at approximately 1 μM PGE$_2$; higher concentrations of PGE$_2$, however, led to a progressive inhibition of the enzyme activity ($\approx 55\%$) with respect to the initial control value (SPM untreated with PGE$_2$). Treatment with progesterone gradually decreased Na$^+$/K$^+$-ATPase activity by about 70%. SPM treated with isomolar concentrations of PGE$_2$ plus progesterone showed a decrease in the enzyme activity throughout the range of concentrations used.

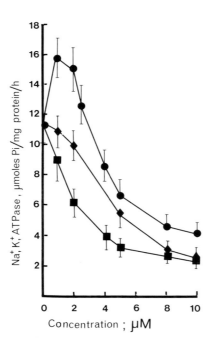

FIG. 1. Effect of prostaglandin E$_2$ (PGE$_2$) (●—●), progesterone (■—■) and isomolar concentrations of PGE$_2$ plus progesterone (◆—◆) on rat brain synaptosomal plasma membrane (SPM)-bound Na$^+$/K$^+$-ATPase activity. Aqueous solutions of the compounds were preincubated with SPM (0.2 mg/ml) in a medium consisting of 20 mM Tris.HCl/20 mM KCl, pH 7.4, plus 50 μM indomethacin, for 1 h at 25 °C. Enzyme activity was estimated as described in the Materials and Methods section. Values are means ± SD of three different experiments.

To investigate whether the effects of PGE_2 and progesterone on Na^+/K^+-ATPase activity are consistent with an effect on the physicochemical characteristics of the membrane, and to eliminate the possibility that these components interact directly with the protein molecules to cause an irreversible change in their activities, we removed PGE_2 and progesterone from the membranes by incubating SPM enriched with PGE_2 and progesterone with fatty acid-free serum albumin. The functional effects were fully reversible. Thus these compounds do not irreversibly change the Na^+/K^+-ATPase activity and their combined presence in the membrane causes a modulation of the enzyme activity. Because of the marked structural differences between PGE_2 and progesterone, the two compounds probably do not bind to the same specific sites on SPM, and the decreased activity of Na^+/K^+-ATPase in the presence of isomolar concentrations of PGE_2 and progesterone (Fig. 1) may therefore be mediated through changes in the membrane fluidity.

Membrane fluidity was measured by the steady-state fluorescence polarization method using 1,6-diphenyl-1,3,5-hexatriene (DPH) as a fluorophore. The fluorescence anisotropy of DPH or, more rigorously, the rotational relaxation time, indicates the mobility of the probe and thus reflects the ordering of the membrane core. The effects of temperature on the fluorescence anisotropy parameter, $[(r_0/r) - 1]^{-1}$, of DPH in SPM are illustrated by representative Arrhenius plots in Fig. 2. The increase in temperature produces a concomitant diminution in the $[(r_0/r) - 1]^{-1}$ values, which means an increase in membrane fluidity. However, the evolution of the fluidity was not linear; a thermotropic transition temperature was observed at $23.5 \pm 1.2\,°C$ in untreated SPM, which separates two domains where the increase in fluidity is directly proportional to the variation in temperature. Treatment of SPM with PGE_2 ($10\,\mu M$) produced a statistically significant ($P < 0.01$, Student's t-test) decrease in $[(r_0/r) - 1]^{-1}$ by comparison with untreated (control) SPM. It must be realized that the corresponding increase in fluidity is constant over the full range of temperatures studied. Furthermore, the thermotropic transition temperature was reduced to $18.1 \pm 1.1\,°C$. On the other hand, treatment of SPM with progesterone ($10\,\mu M$) produced a statistically significant ($P < 0.01$) increase in $[(r_0/r) - 1]^{-1}$ as compared to untreated (control) SPM, while the thermotropic transition temperature was elevated to $34.6 \pm 1.9\,°C$, which is consistent with a decrease in membrane fluidity. A considerable decrease in membrane fluidity was also observed in SPM treated with isomolar concentrations of PGE_2 ($10\,\mu M$) plus progesterone ($10\,\mu M$) as compared to untreated (control) SPM, with the thermotropic transition temperature increased to $32.4 \pm 1.6\,°C$.

The temperature dependence of SPM-bound Na^+/K^+-ATPase activity is shown in Fig. 3. Arrhenius plots revealed a transition temperature at $23.1 \pm 1.4\,°C$, which was reduced to $17.8 \pm 1.1\,°C$ in PGE_2 ($2\,\mu M$)-treated SPM and elevated to $32.6 \pm 1.9\,°C$ in progesterone ($2\,\mu M$)-treated SPM. An Arrhenius transition temperature at $29.3 \pm 1.7\,°C$ was observed in SPM treated with

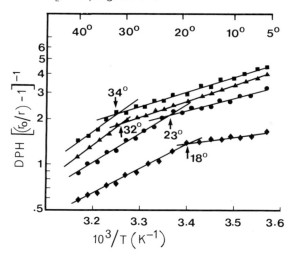

FIG. 2. Temperature dependence of the fluorescence anisotropy of 1,6-diphenyl-1,3,5-hexatriene (DPH) in control SPM (●—●) and in SPM treated with PGE₂ (10 µM) (♦—♦), progesterone (10 µM) (■ — ■), and PGE₂ (10 µM) plus progesterone (10 µM) (▲ — ▲). Experimental details are given in the text. The ordinate is the fluorescence anisotropy and the abscissa is a reciprocal of the absolute temperature. This experiment is representative of three that were performed. The straight lines were fitted by the method of least squares.

isomolar concentrations of PGE_2 (2 µM) plus progesterone (2 µM). What is particularly significant in this study is that the observed transition temperatures for Na^+/K^+-ATPase correspond closely to the thermotropic transitions of the lipid phase separations in Fig. 2. These results suggest that microscopic structural changes in the association between membrane-bound Na^+/K^+-ATPase and its associated lipids are induced by PGE_2 and progesterone.

Further evidence for modulations in SPM fluidity induced by PGE_2 and progesterone was obtained from their effects on the allosteric inhibition of Na^+/K^+-ATPase activity by fluoride (F^-). Figure 4 shows the curves obtained when the relative rates of enzymic activity were plotted against different concentrations of F^- in control SPM and in SPM preincubated with PGE_2 (10 µM), progesterone (10 µM), and isomolar concentrations of PGE_2 (10 µM) plus progesterone (10 µM). The Hill coefficient (slope) for the control SPM was 1.85 ± 0.12, indicating the presence of cooperativity. This value was increased to 2.31 ± 0.19 in SPM treated with progesterone (10 µM). In contrast, after treatment of SPM with PGE_2 the enzyme cooperativity was abolished ($h = 0.95 \pm 0.05$), whereas after treatment of SPM with isomolar concentrations of PGE_2 plus progesterone the enzyme cooperativity was reduced to 1.43 ± 0.09. These results suggest that PGE_2 causes an increase in the fluidity of the annular lipids around the Na^+/K^+-ATPase, while progesterone has an opposite effect.

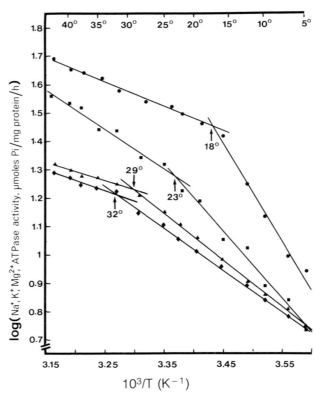

FIG. 3. Effect of temperature on the activity of SPM-bound Na^+/K^+-ATPase in control SPM ($\blacksquare$—$\blacksquare$) and in SPM treated with PGE_2 (2 μM) ($\bullet$—$\bullet$), progesterone (2 μM) ($\blacklozenge$—$\blacklozenge$), and PGE_2 (2 μM) plus progesterone (2 μM) ($\blacktriangle$—$\blacktriangle$). Each point represents the average value of duplicate determinations from a typical experiment which was repeated three times. The straight lines were fitted by the method of least squares.

However, after exposure of SPM to PGE_2 plus progesterone, it was observed that the rigidifying effects of progesterone prevailed.

The increased activity of Na^+/K^+-ATPase induced by low concentrations of PGE_2 (up to 3 μM) may be due to increased fluidity of the annular lipids, resulting in an increase in the conformational flexibility of the enzyme, achieved by a relief of the physical constraint imposed by the bilayer on the protein molecule. The decreased activity of the Na^+/K^+-ATPase, compared to the control value, in SPM treated with high concentrations of PGE_2 (up to 10 μM) is probably due to the fluidizing effects of PGE_2 on the bulk lipids of SPM, or to displacement of the annular lipids from around the enzyme molecules (Deliconstantinos et al 1989b). The decreased activity of Na^+/K^+-ATPase produced by progesterone is presumably due to the decreased fluidity either

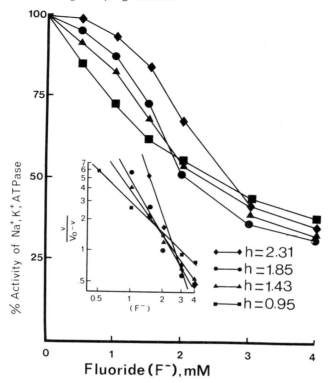

FIG. 4. Effect of fluoride (F^-) on the reaction rate of the SPM-bound Na^+/K^+-ATPase in control SPM ($\bullet$—$\bullet$) and in SPM treated with PGE₂ (10 μM) ($\blacksquare$ — $\blacksquare$), progesterone (10 μM) ($\blacklozenge$—$\blacklozenge$), and PGE₂ (10 μM) plus progesterone (10 μM) ($\blacktriangle$ — $\blacktriangle$). The insert shows Hill plots of the same data. The corresponding Hill coefficients (h) are as indicated. The correlation coefficients (r^2) for the straight lines in the insert are >0.95. V is the reaction velocity and V_0 is the rate of the reaction in the absence of F^-. Points in the curves drawn are mean values of duplicate determinations from a typical experiment which was repeated three times.

of the bulk membrane lipids or of the annular lipids (see Lee 1988) of the enzyme, induced by this hormone.

In addition to altering Na^+/K^+-ATPase activity, changes in membrane fluidity brought about by PGE₂ and/or progesterone may also affect the functioning of other integral enzymes in neuronal membranes. For instance, we have already shown that the correct interaction (coupling) of serotonergic receptors with the integral membrane enzyme adenylate cyclase may be affected by alterations in membrane fluidity (Papaphilis & Deliconstantinos 1980). Binding of PGE₂ to specific membrane receptors coupled to adenylate cyclase in the hypothalamus may be a necessary step for LHRH release (Ojeda et al 1979). Progesterone may inhibit the release of LHRH through a putative non-genomic mechanism, by inhibiting the effects of PGE_2 on the adenylate cyclase enzyme system in the hypothalamus.

Acknowledgements

The technical assistance of Vassiliki Villiotou and Christos Fasitsas is greatly appreciated. This work was supported by funds from the Medical School, University of Athens.

References

Alivisatos SGA, Deliconstantinos G, Theodosiadis G 1981 Specificity of binding of cholesterol, steroid hormones and other compounds in synaptosomal plasma membranes and their effects on ouabain sensitive ATPase. Biochim Biophys Acta 643:650–658

Bernheim HA, Gilbert TM, Stitt JT 1980 Prostaglandin E levels in third ventricular cerebrospinal fluid of rabbits during fever and changes in body temperature. J Physiol (Lond) 301:69–78

Brown ML, Marshall LA, Johnston PV 1984 Alterations in cerebral and microvascular prostaglandin synthesis by manipulation of dietary essential fatty acid. J Neurochem 43:1392–1400

Carlson JC, Gruber MY, Thompson JE 1983 A study of the interaction between progesterone and membrane lipids. Endocrinology 113:190–194

Chan L, O'Malley BW 1976 Mechanism of action of the sex steroid hormones (3 parts). N Engl J Med 294:1322–1430

Chiu EKY, Richardson JS 1985 Behavioral and neurochemical aspects of prostaglandins in brain function. Gen Pharmacol 16:163–175

Deliconstantinos G 1988 Structure activity relationship of cholesterol and steroid hormones with respect to their effects on Ca^{2+}-stimulated ATPase and lipid fluidity of synaptosomal plasma membranes from dog and rabbit brain. Comp Biochem Physiol 89B:585–594

Deliconstantinos G, Fotiou S 1986 Sex steroid and prostaglandin interactions upon the purified rat myometrial plasma membranes. Mol Cell Endocrinol 45:149–156

Deliconstantinos G, Kopeikina-Tsiboukidou L, Villiotou V 1987 Evaluation of membrane fluidity effects and enzyme activities alterations in adriamycin neurotoxicity. Biochem Pharmacol 36:1153–1161

Deliconstantinos G, Kopeikina-Tsiboukidou L, Ramantanis G 1988 Evoked effects of PGE_2 and PGA_2 on lipid fluidity and Ca^{2+}-stimulated ATPase of Walker-256 tumor microsomal membranes. Ann NY Acad Sci 551:245–248

Deliconstantinos G, Kopeikina-Tsiboukidou L, Villiotou V 1989a Evoked effects of cholesterol binding on integral proteins and lipid fluidity of dog brain synaptosomal plasma membranes. Biochem Cell Biol 67:16–24

Deliconstantinos G, Kopeikina-Tsiboukidou L, Ramantanis G 1989b PGE_2 and PGA_2 affect the allosteric properties and the activities of calmodulin-dependent guanylate cyclase and Ca^{2+}-stimulated ATPase of Walker-256 tumour microsomal membranes. Anticancer Res 9:753–760

Duval O, Durant S, Homo-Delarche F 1983 Non-genomic effects of steroids. Interaction of steroid molecules with membrane structures and functions. Biochim Biophys Acta 737:409–442

Hedqvist P 1976 Prostaglandin action on transmitter release at adrenergic neuroeffector junction. Adv Prostaglandin Thromboxane Res 1:357–363

Kontos HA 1981 Regulation of the cerebral circulation. Annu Rev Physiol 43:397–407

Kopeikina-Tsiboukidou L, Deliconstantinos G 1986 Calcium-induced membrane metabolic alterations modify the sex steroids binding to dog brain synaptosomal plasma membranes. Int J Biochem 18:774–784

Kopeikina-Tsiboukidou L, Deliconstantinos G 1989 Calmodulin selectively modulates the guanylate cyclase activity by repressing the lipid phase separation temperature in the inner half of the bilayer of rat brain synaptosomal plasma membranes. Neurochem Res 14:119–127

Lee A 1988 Annular lipids and the activity of the calcium-dependent ATPase. In: Aloia RC et al (eds) Advances in membrane fluidity. Alan R Liss, New York, vol 2:111–139

Malet C, Scherrer H, Saavedra JM, Dray F 1982 Specific binding of (^{3}H)prostaglandin E₂ to brain membranes and synaptosomes. Brain Res 236:227–233

Manevich EM, Lakin KM, Archakou AI et al 1985 Influence of cholesterol and prostaglandin E₁ on the molecular organization of phospholipids in the erythrocyte membrane. A fluorescent polarization study with lipid-specific probes. Biochim Biophys Acta 815:455–460

Ojeda SR, Negro-Vilar A, McCann M 1979 Release of prostaglandin E₂ by hypothalamic tissue: evidence of their involvement in catecholamine-induced luteinizing hormone-releasing hormone release. Endocrinology 104:617–624

Papaphilis A, Deliconstantinos G 1980 Modulation of serotonergic receptors by exogenous cholesterol in the dog brain synaptosomal plasma membrane. Biochem Pharmacol 29:3325–3327

Shinitzky M, Barenholz Y 1978 Fluidity parameters of lipid regions determined by fluorescence polarization. Biochim Biophys Acta 515:367–394

Sokolovsky M, Egozi Y, Avissar S 1981 Molecular regulation of receptors: interaction of β-estradiol and progesterone with the muscarinic system. Proc Natl Acad Sci USA 78:5554–5558

Towle AC, Sze PY 1983 Steroid binding to synaptic plasma membrane: differential binding of glucocorticoids and gonadal steroids. J Steroid Biochem 18:135–143

Wolfe LS, Mamer OA 1975 Measurement of prostaglandin F₂α levels in human cerebrospinal fluid in normal and pathological conditions. Prostaglandins 9:183–192

DISCUSSION

Kordon: Do you think that in for instance the protein kinase C dependent phosphorylation of cells, which markedly affects the binding of PGE₂, the methods you described could be used to determine the site where, or the manner in which, something is rigidified in the system?

Deliconstantinos: We know that when protein phosphorylation occurs via a protein kinase, there are changes in membrane fluidity (Mullin & McGinn 1987). We have seen this after applying epidermal growth factor (EGF) to synaptosomal plasma membranes of rat brain tissue (Deliconstantinos et al 1988). This growth factor, we believe, is able to increase the fluidity of the membrane through phosphorylation by protein kinases. There is now evidence for specific membrane receptors for PGE₁ and PGF₂α on the luteal cell surface, and these receptors are able to undergo endocytosis (Chegini et al 1984). We can therefore suggest that an increase in the activity of protein kinase by PGE_2 could increase the membrane fluidity, or, alternatively, that PGE_2 increases the protein kinase activity by increasing the membrane fluidity.

Kordon: You made the suggestion that GnRH (LHRH) may be down-regulated by progesterone by this mechanism. In fact, in a perfusion system similar to the one presented by Domingo Ramirez, in many instances you do not see a down-regulation of GnRH but a stimulation, so evidently the situation is not a simple one.

Deliconstantinos: I used isolated membranes, so I was unable to see receptor-mediated endocytosis; you need to use cells to observe that. With our membrane system we showed that progesterone increased the rigidity of the membrane lipid bilayer, which leads to an increased expression of 'silent' receptors, or 'cryptic' receptors, for PGE_2 (or perhaps we should say an increase in specific binding sites, rather than receptors); and this then results in an increased binding of PGE_2.

McEwen: You have demonstrated that the myometrial plasma membrane shows the opposite change in fluidity, namely an *increase in fluidity* with progesterone, whereas you found an increase in *rigidity* in synaptosomal membranes. Is anything known about the differences in the lipid composition of these membranes which could explain these different results?

Deliconstantinos: Fluidity depends on the lipid composition, and especially on the cholesterol content of the membrane. The ratio between cholesterol and phospholipid in rat brain synaptosomal plasma membranes is 0.7 in my preparation; it can vary between 0.6 and 0.75, depending on the age of the animals. But in myometrial plasma membranes this ratio is less than 0.4. The fluidity depends on the amount of cholesterol in the biomembranes. Progesterone behaves similarly to cholesterol; that is to say, progesterone decreases the membrane fluidity.

Baulieu: Can you manipulate the membrane system and introduce more cholesterol into the membrane?

Deliconstantinos: Yes. You can increase the ratio of cholesterol to phospholipids in biomembranes up to 2:1. You can prepare liposomes with a ratio of cholesterol to phospholipids of 2:1 and then enrich the membranes with cholesterol.

Baulieu: So, the percentage of cholesterol in relation to phospholipid is critical for fluidity. When you measure fluidity changes produced by progesterone or other steroids in liposomes, do you find that these changes correlate with the cholesterol content?

Deliconstantinos: Yes; we prepare liposomes using different concentrations of cholesterol and phospholipid and when we incorporate progesterone or prostaglandins we observe changes in fluidity of the liposomes which correlate with the ratio of cholesterol to phospholipid. The changes in the fluidity of the liposomes, estimated by fluorescence polarization of the DPH, depend on the cholesterol content of the liposomes, and the effects of progesterone and PGE$_2$ are more marked at higher cholesterol concentrations.

Simmonds: Would such increases in fluidity in neuronal membranes explain the enhanced spread of oxytocin receptors that Bruce McEwen described in the ventromedial nucleus of the hypothalamus after the addition of progesterone? It may depend on whether those oxytocin receptors are already inserted in the neuronal plasma membrane and are simply spreading out, or whether they are spreading via an intradendritic transport system, from which they are subsequently inserted into the plasma membrane.

Deliconstantinos: Yes, and I think that both these systems work in parallel. I believe the increase in the apparent number of oxytocin receptors in the uterus in the presence of progesterone is produced both by the synthesis of receptor mRNA, and by the appearance of previously cryptic oxytocin receptors as a result of an increase in membrane fluidity.

Glowinski: There is now evidence that arachidonic acid or its metabolites may influence several aspects of neurotransmission processes. This includes the sensitivity of some receptors localized on astrocytes or on neurons and also the reuptake processes for glutamate on astrocytes or neurons (Barbour et al 1989). Indeed, you observed a similarity between the effects of progesterone and those of metabolites of arachidonic acid (such as PGE$_2$). This is a nice idea, but you have to take into consideration the fact that prostaglandins are synthesized in astrocytes but not in neurons. Therefore, if one is working on neurons in culture without astrocytes, arachidonic acid can be formed through the activation of phospholipase A$_2$ but cannot be metabolized into prostaglandins. In addition, when you are looking at responses mediated by steroid compounds you may have to do parallel experiments to determine if, when phospholipase A$_2$ activity is blocked by mepacrine or glucocorticoids to prevent the formation of arachidonic acid, the steroid still acts—for instance, changing the response mediated by GABA receptors. Therefore I would like to know if experiments have been done to determine if steroids have very rapid effects on the formation of arachidonic acid and its metabolites. I would also like to hear information on the persistence (or not) of the effects of steroid hormones on the different models discussed during this meeting, after inhibition of the formation of arachidonic acid by inhibitors of phospholipase A$_2$.

Majewska: I have done experiments in which the phospholipase A$_2$ inhibitor mepacrine was tested for effects on GABA$_A$ receptors. I found that mepacrine, which is quite lipophilic and binds strongly to membranes, itself decreases muscimol binding to the receptors. I also found that unsaturated fatty acids (one type of product of phospholipase A$_2$ activity) decrease muscimol binding to the receptor, whereas saturated fatty acids increase the binding. It is unlikely that steroid-mediated effects on the GABA$_A$ receptor are mediated via activation of phospholipase A$_2$, because many of these effects are observed in incubation media lacking calcium, which is essential for the activity of this enzyme.

Deliconstantinos: When we increase the rigidity of the lipid bilayer of the membrane with rigidifying agents we find a decrease in the activity of phospholipase A_2 (Kannagi & Koizumi 1979). This means that we have decreased the rate of release of arachidonic acid, which means a decrease in the production of prostaglandins (Irvine 1982). We have shown that prostaglandins are scavengers of free radicals. We believe that one reason that progesterone increases membrane rigidity is that it acts like cholesterol, becoming incorporated between the phospholipid molecules in lipid membranes. We think the resulting increased rigidity inhibits the production of prostaglandins, which will lead to reduced scavenging of free radicals, which could result in a further increase in the rigidity of the membrane.

Glowinski: Phospholipase A_2 is activated by calcium, so there might be an interaction with the steroid at this point.

Deliconstantinos: There is a phospholipase A_2 which is calcium dependent, and another phospholipase that is Ca^{2+} independent (Wong & Cheung 1979, Burch et al 1986).

Glowinski: Perhaps the calcium sensitivity of the enzyme is changed by the steroid hormone (progesterone). Alternatively, the steroid hormone acts on lipocortin metabolism, since lipocortins regulate the activity of phospholipase A_2.

McEwen: Lipocortin is a glucocorticoid-inducible inhibitor of phospholipase A_2 that has been identified at least in macrophages. There is some question whether it exists in the brain.

Deliconstantinos: When I use calcium in these experiments, I use calcium as a rigidifying agent, to show that in the presence of a lipid bilayer there is an increase in the binding of steroids, or of prostaglandins, and to show that by changing the membrane fluidity there are more receptors for progesterone and PGE_2 in the surface of the membrane. I did not use calcium to induce changes in phospholipase A_2.

Kordon: In answer to Jacques Glowinski's question, we have blocked the arachidonic acid cascade in pituitary cells not with mepacrine, because of its side-effects, but with eicosatetraynoic acid (ETYA), a non-hydrolysable analogue of arachidonic acid. We then checked hormone release from dispersed rat pituitary cells in the presence or absence of steroid. We never saw an effect of ETYA on any of those parameters (Bihoreau et al 1990). Hence, the hypothesis that sensitivity of pituitary cells towards neurotransmitters or steroids could be regulated by arachidonic acid metabolites could not be confirmed, in our hands.

Hall: On the question of phospholipase A_2 inhibition, the 21-aminosteroids, which lack glucocorticoid activity (Braughler et al 1988), inhibit the release of arachidonic acid from cultured pituitary cells that is stimulated by the induction of lipid peroxidation or by treatment with iodoacetate, but they do not inhibit phospholipase A_2 activity in platelets.

Ramirez: Dr Sergio Ojeda, a former student of mine from Chile, showed that oestrogen injected systemically stimulates the production of prostaglandin E$_2$ in the pubertal rat hypothalamus (Ojeda & Campbell 1982). He measured several types of prostaglandin and one specific type was increased by oestrogen, namely PGE$_2$.

In our superfusion system, in which we have a preparation of hypothalamus from an ovariectomized rat treated with oestrogen, progesterone is a powerful releaser of LHRH (see my paper). This effect can be blocked by indomethacin, which is an inhibitor of prostaglandin synthesis. We have also shown that progesterone releases PGE$_2$ from this hypothalamic preparation. So, there is clearly some interaction between steroid and prostaglandin here.

However, in binding studies we always have to be very careful to distinguish non-specific from specific binding of any ligand. In your experiments, Professor Deliconstantinos, you are dealing with a very different concept, namely total binding of ^{3}H-labelled PGE$_2$ without considering non-specific binding. Do I have to take home the idea that total binding is the important element that we have to consider in the analysis of binding data, or must we still be careful about the distinction between specific and non-specific binding? These are operational definitions, I admit, but if I were to use tritiated progesterone to detect steroid binding to membranes in the central nervous system, and I wanted to use the classical operational definition of specific versus non-specific, it would be impossible to do these experiments, because ^{3}H-labelled progesterone shows high non-specific binding.

Deliconstantinos: Some studies deal with specific binding of a ligand. When the idea is to show this specific binding, people incubate membranes and a small amount of ligand, only a few nanomoles, and they see specific binding at the picomolar level. But when they want to see functional changes, they add ligand by the spoonful, as it were, because you cannot see functional effects with a few picomoles of progesterone. The functional changes observed in the present study are specific effects and the total binding, which I showed, is the binding in nanomoles which is able to cause functional changes; these are clearly specific changes, because they are time and concentration dependent.

Baulieu: We showed that GnRH neurons do not have intracellular progesterone receptors (Sterling et al 1984). Surrounding the GnRH-synthesizing neurons are progesterone receptor-containing neurons, demonstrable by immunological double-labelling, because the progesterone receptor is nuclear and GnRH is found in the cytoplasm. So when speculating about the release of GnRH and the mechanism of action of progesterone, we must remember that there is cellular heterogeneity and should not rely only on studies of brain homogenates.

Joubert-Bression: Did you notice any variation in the number of PGE$_2$ receptors when working in the physiological range of progesterone concentrations, namely 10^{-8} M? If you studied this during the physiological cycle (the oestrous cycle), you might be able to see changes in the number of PGE_2 binding sites.

Deliconstantinos: We can estimate progesterone concentrations in the blood, but we do not actually know the amount of progesterone within the membranes—for instance, in the myometrial membranes of the uterus. We know that steroids accumulate in membranes, so we have to ask what is a physiological concentration; it may be 10^{-8} M in the blood, but we don't know the concentration in the membranes. It could be much higher as a result of accumulation in membranes. There could be an increased concentration in the blood, but the same amount of progesterone or oestrogen in the membranes as before, because the membrane can retain steroid.

Joubert-Bression: The answer is to look during the oestrous cycle. If you found changes in the receptor number at the time of the progesterone peak, this might have physiological relevance.

Deliconstantinos: Yes, or if there are changes in the activity of the receptors, due to alterations of the membrane lipid bilayer fluidity.

Majewska: Some effects of steroids on, for example, GABA receptors are observed very quickly, in a fraction of a second. Can the interaction of a steroid with lipid in the neuronal plasma membrane explain phenomena which occur so rapidly? Can fluidity changes have such very rapid effects?

Deliconstantinos: Yes. We believe that the first key event is the change in membrane fluidity, which alters the microenvironment of the receptor immediately after the ligand binds. For example, when a muscarinic acetylcholine receptor interacts with a steroid, the direct initial event is, in our view, the change in fluidity of the annular lipids (Lee 1988) of that muscarinic receptor.

Kordon: I am not quite ready to take home the concept of total binding, as Domingo said, but this concept may have some value for a few ligands which may stick to the membrane in a relatively non-specific, receptor-independent manner and have biophysical effects on that membrane. Those may not necessarily be physiological ligands, but we should be aware of the possibility when we work with such ligands.

References

Barbour B, Szatkowski M, Ingledew N, Altwell D 1989 Arachidonic acid induces a prolonged inhibition of glutamate uptake into glial cells. Nature (Lond) 342:918–920

Bihoreau C, Rasolonjanahary R, Gerozissis K, Clauser H, Kordon C 1990 Arachidonate metabolism in the anterior pituitary: effect of arachidonate inhibitions on basal or stimulated secretion of PRL, GH and LH. II. Hormone release from dispersed pituitary cells. J Neuroendocrinol, in press

Braughler JM, Chase RL, Neff GL et al 1988 A new 21-aminosteroid antioxidant lacking glucocorticoid activity stimulates ACTH secretion and blocks arachidonic acid release from mouse pituitary tumor (A + T-20) cells. J Pharmacol Exp Ther 244:423–427

Burch RM, Luini A, Axelrod J 1986 Phospholipase A$_2$ and phospholipase C are activated by distinct GTP-binding proteins in response to α_1-adrenergic stimulation in FRTL 5 thyroid cells. Proc Natl Acad Sci USA 83:7201–7205

Chegini N, Rao CV, Cobbs G 1984 A quantitative electron microscope autoradiograph study on [^{3}H]PGE$_1$ and F$_{2\alpha}$ internalization in bovine luteal slices. Mol Cell Endocrinol 38:117–129

Deliconstantinos G, Kopeikina L, Villiotou V, Hadjiminas J 1988 Receptor-mediated changes of the membrane fluidity induced by EGF in rat brain synaptosomal plasma membranes. Advanced Study Institute. Vascular endothelium: receptor and transduction mechanism. Porto Carras, Neos Marmaras, Halkidiki, Greece, June 18–29

Irvine RF 1982 How is the level of free arachidonic acid controlled in mammalian cells? Biochem J 204:3–16

Kannagi R, Koizumi K 1979 Effect of different physical states of phospholipid substrates on partially purified platelet phospholipase A$_2$ activity. Biochim Biophys Acta 556:423–433

Lee A 1988 Annular lipids and the activity of the calcium-dependent ATPase. In: Aloia RC et al (eds) Advances in membrane fluidity. Alan R Liss, New York, vol 2:111–139

Mullin JM, McGinn MT 1987 The phorbol ester, TPA, increases transepithelial epidermal growth factor flux. FEBS (Fed Eur Biochem Soc) Lett 221:359–364

Ojeda SR, Campbell WB 1982 An increase in hypothalamic capacity to synthesize PGE$_2$ precedes the first preovulatory surge of gonadotropins. Endocrinology 111:1031–1037

Sterling RJ, Gasc JM, Sharp PJ, Tuohimaa P, Baulieu EE 1984 Absence of nuclear progesterone receptor in LH releasing hormone neurones in laying hens. J Endocrinol 102:R5–R7

Wong PYK, Cheung WY 1979 Calmodulin stimulates human platelet phospholipase A$_2$. Biochem Biophys Res Commun 90:473–480

Steroids and neuronal destruction or stabilization

Edward D. Hall

Central Nervous System Diseases Research Unit, The Upjohn Company, Kalamazoo, MI 49001, USA

Abstract. Extensive work has indicated that glucocorticoid steroids may play a role in promoting age-related central neuronal degeneration. It has also been shown that glucocorticoid supplementation may intensify acute post-ischaemic neuronal necrosis and that prior adrenalectomy is protective. A glucocorticoid inhibition of injury-induced axonal reactive sprouting has also been reported. The mechanism of this deleterious effect on chronic or acute neuronal degeneration and regenerative responses is thought to involve specific glucocorticoid receptors either on susceptible nerve cells or on adjacent glial cells. However, other studies have shown that intensive short-term glucocorticoid treatment may attenuate post-traumatic and post-ischaemic central neuronal damage. Anterograde degeneration of motor nerve fibres can also be retarded by intensive glucocorticoid pretreatment. The mechanism of these high dose protective effects appears to involve an intrinsic ability of certain glucocorticoids to inhibit oxygen free radical-induced lipid peroxidation, a phenomenon that may be fundamentally involved in neuronal degeneration. Recently, steroid analogues which lack glucocorticoid receptor affinity have been shown to duplicate the antioxidant and cerebroprotective actions of the glucocorticoids in models of neuronal damage. Thus, the deleterious and protective effects of steroids on neuronal viability depend on two different mechanisms, separable by dose, duration of treatment, specific situation and chemical structure.

1990 Steroids and neuronal activity. Wiley, Chichester (Ciba Foundation Symposium 153) p 206–219

Deleterious effects of glucocorticoid steroids on neuronal survival

Role of glucocorticoid steroids in age-related neuronal degeneration

The first suggestion that glucocorticoid steroids might have deleterious effects on neuronal survival came from the work of Landfield and colleagues (1978) who showed in rats a significant positive correlation between progressive age-related neuronal loss in the hippocampus and elevations in plasma corticosterone concentration. They went on to show that adrenalectomy forestalled the loss of hippocampal neurons (Landfield et al 1981). These findings were replicated by Sapolsky et al (1985) who postulated that cumulative glucocorticoid exposure over the lifespan may enhance age-dependent loss of central neurons (at least in the hippocampus) and that prolonged stress, by further elevating steroid levels, could accelerate brain ageing.

Sapolsky and coworkers have shown that corticosterone can exacerbate the hippocampal neurodegenerative effects of either the ATP depleting agent 3-acetylpyridine or the excitotoxin kainic acid, whereas adrenalectomy affords partial protection (Sapolsky 1985).

Two potential explanations for the hippocampal toxicity of glucocorticoid steroids have been put forward, both of which centre on a glucocorticoid receptor mechanism. Indeed, the selective vulnerablity of the hippocampus is probably due to the high concentration of glucocorticoid receptors in that brain region (McEwen et al 1969). The first proposed mechanism, suggested by Sapolsky, relates to his finding that corticosterone can impair glucose utilization by hippocampal neurons. Administration of the sugar mannose, whose uptake by hippocampal neurons is not impaired by glucocorticoids, results in protection of hippocampal neurons against the exacerbation of kainic acid toxicity by corticosterone (Sapolsky 1986). The second mechanism for glucocorticoid neurotoxicity, advanced by Landfield's group, is based on the recent elegant electrophysiological evidence that corticosterone acts to increase intracellular calcium levels in hippocampal pyramidal neurons (Kerr et al 1989). They found that in hippocampal slices from adrenalectomized rats the calcium-dependent afterhyperpolarization of pyramidal neurons is reduced in comparison to that observed in normal rats. Also, the calcium action potential amplitude and duration are lower than normal in adrenalectomized animals. Consistent with this possible modulatory effect of glucocorticoids on neuronal calcium conductance is our finding that treatment of cats with the glucocorticoid methylprednisolone for one week increases the amplitude of the calcium-based afterdepolarization in spinal motor neurons (Hall 1982). Furthermore, similar glucocorticoid treatment increases the post-tetanic repetitive discharge of motor nerve terminals, a phenomenon also related to inward calcium fluxes (Riker et al 1975). Thus, there is ample evidence that glucocorticoids can augment stimulation-induced inward calcium movement. In view of the well-known cytotoxic effects of elevated intracellular free calcium levels, the continuous presence of glucocorticoids could promote neuronal ageing by this mechanism, as well as by an impairment of glucose metabolism. If both mechanisms are mediated via glucocorticoid receptors, it follows that the hippocampus, with its high concentration of glucocorticoid receptors, would show the greatest sensitivity to glucocorticoid neurotoxicity of the different brain regions.

Glucocorticoid exacerbation of ischaemic neuronal damage

In addition to a possible role in age-related neuronal damage, glucocorticoids have been shown to worsen acute post-ischaemic neuronal necrosis. Sapolsky

& Pulsinelli (1985), using a rat model of temporary global ischaemia, have shown that prior adrenalectomy reduces post-ischaemic neuronal damage in cerebral cortex, striatum and all regions of the hippocampus by comparison with intact animals, whereas corticosterone supplementation enhances neuronal necrosis. Similarly, we have observed that acute high dose treatment with methyl-prednisolone increases post-ischaemic loss of hippocampal CA1 cells in a gerbil model of global ischaemia (E. D. Hall & K. E. Pazara, unpublished results). Yet, a glucocorticoid worsening of brain damage subsequent to global ischaemia may not be generalizable to models of focal brain ischaemia. Braughler & Lainer (1986) have reported that high doses of methylprednisolone can improve the survival of gerbils subjected to a severe focal ischaemic insult. This effect is correlated with an improved neuronal survival in cortex, but not hippocampus (E. D. Hall & K. E. Pazara, unpublished results).

Sapolsky & Pulsinelli (1985) have speculated on several possible explanations for the detrimental action of glucocorticoids on global ischaemia-induced neuronal necrosis. One which they have tended to dismiss prematurely has to do with the potential for glucocorticoid steroids to increase plasma glucose levels, leading to an exacerbation of ischaemic brain lactic acidosis. Several reports have now shown that elevated levels of plasma glucose enhance ischaemic brain damage. A footnote in the paper of Sapolsky & Pulsinelli (1985) shows that the plasma glucose levels in their corticosterone-supplemented rats were double those in the adrenalectomized animals. In support of this view, another group has shown definitively that chronic pretreatment of rats with the potent glucocorticoid dexamethasone aggravates post-ischaemic brain damage by inducing hyperglycaemia (Koide et al 1985). The finding by Sapolsky & Pulsinelli (1985) that the worsening of ischaemic brain damage by glucocorticoids does not correlate with the density of glucocorticoid receptors in different brain regions is consistent with a mechanism that is independent of brain steroid receptors.

Glucocorticoid impairment of lesion-induced axonal sprouting and synaptogenesis

An additional deleterious effect of glucocorticoids on the nervous system has been documented. Scheff & Cotman (1982) have shown that corticosterone treatment of rats significantly impairs axonal sprouting and synaptogenesis in the hippocampus after lesions of the entorhinal cortex. Astrocytes appear to hypertrophy in lesioned and glucocorticoid-treated rats. For this reason, these investigators suggest that sustained treatment (as against acute treatment) of neural injury (see below) with glucocorticoids can potentially impair recovery. The mechanism of this effect is unknown, but in view of its occurrence with modest glucocorticoid doses, a receptor-mediated action is suggested.

Beneficial effects of glucocorticoids on neuronal survival

Glucocorticoid steroids in acute central nervous system injury

Perhaps surprising, in view of the deleterious effects of glucocorticoid steroids on neuronal survival in some situations, as already discussed, is the fact that they have been used extensively in the clinical treatment of acute central nervous system trauma, of both spinal cord and brain. The rationale for their use has mainly centred on the expectation that they will reduce post-traumatic spinal cord and cerebral oedema. This is based on the remarkable reduction of peritumoral brain oedema. However, the efficacy of steroids in promoting neurological recovery after CNS injury has been disappointing at best. Many clinicians have concluded that the conventional use of steroids in the acute management of spinal trauma is not beneficial and is fraught with potentially serious side-effects beyond the issues set out here.

Nevertheless, several years ago, we embarked on a pharmacological analysis of the acute effects of high doses of the potent glucocorticoid methylprednisolone (MP) in experimental models of acute CNS injury. Careful attention was paid to possible therapeutic mechanisms beyond oedema reduction and to the dose–response and time–action characteristics which MP would show if it acted via those mechanisms. We have focused our attention mainly on the premise of Demopoulos et al (1972) that the principal molecular basis for post-traumatic neuronal degeneration is lipid peroxidation induced by oxygen free radicals and that proper application of steroids might inhibit this degenerative process.

In an initial study we showed that pretreatment of cats with a single large intravenous dose of MP (sodium succinate salt) served to protect homogenates of uninjured spinal cord, removed one hour after steroid administration, from *in vitro* lipid peroxidation (Hall & Braughler 1981). It was striking to observe that a very large, non-physiological dose of 30 mg/kg was needed for this antioxidant effect, pretreatment with lower doses being ineffective. In a parallel study in which we followed spinal tissue levels of MP resulting from a single large dose over time, the time-course of the lipid 'antioxidant' effect followed the tissue pharmacokinetics closely, indicative of a non-classical mechanism of steroid action (Braughler & Hall 1982). In other words, the steroid has to be present in the spinal tissue in a critical concentration in order for the protection against lipid peroxidation to occur. More recently, MP has been shown to inhibit peroxidation in rat brain synaptosomal membranes directly when present in a 100 μM concentration (Braughler 1985), a level consistent with the peak spinal tissue levels after a 30 mg/kg i.v. dose. Interestingly, the antioxidant potency of different glucocorticoids *in vitro* does not correlate well with their known glucocorticoid potencies. For example, prednisolone, which is only slightly less potent than MP as a glucocorticoid, is only half as potent as a lipid antioxidant.

Hydrocortisone (cortisol), which is the prototypical glucocorticoid, does not inhibit lipid peroxidation, even at very high concentrations.

After the earlier pilot experiments, we and others have shown that a 30 mg/kg dose of MP, given intravenously to pentobarbitone-anaesthetized cats soon after blunt spinal cord injury, can also attenuate post-traumatic lipid peroxidation, as measured by various biochemical indices (see review by Hall & Braughler 1987). In addition to the demonstration of the ability of high doses of MP to inhibit lipid peroxidation *in vitro* and *in vivo*, work in our laboratories and others indicates that a 30 mg/kg i.v. dose of MP can exert several protective actions on the injured spinal cord that no doubt contribute to an attenuation of post-traumatic neuronal degeneration. Many of these, we believe, are secondarily related to inhibition of lipid peroxidation. The list includes the support of energy metabolism, prevention of the development of progressive post-traumatic ischaemia, the reversal of intracellular calcium accumulation, prevention of neurofilament degradation, and inhibition of the formation of vasoactive prostaglandin $F_{2\alpha}$ and thromboxane A_2. Probably related to these beneficial biochemical and physiological actions is the enhancement of the acute recovery of somatosensory evoked potentials. An additional effect of glucocorticoids that may help to augment neurophysiological recovery concerns an increase in spinal neuronal excitability (Hall 1982). The dose–response and time–action characteristics of these beneficial actions are inconsistent with a glucocorticoid receptor mechanism.

On the basis of these findings we have used cats subjected to a moderately severe lumbar spinal cord compression injury to test a dosing regimen involving an initial administration of a 30 mg/kg i.v. bolus, 30 minutes after injury, followed with individual 15 mg/kg i.v. doses, two and six hours later, and then a continuous i.v. infusion of 2.5 mg/kg per hour for the remainder of the first 48 hours after injury. The cats were evaluated by observers unaware of their experimental treatment weekly for four weeks, for walking, running and stair-climbing ability. They were then killed for histological analysis of the spinal injury site. In comparison to cats treated with vehicle after injury, the MP-treated cats have shown significantly higher recovery scores, beginning at two weeks after injury. In addition, a reduction in post-traumatic spinal tissue loss is observed, the degree of which is inversely correlated with the neurological recovery score ($r = -0.88$) (Braughler et al 1987). These studies prove that a glucocorticoid dosing regimen designed to inhibit post-traumatic lipid peroxidation is associated with both enhanced tissue preservation and functional recovery.

Similarly, MP has been shown to enhance the early recovery of mice subjected to a moderately severe concussive head injury (Hall 1985). As with spinal cord injury in cats, the optimal i.v. dose is 30 mg/kg, with smaller and larger doses showing less activity. With a more severe injury, the optimum dose in mice is 60 mg/kg (Hall et al 1987). Such a shift in potency as a function of injury severity is to be expected for a mechanism of action that does not operate via glucocorticoid receptors.

Duplication of cerebroprotective effects of glucocorticoids with a non-glucocorticoid steroid

From the atypical pharmacological characteristics of MP's effects on the injured spinal cord and brain, we postulated that the cerebroprotective action is based upon inhibition of lipid peroxidation and related pathophysiological events and is not glucocorticoid receptor-mediated, as outlined above. We further reasoned that it ought to be possible to design a steroid analogue of MP that would lack the glucocorticoid receptor-based actions while retaining the ability to inhibit lipid peroxidation and protect the injured nervous system. If this were successful, a new class of antioxidant steroids could be developed without the potential for glucocorticoid receptor-mediated side-effects (such as diabetic problems, immunosuppression and infection, impaired wound-healing, gastric ulceration and negative nitrogen balance).

To test this hypothesis we have prepared several MP analogues that lack the 11β-hydroxyl functional group that is essential for glucocorticoid receptor binding. Most of these non-glucocorticoid steroids are either Δ-9,11 or 11α substituted compounds. They have been screened for their ability to inhibit CNS tissue lipid peroxidation (that is, for ability to protect [^{14}C]GABA uptake by rat brain synaptosomes from xanthine/xanthine oxidase-induced peroxidative impairment, superoxide-mediated). The more active compounds in the series are then secondarily screened in a mouse model of severe head injury for the promotion of early neurological recovery (Hall 1985).

The most impressive compound in these assays has been U72099E (17, 21-dihydroxyl-11α-t-butylacetoxy-1,4-pregnadiene-3,20-dione-21-hemisuccinate). It is devoid of glucocorticoid activity, as defined by its inability to inhibit weight gain or to cause thymic involution in mice treated intraperitoneally with up to 100 mg/kg per day for four days. In comparison, a 30 mg/kg dose of MP for the same period causes a complete suppression of weight gain and a 43.5% reduction in thymus weight. Also, U72099E, at concentrations as high as 10^{-5} M, fails to suppress adrenocorticotropin (ACTH) secretion in cultured mouse AtT-20 pituitary cells, whereas MP causes a marked suppression at much lower concentrations.

However, despite its essentially complete lack of these glucocorticoid receptor-mediated activities, U72099E is equally effective as, yet more potent than, MP at protecting rat brain synaptosomes from peroxidation-induced inhibition of synaptosomal [^{14}C]GABA uptake. The optimal in vitro antioxidant concentration is 30 µM for U72099E, compared to 100 µM for MP. A similar enhancement of in vivo cerebroprotective potency has been observed in the severely head-injured mice. Whereas MP, given in a single i.v. dose immediately after concussive head injury, improves the neurological status one hour after trauma (the grip test score) in a dose-related manner, a 60 mg/kg dose is required for a significant effect. On the other hand, U72099E produces a significant enhancement of early recovery at 30 mg/kg (Hall et al 1987). Thus, an excellent correlation between the *in vitro* lipid antioxidant activity and *in vivo* cerebroprotective efficacy and potency for MP and U72099E has been demonstrated, confirming the hypothesis that a non-glucocorticoid steroid could duplicate the protective efficacy of MP in models of neuronal membrane damage and acute CNS injury.

Glucocorticoid preservation of motor nerve function during early degeneration

We have also shown that intensive glucocorticoid pretreatment can retard the post-traumatic degeneration of peripheral motor nerve fibres. Surgical transection of cat hindlimb motor axons at the level of the greater sciatic foramen, followed 48 hours later by an assessment of neuromuscular function in the *in vivo* soleus nerve muscle preparation, has been shown to provide a reproducible model for the study of the early phases of anterograde neuronal degeneration. In this model, the 48 hour degenerating distal motor axons, and the nerve terminals in particular, display subtle defects in neuromuscular transmission and excitability that can be readily quantified by functional neuromuscular testing.

This model has been used to show that seven days of pretreatment (8 mg/kg i.m. daily) with either of the glucocorticoids triamcinolone (Hall et al 1983) or methylprednisolone (Hall & Wolf 1984) can significantly preserve the ability of the degenerating soleus nerve terminals to transmit single and repetitive impulses. Studies in rats in another laboratory have shown a similar preservation of phrenic motor nerve terminal structure and function during early degeneration of triamcinolone pretreatment (Drakontides 1982).

After the subsequent discovery of the intrinsic lipid antioxidant properties of at least some glucocorticoids (Hall & Braughler 1981, Braughler 1985), we decided to investigate whether pretreatment with a *bona fide* antioxidant could similarly retard the anterograde degeneration process. As predicted, we found that a five-day dosing regimen with a combination of the lipid peroxidation inhibitor D-α-tocopherol (200 I.U. orally per day) and selenium (50 µg orally per day; a co-factor for the lipid hydroperoxide-scavenging enzyme glutathione peroxidase) attenuated 48 hour degeneration of cat soleus motor axons even more effectively than the glucocorticoid steroids (Hall 1987). This demonstration strongly implies that lipid peroxidation may be a fundamental mechanism of anterograde degeneration and that the glucocorticoid steroids are probably effective in this context, as they are in the context of acute CNS injury, by acting as lipid antioxidants.

Summary

In summary, glucocorticoids appear to have complicated effects on neuronal survival in relation to ageing or injury. In the context of ageing, endogenous glucocorticoids may play an important role in age-related neuronal degeneration, probably via a glucocorticoid receptor mechanism that triggers impaired glucose utilization and/or increased intracellular free calcium concentrations. In contrast, in acute neuronal injury or ischaemia, pharmacological glucocorticoid administration may be either deleterious or protective. The deleterious action is probably dependent in part on peripheral glucocorticoid receptor mechanisms that require further definition. On the other hand, the basis for the protective action is clearly independent of glucocorticoid receptors and involves instead an inhibition of oxygen free radical lipid peroxidation after injury.

References

Braughler JM 1985 Lipid peroxidation-induced inhibition of gamma aminobutyric acid uptake by rat brain synaptosomes: protection by glucocorticoids. J Neurochem 44:1282–1288

Braughler JM, Hall ED 1982 Correlation of methylprednisolone levels in cat spinal cord with its effects on spinal lipid peroxidation, ($Na^+ + K^+$)-ATPase activity and motor neuron function. J Neurosurg 56:838–844

Braughler JM, Lainer MJ 1986 The effects of large doses of methylprednisolone on neurological recovery and survival in a gerbil stroke model. Cent Nerv Syst Trauma 3:153–162

Braughler JM, Hall ED, Means ED, Anderson DK 1987 Evaluation of an intensive CNS injury dosing regimen of methylprednisolone sodium succinate in experimental spinal cord injury. J Neurosurg 67:102–105

Demopoulos HB, Milvy P, Kakari S, Ransohoff J 1972 Molecular aspects of membrane structure in cerebral edema. In: Reulen HJ, Schurmann K (eds) Steroids and brain edema. Springer-Verlag, New York, p 29–40

Drakontides AB 1982 The effect of glucocorticoid treatment on denervated rat hemidiaphragm. Brain Res 239:175–189

Hall ED 1982 Glucocorticoid effects on central nervous excitability and synaptic transmission. Int Rev Neurobiol 23:165–195

Hall ED 1985 High dose glucocorticoid treatment improves neurological recovery in head-injured mice. J Neurosurg 62:882–887

Hall ED 1987 Intensive antioxidant pretreatment retards motor nerve degeneration. Brain Res 413:175–178

Hall ED, Braughler JM 1981 Acute effects of intravenous glucocorticoid pretreatment on the *in vitro* peroxidation of cat spinal cord tissue. Exp Neurol 73:321–324

Hall ED, Braughler JM 1987 Non-surgical management of spinal cord injuries: a review of studies with the glucocorticoid steroid methylprednisolone. Acta Anaesthesiol Belg 38:405–409

Hall ED, Wolf DL 1984 Methylprednisolone preservation of motor nerve function during early degeneration. Exp Neurol 84:715–720

Hall ED, Riker WF, Baker T 1983 Beneficial action of glucocorticoid treatment on neuromuscular transmission during early motor nerve degeneration. Exp Neurol 79:488–496

Hall ED, McCall JM, Chase RL, Yonkers PA, Braughler JM 1987 A nonglucocorticoid steroid analog of methylprednisolone duplicates its high-dose pharmacology in models of central nervous system trauma and neuronal membrane damage. J Pharmacol Exp Ther 242:137–142

Kerr DS, Campbell LW, Hao S-Y, Landfield PW 1989 Corticosteroid modulation of hippocampal potentials: increased effect with aging. Science (Wash DC) 245:1505–1509

Koide T, Wieloch T, Siesjö BK 1985 Chronic dexamethasone pretreatment aggravates ischemic brain damage by inducing hyperglycemia. J Cereb Blood Flow Metab 5 (Suppl 1):S251

Landfield PW, Waymire JC, Lynch G 1978 Hippocampal aging and adrenocorticoids: quantitative correlations. Science (Wash DC) 202:1098–1102

Landfield PW, Baskin RK, Pitler TA 1981 Brain aging correlates: retardation by hormonal-pharmacological treatments. Science (Wash DC) 214:581–584

McEwen BS, Weiss JM, Schwartz LS 1969 Uptake of corticosterone by rat brain and its concentration by certain limbic structures. Brain Res 16:227–241

Riker WF, Baker T, Okamoto M 1975 Glucocorticoids and mammalian motor nerve excitability. Arch Neurol 32:688–694

Sapolsky RM 1985 A mechanism for glucocorticoid toxicity in the hippocampus: increased neuronal vulnerability to metabolic insults. J Neurosci 5:1228–1232

Sapolsky RM 1986 Glucocorticoid toxicity in the hippocampus: reversal by supplementation with brain fuels. J Neurosci 6:2240–2244

Sapolsky RM, Pulsinelli WA 1985 Glucocorticoids potentiate ischemic injury to neurons: therapeutic implications. Science (Wash DC) 229:1397–1399

Sapolsky RM, Krey LC, McEwen BS 1985 Prolonged glucocorticoid exposure reduces hippocampal neuron number: implications for aging. J Neurosci 5:1222–1227

Scheff SW, Cotman CW 1982 Chronic glucocorticoid therapy alters axonal sprouting in the hippocampal dentate gyrus. Exp Neurol 76: 644–654

DISCUSSION

McEwen: In response to your point about the hyperglycaemia that results from raised glucocorticoid levels, during neuronal damage, I would like to stress that although plasma glucose levels may increase when glucocorticoid levels are increased, at the same time the glucocorticoids may block the uptake of glucose into nerve cells, so there won't necessarily be high levels of glucose inside nerve cells. Indeed, if intracellular glucose levels aren't high enough the cell may not be able to maintain energy production. Thus, to say that glucocorticoids cause hyperglycaemia which exacerbates ischaemic brain lactic acidosis is not a sufficient explanation for their effects. We know that after hypoxia there is a massive release of excitatory amino acids, and this is the reason that Sapolsky and Pulsinelli drew the parallel of transient ischaemia with the application of exogenous excitatory amino acids to the hippocampus. As Ed Hall said, the damage produced by kainic acid *in vivo* could be prevented by giving glucose or metabolizable sugars (Sapolsky 1986), and this could also be achieved *in vitro*.

Hall: The lactic acid accumulation doesn't necessarily have to occur only in the neurons; lactic acid could also be accumulated by the adjacent glial cells, or there might be extracellular acidosis.

McEwen: In Sapolsky's studies on the effects of glucocorticoids on glucose uptake by neurons and glial cells in culture, only hippocampal cell glucose uptake was significantly inhibited by glucocorticoids, and both neuronal and non-neuronal hippocampal cells were affected. So perhaps in the hippocampus even the glial cells are following the same mechanisms for glucocorticoid-induced cell damage. And, incidentally, this is another argument for the existence of specialized glial cells.

Hall: Another point is that Sapolsky and Pulsinelli saw exacerbation by corticosterone of ischaemic brain damage in all areas of the brain, not just the hippocampus. Thus, the effect does not correlate with glucocorticoid receptor population. I am not convinced that hyperglycaemia doesn't play some role in the glucocorticoid exacerbation of post-ischaemic brain damage. Salpolsky and Pulsinelli did point out (1985) that in corticosterone-treated rats the blood glucose levels were twice as high as those of adrenalectomized animals.

McEwen: I agree with you that glucocorticoids are not entirely bad for the nervous system! We have recently found that after adrenalectomy and consequent glucocorticoid loss, neurons in the rat dentate gyrus begin to die within 3–7 days. Most of the destructive effects of glucocorticoids that we have seen are in the Ammon's horn, but the dentate gyrus shows a dependency upon adrenal steroids; if you take adrenal steroids away the neurons die and if you give very low doses of corticosterone, aldosterone or even dexamethasone after adrenalectomy, cell death is prevented. We don't know the significance of this finding but it highlights the point that your adrenals are not entirely bad for you.

Hall: If you think about the data carefully, you can see that the deleterious and beneficial effects of glucocorticoids on the nervous system are separable in terms of dose, duration of exposure and mechanism of action.

de Kloet: Dr Sapolsky's hypothesis, which states that high levels of corticosterone facilitate brain ageing because the neurons, particularly in the hippocampus, are metabolically compromised so that they cannot withstand excessive excitatory signals, is attractive in its simplicity (Sapolsky et al 1986). However, when one tries to understand the mechanistic details of how glucocorticoids actually achieve this effect, there are a number of paradoxes which are not so easy to understand. Bruce McEwen mentioned one such paradox. Neurons in the hippocampal dentate gyrus die after adrenalectomy, while those in the CA1 field do not. On the other hand, when animals are exposed to levels of glucocorticoids high enough to cause hippocampal neuronal death in the CA1 field, other neurons, in the dentate gyrus, survive and do not show signs of degeneration.

Glucocorticoids are surely beneficial when they are secreted in response to stress, because they transiently suppress excitability of the target cell and this is a protective mechanism which gives the cell the opportunity to restore its function before the next challenge occurs. Thus it is inappropriate to say that high glucocorticoid levels are damaging. On the contrary, high glucocorticoid levels are apparently needed for adaptation. For the brain it is important to view such effects in the context of the various corticosteroid receptor types and other aspects of neural functioning, such as those underlying behavioural states.

Hall: I agree that there are a number of problems with Dr Sapolsky's hypothesis and although I think his work is very interesting a lot of questions remain unanswered. His experiments with corticosterone and hydrocortisone are complicated by the fact that these two steroids have both glucocorticoid and mineralocorticoid activity. I would like to know if Bruce McEwen or Dr Sapolsky have looked at the effect on the hippocampus of chronic exposure to a steroid that has purely glucocorticoid activity (such as dexamethasone).

McEwen: Those would be difficult experiments to do, because you would need 12 weeks of exposure.

Lambert: MK-801, which blocks NMDA-mediated responses, has protective effects against neurodegeneration induced by ischaemic insult, so is it possible that high doses of glucocorticoids could have an effect on NMDA receptors?

Hall: We have looked at this, because the antagonism of NMDA-mediated responses is another avenue by which to protect against post-ischaemic or post-traumatic neuronal damage. We have looked at the ability of our non-glucocorticoid steroids to antagonize excitatory amino acids and neither U72099E nor 21-aminosteroids antagonize quisqualate-, kainate- or NMDA-induced seizures in mice, even using subcutaneous doses as high as 50 mg/kg. We have not looked at the effects of these compounds on binding of ligands to excitatory amino acid receptors, but I think it's clear that neither glucocorticoids nor the non-glucocorticoid steroids that we have studied act as antagonists at these receptors.

Kubli-Garfias: Do you know anything about the mechanism through which corticosteroids exert their antioxidant effects? Superoxide dismutase and other enzymes protect against the deleterious effects of oxgyen radicals, so is there any connection between corticosteroids and those enzymes?

Hall: Harry Demopoulos, who originally postulated that glucocorticoids might protect against CNS injury by inhibiting lipid peroxidation (Demopoulos et al 1972), has suggested that glucocorticoids may intercalate within the lipid bilayer. Dr Makriyannis has talked about this sort of incorporation but I don't know if, or how, glucocorticoids do this. By incorporating into the membrane, glucocorticoids might affect membrane fluidity and so decrease the ability of peroxidized fatty acids to move around and steal each other's electrons. That is a very simplistic theory but it's the best I can propose at this time. Using fluorescence spectroscopy, we have shown that 21-aminosteroids do decrease membrane fluidity. In addition, they have the ability to scavenge lipid peroxyl radicals and some ability to scavenge for oxygen radicals, so they are probably better antioxidants than the glucocorticoids. The glucocorticoid antioxidant effect is less specialized and probably just involves incorporation into the membrane and direct protection of phospholipids from free radical attack.

Feldman: I think Dr Sapolsky has done experiments with corticosterone in rats, and in monkeys that are extremely stressed (Uno et al 1989). High levels of hydrocortisone are produced and there is extensive damage in the hippocampus. There are thousands of patients who receive glucocorticoid treatment for months or longer periods, yet I am not aware that any of them suffer mental impairment; if they suffered damage in the hippocampus similar to that seen in experimental animals you would expect to see some loss of short-term memory, for example. Most patients on long-term glucocorticoid therapy are given prednisone or dexamethasone, not corticosterone or hydrocortisone, so this difference might be the reason why we do not see these side-effects.

Hall: Dr de Kloet is right to be concerned about how much we really understand the effects of glucocorticoids, and we don't know to what extent a steroid with only glucocorticoid activity would cause chronic degeneration of the brain. I agree that there's much we don't know about that particular issue.

de Kloet: Another paradox which has not been resolved is that a chronically elevated glucocorticoid level causes down-regulation of glucocorticoid receptors, which is essentially an adaptive response. You could argue that animals with decreased glucocorticoid receptor levels would be able to respond less efficiently to episodic changes in glucocorticoid level. This is possible, but it has not been investigated. At present there are only theories and assumptions, but no facts.

Hall: I would agree with that.

McEwen: Glucocorticoids don't by themselves kill cells, so we have to consider what else might be contributing. Other factors might include excitatory amino acids, the ongoing activity of the neurons, calcium levels in the neurons, or the types and quantities of other neurotransmitters that are being released. It seems to me that the specific behavioural state of the animal or person is important in determining the nature of the 'permissive' effect of glucorticoids. In the stress experiment using vervet monkeys that Shaul Feldman referred to, the primates were subjected to a considerable amount of social stress in that they were continuously beaten by more dominant animals. This is one of the most pernicious and continuous forms of stress to which an animal can be exposed and is different from the types of stress that humans are subjected to where they have some control over their situation. I think the fact that the glucocorticoids don't kill neurons by themselves means that we have to consider other aspects, such as neural activity and the behaviour of the animal, if we are to understand the nature and degree of the effects of glucocorticoids.

Hall: Experiments that Sapolsky has done, both *in vitro* and *in vivo*, on the exacerbation of hippocampal neural damage by kainic acid and paraquat, have shown that the glucocorticoid hydrocortisone by itself did not have a negative effect on the neurons; the deleterious effect was manifested only when another neurotoxin was also present.

Makriyannis: Do you test for free radical formation, Dr Hall?

Hall: My colleague Dr J.M. Braughler at Upjohn tests for lipid radical formation by the thiobarbituric acid (i.e. malonyldialdehyde) method.

Deliconstantinos: The assessment of oxygen free radical formation by estimating malonyldialdehyde (MDA) formation is not sufficiently sensitive, or selective, to show that oxygen free radicals are being formed.

To show that glucocorticoids can act as scavengers, you must show that they can do so in a simple system in addition to showing that they can be incorporated into the membrane and inhibit lipid peroxidation. You could for example use cytochrome c and H_2O_2 to generate oxygen radicals; then you could see if the glucocorticoids are scavengers. If they do act as scavengers you need to determine whether they are traps, or quenchers, or whether they inhibit the production of the oxygen free radicals. Glucocorticoids may inhibit the formation of MDA but this does not necessarily mean that they inhibit oxygen radical formation, because they may inhibit prostaglandin production, and MDA is one of the by-products of prostaglandin synthesis.

Hall: In our experiments we removed brain tissue from the injured animal and determined the extent of peroxidation in the *ex vivo* tissue samples by measuring malonyldialdehyde. To further study the antioxidant mechanism of action of the non-glucocorticoid steroids, Dr Braughler has also used 2,2-azobis(2,4-dimethylvaleronitrile) to cause the formation of linoleic acid hydroperoxide at a fixed rate. He has shown that the rate of this peroxidation is inhibited by the 21-aminosteroids (Braughler & Pregenzer 1989). So we have looked at peroxidation in a fairly detailed way.

Makriyannis: Do you think that the scavenging glucocorticoid and non-glucocorticoid steroids will be of therapeutic use?

Hall: We are at present mainly interested in acute trauma and ischaemia, and our initial clinical trials with the 21-aminosteroid U74006F (tirilazad mesylate) will be designed to test its beneficial effects after acute head injuries, spinal injury, subarachnoid haemorrhage and stroke. As you might imagine, we have thought a great deal about the possible efficacy that a potent antioxidant like U74006F might have against a variety of CNS and non-CNS diseases that may involve oxygen radicals.

Makriyannis: Are these compounds more effective than vitamin E?

Hall: We have compared the abilities of 21-aminosteroids and vitamin E to reduce neuronal damage after ischaemia in the gerbil. Vitamin E (five months of a four-fold dietary supplementation) protects against damage in those brain regions that show the mildest amount of cell loss after ischaemia (e.g. medial cerebral cortex). The 21-aminosteroids have greater protective powers than vitamin E in more severely damaged brain regions, so I think these steroids have advantages over the traditionally used antioxidants.

Makriyannis: Many drug companies are interested in developing radical scavengers, but to my knowledge none have been marketed.

Hall: That's correct. We have started phase II clinical trials in moderate and severe head injury, but as yet none of the compounds is ready for the market place.

Ramirez: The neurotoxic effects of MPTP (1,2,3,6-tetrahydro-1-methyl-4-phenylpyridine) may be due to production of radicals by its active metabolite 1-methyl-4-pyridinium, MPP^+. Do the 21-aminosteroids and the antioxidant U74006F protect against the neurotoxicity of this compound?

Hall: We have looked at dopamine depletion caused by MPTP in three different strains of mice. Although mice are not the best animals in which to study MPTP toxicity, the compound is toxic when given in high doses (30 mg/kg i.p., twice daily for three days). U74006F does protect against MPTP-induced dopamine depletion in CF1 and Swiss Webster mice, but not in C57 mice, which are a better model. I don't understand why the drug is effective in some strains but not in others, unless in mice MPTP does not exert its effects through free radical production. Others have suggested that excitatory amino acids may be more important than free radical production in mediating the neurotoxicity of MPTP, which the 21-aminosteroids and U72099E do not directly antagonize.

Joubert-Bression: In Cushing's syndrome, levels of hydrocortisone are raised. Is anything known about the cause of neuronal death in these patients?

Hall: No; I don't know if there is in fact overt neuronal damage associated with Cushing's syndrome.

Dubrovsky: There have been reports of brain atrophy in Cushing's disorders (Heinz et al 1977, Okuno et al 1980) but no systematic studies have been done.

References

Braughler JM, Pregenzer JF 1989 The 21-aminosteroid inhibitors of lipid peroxidation: reactions with lipid peroxyl and phenoxyl radicals. Free Rad Biol Med 7:125–130

Demopoulos HB, Milvy P, Kakari S, Ransohoff J 1972 Molecular aspects of membrane structure in cerebral edema. In: Reulen HJ, Schurmann K (eds) Steroids and brain edema. Springer-Verlag, New York, p 29–40

Heinz ER, Martinez J, Haenggeli A 1977 Reversibility of cerebral atrophy in anorexia nervosa and Cushing's syndrome. J Comput Assist Tomogr 1:415–418

Okuno T, Ito M, Konishi Y, Yoshioka M, Nakano Y 1980 Cerebral atrophy following ACTH therapy. J Comput Assist Tomogr 4:20–23

Sapolsky RM 1986 Glucocorticoid toxicity in the hippocampus: reversal by supplementation with brain fuels. J Neurosci 6:2240–2244

Sapolsky RM, Pulsinelli WA 1985 Glucocorticoids potentiate ischemic injury to neurons: therapeutic implications. Science (Wash DC) 229:1397–1399

Sapolsky RM, Krey LM, McEwen BS 1986 The neuroendocrinology of stress and aging: the glucocorticoid cascade hypothesis. Endocr Rev 7:282–301

Uno H, Tarara R, Else JG, Suleman MA, Sapolsky RM 1989 Hippocampal damage associated with prolonged and fatal stress in primates. J Neurosci 9:1705–1711

General discussion II

Sex differences in GABA-mediated responses

Johnston: We and other workers have done some studies on stress-induced changes in $GABA_A$ receptors and have found that these receptors are rapidly regulated. For example, injecting rats with saline can increase the density of $GABA_A$ receptors in the forebrain (Maddison et al 1987). We have looked at the effect of a swim stress on $GABA_A$ receptors in mouse forebrain. The mice swim in warm water (32 °C) for three minutes. This produces an analgesia that is relatively insensitive to naloxone and therefore not solely opiate mediated. The analgesia persists for 30 minutes. If you kill the mice immediately after the three-minute swim you find that the $GABA_A$ receptor density in the forebrain has been up-regulated by about 70%; the low affinity GABA receptors are increased in greater proportion than the high affinity sites. If you kill the mice half an hour after the swim stress, you find that the number of receptors has returned to control levels, so there's a correlation between the up-regulation and the analgesia (Skerritt et al 1981).

Recently we found that these effects of swim stress are more pronounced in female than in male adult QS mice (M. Akinci & G. A. R. Johnston, unpublished results). This led us to look for other reports of differences between male and female GABA receptors. We found that there's a great deal of information about such differences but generally nobody seems to comment on them and the information tends to be buried among the experimental details. For example, we normally administer the GABA antagonist picrotoxin intravenously, and were trying to find what dose should be used for an intraperitoneal injection. When we found this information we noticed that the authors mentioned that female mice and rats are more sensitive than males to picrotoxin antagonism of responses to GABA but that if you remove the gonads the sexes are equally sensitive (Pericic et al 1985). Again, the benzodiazepine diazepam, which enhances responses to GABA, has been reported to decrease plasma corticosterone levels in female but not male rats (Pericic et al 1985). George Fink and his colleagues (1982) reported that higher doses of alphaxalone are needed to produce surgical anaesthesia in male rats than in female rats, and oestrogen treatment reduces the dose required in males to that which is effective in females. There is a rather provocative point in a paper by Pericic et al (1985) that male rats may have a 'more powerful GABA system' than female rats. Male Wistar rats appear to be less 'emotional and aggressive' than female rats of the same age housed in the same environment. It's interesting that benzodiazepines are prescribed much more frequently for women than they are for men. That may result from bias among medical practitioners, or it could reflect the fact that females may be more sensitive to benzodiazepines than males.

Majewska: I agree; females may be better able to adapt to their environment!

Olsen: We have found that female rats are more sensitive to treatment with the experimental convulsant drug pentylenetetrazol, which is a $GABA_A$ receptor-chloride channel antagonist. We have looked at the binding to the GABA receptor of muscimol, flunitrazepam, and *t*-butylbicyclophosphoro-thionate (TBPS), but have not found the binding, or steroid modulation of that binding, to be different in brain membranes or tissue sections from any region of male and female rats. However, the *in vivo* sensitivity to various GABAergic drugs such as benzodiazepines, barbiturates and ethanol is different in male and female rats, and ovariectomy causes female sensitivity to become more like that of males (N. Kokka, D. Sapp, U. Witte & R. W. Olsen, unpublished results, and the results of Professor Johnston mentioned above).

McEwen: To what extent could these various differences be due to differences in liver metabolism?

Johnston: Most of the effects that have been reported are almost instantaneous; they don't take a long time to develop. Picrotoxin-induced seizures are immediate, the swim stress has effects within a few minutes, and the induction of surgical anaesthesia takes only a few minutes.

McEwen: A metabolic difference between the sexes would tend to be manifested as a change in the duration of an effect, so these differences are probably not due to metabolic variations.

Dubrovsky: There is a female/male sex ratio of 1.6 to 1.0 in the incidence of depression (Weissman & Klerman 1977). Contrary to expectation, the relationship of the neuroendocrine systems to the depressed state is inconsistent for both women and men.

To what extent intrauterine hormones influence the growing fetus remains to be assessed. There has been a big upsurge of interest and work in this field. Hormonal actions appear to affect a wide range of a subject's characteristics. According to Geschwind & Galaburda (1987), left-handedness is just one indication of the slight difference in human talents brought about by changing levels of sex hormones *in utero*. Too much testosterone will slow the growth of the left side of the brain, which mainly controls the contralateral, right side of the body. As speech functions are also lateralized toward the left hemisphere, insufficient development will cause not only left-handedness, but also language problems. Coupled with this, Geschwind & Galaburda (1987) describe a higher susceptibility to migraine, epilepsy and diseases of the immune system associated with left-handedness. All disturbances could be traced back to the effects of sex hormones in the unborn child.

Majewska: The sensitivity to anaesthesia could vary during the oestrous cycle. When the level of progesterone is high, the level of tetrahydroprogesterone will probably be high, so there would be a lower threshold for anaesthesia then.

Martini: The majority of metabolic differences between males and females seem to be due to the different 'organization' of the patterns of growth hormone secretion in the two sexes. It might be worth investigating whether sexual differences in GABA receptor functioning might also result from the sexual dimorphism in growth hormone secretion.

Hall: We discovered a rather striking sexual difference in our experiments on ischaemia in the gerbil. We usually use male gerbils but for a time we could obtain only females. When we looked at the amount of post-ischaemic degeneration in the cortex and CA1 areas after a three-hour period of unilateral carotid occlusion we found to our surprise that the degree of cell loss in the females was dramatically less than it was in males. Although there are some subtle circulatory differences between male and female gerbil brains, we found that blood flow during and after ischaemia is the same in male and female gerbils. Because we favour the theory that free radicals are the pre-eminent cause of ischaemic damage, we think that oestradiol or oestriol may act as antioxidants. In fact these two steroids have a significant ability to inhibit lipid peroxidation *in vitro* (Vladimirov et al 1973). Also, the same difference has been found to exist between male and female rats. A number of eminent people work in the field of ischaemia, so it surprises me that no such difference has been reported before now. I have asked neurologists whether women who have strokes suffer less neuronal damage or have better prospects of recovery than men, but most strokes in women occur after the menopause, when the difference might no longer be evident.

Lambert: In females, GABA-potentiating steroids activate chloride channels, which could clamp the membrane potential at the chloride reversal potential, so that NMDA receptors are not freed of the magnesium block of the cation channel which would otherwise unblock as a consequence of depolarization.

Hall: That's a possible explanation. In our experiments the animals are highly anaesthetized during ischaemia and then allowed to recover. Clinical manifestations of ischaemia, such as circling behaviour, torso curvature or seizures during the period of carotid occlusion, do not seem to differ between male and female gerbils.

Johnston: There are clinical conditions that show sex differences. Anorexia nervosa, which is associated with high levels of plasma cortisol, has a higher incidence in women than in men (Brambilla et al 1985). Also, women are more frequently diagnosed than men as suffering from depression, and hypercortisolaemia can induce symptoms of depression (Carpenter & Gruen 1982, Dohrenwend & Dohrenwend 1976).

Feldman: Hypercortisolaemia is a result, not a cause of depression.

Dubrovsky: Hypercortisolaemia was considered to be an epiphenomenon of low catecholamine levels and was hypothesized to occur in depression; this view has now been overtaken by new neuropharmacological data (see my paper, p 240) and by behavioural and clinical evidence indicating that adrenal steroids can significantly affect behaviour, especially depressive syndromes in Cushing's disorders. Moreover, studies in depressed patients show that corticotropin releasing factor (CRF) produced a blunt response in ACTH release (Gold et al 1984). Basal ACTH values were normal in all patients tested (60 drug-free subjects). Notwithstanding these results, depressed patients tended to have higher mean ($\pm$ SD) basal cortisol values: 4.2 ± 1.1 versus $1.9 \pm 0.4\,\mu g/dl$ (Gold et al 1984). These data, plus clinical results showing that the depression observed frequently in Cushing's patients is relieved by adrenal suppression (Kramlinger et al 1985), suggest a pathophysiological role for adrenal steroids in depression. In our own experience, adrenal suppression with ketoconazole in five cases of severe depression resulted in noticeable mood and behaviour improvement within 24 hours of the initiation of treatment. That is, the recovery process has qualitatively and quantitatively significant differences from treatment with tricyclics. But the adrenals produce a multitude of hormones, so we believe that a balance between them finally determines their effects. As a matter of fact, a recent report (Ponsart et al 1987) suggests that the diagnostic performance of the basal free cortisol/18OHDOC ratio in endogenous depression is as reliable as the dexamethasone suppression test. Thus a simple procedure based on hormonal ratios can be of value in clinical psychiatry.

McEwen: There are two kinds of differences between sexes that affect brain functioning. Activational effects are those in which the presence of the gonads and the different levels of the different sex hormones alter brain functioning. The other type of effects are developmental or organizational effects which tend to be seen even after removal of the gonads and consequent loss of the gonadal steroids. The effects we have been discussing, where after gonadectomy or oestrogen treatment of the male the difference between the sexes is no longer apparent, are activational effects. The difference between the incidence of depression in men and women may be more likely to result from organizational or developmental differences between the sexes, which tend to survive changes in gonadal hormone levels. We have to bear this in mind, even though we don't have experimental results.

References

Brambilla F, Cavagnini F, Invitti C et al 1985 Neuroendocrine and psychopathological measures in anorexia nervosa: resemblances to primary affective disorders. Psychiatry Res 16:165–176

Carpenter WT, Gruen PH 1982 Cortisol's effects on human mental functioning. J Clin Psychopharmacol 2:91–101

Dohrenwend BP, Dohrenwend BS 1976 Sex differences and psychiatric disorders. Am J Sociology 81:1447–1454

Fink G, Sarkar DK, Dow RC et al 1982 Sex difference in response to alphaxalone anaesthesia may be oestrogen dependent. Nature (Lond) 298:270–272

Geschwind N, Galaburda AM 1987 Cerebral lateralization: biological mechanisms, associations and pathology. MIT Press, Boston, MA

Gold PW, Chrousos G, Kellner Ch et al 1984 Psychiatric implications of basic and clinical studies with corticortropin-releasing factor. Am J Psychiatry 141:619–627

Kramlinger KG, Peterson GC, Watson PK, Leonard LJ 1985 Metyrapone for depression and delirium secondary to Cushing's syndrome. Psychosomatics 26:67–71

Maddison JE, Dodd PR, Johnston GAR, Farrell GC 1987 Brain γ-aminobutyric acid receptor binding is normal in rats with thioacetamide-induced hepatic encephalopathy despite elevated plasma γ-aminobutyric acid-like activity. Gastroenterology 93:1062–1068

Pericic D, Manev H, Lakic N 1985 Sex differences in the response of rats to drugs affecting GABAergic transmission. Life Sci 36:541–547

Ponsart ED, Ansseau M, Saloy J et al 1987 Diagnostic performance of basal free cortisol 18-hydroxy-11-deoxycorticosterone (18OHDOC) ratio in endogenous depression: comparison with the dexamethasone suppression test. Biol Psychiatry 22:947–956

Skerritt JH, Trisdikoon P, Johnston GAR 1981 Increased GABA binding in mouse brain following acute swim stress. Brain Res 215:398–403

Vladimirov YA, Sergeev PV, Seifulla RD, Rudnev YN 1973 Effects of steroids on lipid peroxidation in liver mitochondrial membranes. Molekulyarnaya Biologiya 7:247–253

Weissman MM, Klerman GL 1977 Sex differences and the epidemiology of depression. Arch Gen Psychiatry 34:98–111

Steroids in relation to epilepsy and anaesthesia

T. Bäckström*, K. W. Gee†, N. Lan†, M. Sörensen‡ and G. Wahlström°

Departments of Gynecology*, Physiology* and Pharmacology°, Universities of Umeå and Uppsala, Sweden, School of Pharmacy†, University of Southern California, Los Angeles, USA, and Anesthesia‡, Hvidovre Hospital, Copenhagen, Denmark

Abstract. Increasing numbers of reports indicate direct effects of ovarian steroids on the central nervous system. Effects of progesterone and its metabolites on brain excitability in humans and in experimental animals have been studied. Anti-epileptic effects have been shown in cats and in women with partial epilepsy and well-defined epileptic foci. The reduced progesterone metabolite 5α-pregnan-3α-ol-20-one and its 5β analogue also decreased the epileptic activity resulting from a penicillin-induced cortical focus in cats. 5α-Pregnan-3α-ol-20-one protected mice against metrazol-, bicuculline- and picrotoxin-induced seizures but not against electroshock- and strychnine-induced seizures. Progesterone, 5α-pregnan-3α-ol-20-one and 5β-pregnan-3α-ol-20-one also induce anaesthesia in humans and animals; in a rat model of anaesthesia 5α-pregnan-3α-ol-20-one was eight times more potent than methohexitone (the most potent anaesthetic barbiturate). Anaesthesia with loss of the eyelash reflex was observed in humans 75–90 seconds after the intravenous injection of 5β-pregnan-3α-ol-20-one in lipid emulsion. The *in vivo* production and brain distribution of centrally active steroids has also been studied in relation to the phases of the ovarian and menstrual cycle. A subset of women with epilepsy show changes in seizure frequency in relation to hormonal variations during the menstrual cycle. In the luteal phase when progesterone levels are high the number of generalized seizures is low. It is possible that progesterone and its metabolites play a role in epileptic seizures and also in the premenstrual syndrome.

1990 Steroids and neuronal activity. Wiley, Chichester (Ciba Foundation Symposium 153) p 225–239

It is well known that some women show variations in mental and neurological symptoms in relation to different phases of the menstrual cycle (Laidlaw 1956, Bäckström et al 1983a). As the menstrual cycle is regulated by the production of pituitary gonadotropins and ovarian steroids, it is conceivable that there is a relationship between hormone production and the variation in CNS symptoms. In this respect we discuss some of the clinical and experimental data which point to effects of progesterone and its metabolites in epilepsy and anaesthesia.

Effects of progesterone and its metabolites on brain excitability

Progesterone given intravenously in doses of 400–600 mg induces sleep/anaesthesia in humans (Merryman et al 1954) as well as in animals (Gyermek et al 1968). In ovariectomized cats, progesterone at plasma levels found during pregnancy can significantly decrease the frequency of epileptic spikes from a penicillin-induced epileptic focus (Landgren et al 1978). In women with partial epilepsy and well-defined epileptic foci, progesterone significantly reduces the spike frequency as measured on a continuous EEG. When progesterone was infused to achieve plasma levels observed during the luteal phase of the menstrual cycle, four out of seven female epileptic patients were shown to have a significant reduction in the spike frequency. The women with low plasma binding of progesterone showed the best response to the progesterone infusion, whereas those with the highest plasma binding had no response to the infusion (Bäckström et al 1984).

Progesterone metabolites that are reduced at the C-5 position are very potent in their CNS depressant action, particularly C-5 reduced steroids with a 3α-hydroxyl group (Gyermek et al 1968). When tested for its anaesthetic potency in a well-defined rat model (Wahlström 1966), 5α-pregnan-3α-ol-20-one was about eight times more potent, on a weight basis, than methohexitone, the most potent barbiturate known (Norberg et al 1987). The 5α-reduced derivative of progesterone seems to be a more potent anaesthetic than the 5β isomer. Young rats require higher doses of these steroids than older rats for induction of anaesthesia (Norberg et al 1987).

We have also injected 5β-pregnan-3α-ol-20-one in lipid emulsion into humans. Loss of the eyelash reflex was induced 75–90 seconds after an injection of 0.4–0.6 mg/kg body weight (Carl et al 1990).

In a cat model of epilepsy with an artifical epileptic focus, induced by applying penicillin to the cerebral cortical surface, 5α-pregnan-3α-ol-20-one and 5β-pregnan-3α-ol-20-one can totally inhibit the epileptic activity with a very short latency period. Both derivatives were more potent in their anti-epileptic action than clonazepam on a weight basis (Landgren et al 1987). In *in vitro* assays, we have found that 5α-pregnan-3α-ol-20-one is more potent than clonazepam in its ability to influence GABA$_A$ receptor-linked chloride channel opening (Gee 1988). In mice the 5α metabolite inhibits convulsions induced by metrazol, (+)-bicuculline and picrotoxin, with maximum potency against (+)-bicuculline-induced seizures. No effects were seen against maximal electroshock- and strychnine-induced seizures (Belelli et al 1989). These rapid effects of 5α-pregnan-3α-ol-20-one may well be mediated via actions on the GABA$_A$ receptor–chloride ionophore complex (Gee 1988).

In vivo production of CNS-active progesterone metabolites

Centrally active steroids are produced by the ovary in both humans and lower mammals. Progesterone is synthesized by the corpus luteum in a well-known cyclical pattern; the hormone reaches a 20-fold higher concentration during the luteal phase than in the follicular phase. 5α-Pregnane-3,20-dione (5α-DHP), a precursor of 5α-pregnan-3α-ol-20-one, is also produced by the human corpus luteum and varies in its plasma concentrations during the menstrual cycle (Bäckström et al 1986). 5α-Pregnan-3α-ol-20-one has been measured in ovarian tissue in rats and shows clear fluctuations with the ovarian cycle (Ichikawa et al 1974). During human pregnancy, 5α-pregnane-3,20-dione increases in concentration about 10 times, to reach a level that is about one-third of the plasma progesterone concentration (Löfgren et al 1988). The concentration in fetal blood is about 10 times the concentration in maternal plasma. In plasma, progesterone is bound to transcortin and albumin; it is generally considered that the unbound fraction exerts the hormonal effects on peripheral organs (Lipsett 1988). The 5α-reduced progesterone metabolites are not known to bind specifically to plasma-binding proteins, but will bind to albumin with low affinity (Westphal 1971).

Progesterone distribution in the brain

In rats the concentration of progesterone in the brain varies in parallel with its cyclical production by the ovary (Bixo et al 1986). This variation is especially marked in the cortex, where there is a 300-fold difference in the tissue concentration between the two phases of the ovarian cycle. The concentration varies widely between different brain regions, the highest concentrations being found in the cerebral cortex and hypothalamus (Bixo et al 1986). Anaesthetic doses of progesterone injected intravenously into rats produced brain progesterone concentrations that were 1000 times higher than that observed during the postovulatory phase (Bixo & Bäckström 1990). The ratio of 5α-pregnan-3α-ol-20-one to progesterone was about 100 times higher in brain tissue than in plasma. The enzyme 5α-reductase is present in the brain (Kraulis et al 1975) and the production of 5α-reduced metabolites may be an important factor in the anaesthetic action of progesterone.

Epileptic seizures during the menstrual cycle

A subset of women with epilepsy show a change in seizure frequency with different phases of the menstrual cycle. We studied women with partial epilepsy prospectively throughout a number of menstrual cycles (Bäckström 1976). The seizures were counted by the patient and their relatives. Blood samples were taken at regular intervals for oestradiol and progesterone radioimmunoassay. The frequency of generalized seizures increased in two periods. The first occurred shortly after the rapid decrease in progesterone level during menstruation and the second during the preovulatory rise in oestrogen. During the luteal period with high progesterone levels the number of generalized seizures was very low. A numerical comparison between the follicular and luteal phases showed that a greater number of generalized seizures were occurring during the follicular phase. Also, the number of seizure-free days was lower during the follicular phase (Bäckström 1976). The results indicated an ameliorating effect of factors present during the luteal phase, especially with regard to generalized seizures. The increase in seizure frequency during menstruation could be explained by a rebound effect after a rapid decrease in the anti-epileptic factor premenstrually, similar to what is seen when administration of anti-epileptic drugs is ended abruptly. These findings are in accordance with those reported by Laidlaw (1956), who found a variation in seizure frequency during the menstrual cycle which is similar to our findings.

There are, however, several types of epilepsy of differing aetiology. In patients with petit mal epilepsy, who have another pathogenetic background, we have noted a different cyclical pattern during the menstrual cycle. We have so far investigated four patients and they all have a similar pattern. We have made 24-hour EEG recordings every second day during the menstrual cycle using a portable tape-recorder. These patients have a gradually increasing seizure frequency during the luteal phase, reaching a maximum in the premenstrual phase. When menstruation starts the number of seizures decreases and is low in the follicular phase (Bäckström et al 1983a). This pattern is interesting because it very much resembles the pattern of mood changes in the so-called premenstrual syndrome (Bäckström et al 1983a,b). In patients with this syndrome there is a gradual increase in the severity of adverse moods, such as irritability and depression, during the luteal phase. The symptoms reach a peak in severity during the last five premenstrual days and after the onset of menstrual bleeding the symptoms rapidly disappear. The patients are usually completely free of symptoms 3–4 days after the onset of menstrual bleeding.

Symptom variation in the premenstrual syndrome is related to the presence of the corpus luteum. The symptoms start when the luteal phase starts and end when the luteal phase ends. In anovulatory cycles where no corpus luteum is developed the cyclicity in the mood changes disappears (Hammarbäck & Bäckström 1988). The cyclicity of symptoms continues in patients who are hysterectomized but have their ovaries intact, indicating that the presence of menstruation is not necessary for the cyclical mood changes (Bäckström et al 1981). The nature of the symptom-provoking factor produced by the corpus luteum is, however, still unknown.

Acknowledgements

This study was supported by the Swedish Medical Research Council, project numbers 6862 and 3495.

References

Bäckström T 1976 Epileptic seizures in women in relation to variations of plasma estrogen and progesterone during the menstrual cycle. Acta Neurol Scand 54:321–347

Bäckström T, Boyle H, Baird DT 1981 Persistence of symptoms of premenstrual tension in hysterectomised women. Br J Obstet Gynaecol 88:530–536

Bäckström T, Baird DT, Bancroft J et al 1983a Endocrinological aspects of cyclical mood changes during the menstrual cycle or the premenstrual syndrome. J Psychosom Obstet Gynaecol 2:8–20

Bäckström T, Sanders D, Leask R, Davidson D, Warner P, Bancroft J 1983b Mood, sexuality, hormones and the menstrual cycle. II. Hormone levels and their relationship to the premenstrual syndrome. Psychosom Med 45:503–507

Bäckström T, Zetterlund B, Blom S, Romano M 1984 Effects of continuous progesterone infusion on the epileptic discharge frequency in women with partial epilepsy. Acta Neurologica Scand 69:240–248

Bäckström T, Andersson A, Baird DT, Selstam G 1986 5alpha-pregnane-3,20-dione in peripheral and ovarian vein blood of women of different stages of the menstrual cycle. Acta Endocrinol 111:116–121

Belelli D, Bolger MB, Gee KW 1989 Anticonvulsant profile of the progesterone metabolite 5alpha-pregnan-3alpha-ol-20-one. Eur J Pharmacol 166:325–329

Bixo MB, Bäckström T 1990 Regional distribution of progesterone and 5alpha-pregnane-3,20-dione in rat brain during progesterone induced anaesthesia. Psycho-neuroendocrinology 15:159

Bixo M, Bäckström T, Winblad B, Selstam G, Andersson A 1986 Comparison between pre- and postovulatory distributions of oestradiol and progesterone in the brain of the PMSG-treated rat. Acta Physiol Scand 128:241–246

Carl P, Högskilde S, Nielsen JW, Sörensen M, Lindholm B, Karlen B, Bäckström T 1990 Pregnanolone emulsion. A preliminary pharmacokinetic and pharmacodynamic study of a new intravenous anaesthetic agent. Anesthesiology, in press

Gee KW 1988 Steroid modulation of the GABA/benzodiazepine receptor-linked chloride ionophore. Mol Neurobiol 2:291–317

Gyermek L, Iriarte J, Crabbe P 1968 Structure–activity relationship of some steroidal hypnotic agents. J Med Chem 11:117–125

Hammarbäck S, Bäckström T 1988 Induced anovulation as treatment of premenstrual tension syndrome. A double-blind cross-over study with GnRH-agonist versus placebo. Acta Obstet Gynecol Scand 67:159–166

Ichikawa S, Sawada T, Nakamura Y, Morioka H 1974 Ovarian secretion of pregnane compounds during the estrous cycle and pregnancy in rats. Endocrinology 94:1615–1620

Kraulis I, Foldes G, Traikov H, Dubrovsky B, Birmingham MK 1975 Distribution, metabolism and biological activity of deoxycorticosterone in the central nervous system. Brain Res 88:1–14

Laidlaw J 1956 Catamenial epilepsy. Lancet 2:1235–1237

Landgren S, Bäckström T, Kalistratov G 1978 The effect of progesterone on the spontaneous interictal spike evoked by topical application of penicillin to the cat's cerebral cortex. J Neurol Sci 36:119–133

Landgren S, Aasly J, Bäckström T, Dubrovsky B, Danielsson E 1987 The effect of progesterone and its metabolites on the interictal epileptiform discharge in the cat's cortex. Acta Physiol Scand 131:33–42

Lipsett MB 1988 Steroid hormones. In: Yen SSC, Jaffe RB (eds) Reproductive endocrinology. Saunders, Philadelphia, p 140–153

Löfgren M, Bäckström T, Joelsson I 1988 Decrease in serum concentration of

5alpha-pregnane-3,20-dione prior to spontaneous labor. Acta Obstet Gynecol Scand 67:467–470

Merryman W, Boiman R, Barnes L, Rothchild I 1954 Progesterone 'anaesthesia' in human subjects. J Clin Endocrinol Metab 14:1567–1569

Norberg L, Wahlström G, Bäckström T 1987 The anaesthetic potency of 3alpha-hydroxy-5alpha-pregnan-20-one and 3alpha-hydroxy-5beta-pregnan-20-one determined with an intravenous EEG-threshold method in male rats. Acta Pharmacol Toxicol Scand 61:42–47

Wahlström G 1966 Estimation of brain sensitivity to hexobarbitone in rats by an EEG-threshold. Acta Pharmacol Toxicol 24:404–418

Westphal U 1971 Steroid protein interactions. Springer-Verlag, New York, p 164–225

DISCUSSION

Smith: Your data revealing cyclical hormonal influences on epileptic seizure activity would be consistent with oestradiol having activating effects and progesterone having suppressant effects on neuronal function. You said, however, that in petit mal epilepsy there was an increase in seizures during the premenstrual phase, but in other types of epilepsy the increase occurred during the follicular phase, in mid-cycle. Petit mal epilepsy would thus be correlated with the fall in progesterone concentrations, which would result in decreased GABA function, and the other types of epilepsy with the increase in oestradiol, which would be consistent with the potentiating effects of oestradiol on excitatory amino acid function that I have observed (Smith 1989). So two different mechanisms might be involved: do you have any idea what these mechanisms might be?

Bäckström: The aetiology of petit mal epilepsy is not completely understood and there are several theories about its causation. The latest theory is that petit mal epilepsy is a disease of the cerebral cortex, an area that usually has inhibitory effects on 'activating centres' deeper in the brain. For some reason these inhibitory effects are decreased in petit mal epilepsy. If progesterone or its metabolites have anaesthetic effects in the cerebral cortex, perhaps the progesterone production during the luteal phase might decrease the inhibitory action of the higher centres on the lower activating centres.

Patients with partial epilepsy always have brain damage in the cerebral cortex and epileptic activity is generated from this area of damage—the epileptic focus. From this focus epileptic activity spreads over the cortex, down to deeper centres, and when the epileptic activity spreads over the entire brain a generalized seizure results. Perhaps the pregnane steroids inhibit the activity in the focus. This might explain the observed difference in seizure frequency during the menstrual cycle between petit mal and partial epilepsy. This is of course a speculation and I have no evidence that it is the correct explanation.

Baulieu: You demonstrated that both 5α- and 5β-pregnan-3α-ol-20-one inhibited epileptic activity and had anaesthetic actions. Do you consider 5α- and 5β-pregnanolone to be equipotent and interchangeable?

Bäckström: In our rat model of anaesthesia, both compounds are active, but 5β-pregnan-3α-ol-20-one is less potent than the 5α metabolite but more potent than methohexitone. Incidentally, young rats require higher doses of pregnanolone for anaesthesia.

Baulieu: Can you put the animal to sleep with the 5α metabolite?

Bäckström: We haven't tried that but I think 5α-pregnan-3α-ol-20-one would work. Alphaxalone, the active component of Althesin, which has been used clinically, is a 5α-reduced pregnane steroid.

Baulieu: You have suggested that the cause of premenstrual syndrome might be a factor of luteal origin. Could this be progesterone?

Bäckström: We studied postmenopausal women receiving hormone replacement therapy. These women were given oestrogen for three weeks and during the last 11 days of the cycle they were given a progestogen (lynestrenol) in addition to the oestrogen. The women developed a cyclicity in their moods that was similar to the cyclicity seen in women with premenstrual syndrome. However, other women, who received only oestrogen for three weeks followed by one week without hormone treatment, did not develop any cyclicity in their symptoms (Hammarbäck et al 1985).

Baulieu: So you think a progestin is involved?

Bäckström: Yes, I think so, but we have no knowledge of the mechanism of action.

Martini: You are right to be cautious about the nature of this luteal factor; the corpus luteum produces many compounds in addition to steroids. For example, it produces relaxin, a hormone which possesses insulin-like activity.

McEwen: When you gave oestrogen and progestagens to postmenopausal women you saw cyclicity of mood. Did the occurrence and nature of these mood changes relate to premenopausal susceptibility to mood changes? Did hormone treatment after the menopause re-establish sensitivity in women who were prone to premenstrual syndrome before the menopause?

Bäckström: Yes.

McEwen: So individual differences that existed before the menopause are re-established or re-expressed after the hormone treatment?

Bäckström: In these individuals the severity of the symptoms resulting from postmenopausal hormone replacement therapy was much less than the severity of the symptoms of premenstrual syndrome. Women who had suffered from PMS before the menopause were not specially recruited for the study, but we asked the women recruited whether they had experienced cyclical mood changes. We found that the severity of cyclical mood changes caused by hormone therapy was higher in women who had previously suffered from PMS. However, it has been reported that up to 75% of all women of fertile age notice some kind of cyclical mood changes, but not all of these women suffer from PMS—probably only 5–10% (Andersch et al 1986).

Martini: Is there a gliosis associated with the epileptic focus in your patients?

Bäckström: That would depend on what the cause of the focus was.

Feldman: Partial epilepsy originates from a focus in a particular region in the brain and epileptic foci can thus have different aetiologies. The focus could be a small glioma, an old scar, or a small vascular malformation. Around such lesions there is usually some gliosis, but the aetiologies are different.

Martini: I wonder whether this gliosis could provide a protective mechanism. We have shown that there is a high level of 5α-reductase in glial cells. It is possible that progesterone might be converted to its 5α-reduced metabolites in the glial cells around the focus; these metabolites could inhibit epileptic activity.

Feldman: Epilepsy in pregnancy is one of the most interesting problems in clinical neurology. About a third of the women whose seizures were controlled before pregnancy show increased seizure frequency during pregnancy. This increase is mainly attributable to a decline in plasma anti-epileptic drug levels, so seizures can be controlled again by increasing the dose of the drug.

Some women have seizures for the first time when they become pregnant. This form of epilepsy, epilepsia gravidarum, is thought to be due to metabolic changes that occur during pregnancy; in particular, the high level of oestrogens during pregnancy may lower the epileptic threshold. These women may possess a silent focus, which normally is not active, but becomes epileptogenic when oestrogen levels are increased. In women who were epileptic before pregnancy the combination of the decreased blood levels of anti-epileptic drugs and the high oestrogen level may cause increased seizure frequency.

Bäckström: Epilepsy in pregnancy is diverse and difficult to understand. It has been found that about 40% of women with epilepsy show a decreased frequency of seizures during pregnancy, about 35% show increased seizure frequency, and in some patients there is no change. Attempts have been made to relate the changes in seizure frequency to blood oestradiol concentration. It seems that patients with high oestrogen levels show increased seizure frequency in pregnancy compared to women with low oestrogen levels. These studies are complicated by the fact that the patients have altered absorption of anti-epileptic drugs. Also, because these drugs are teratogenic, the patients are reluctant to take them. They sometimes claim to be taking them but if you measure plasma concentrations you find no drugs in their blood (Janz et al 1982).

Feldman: Non-compliance with treatment is the most common cause of uncontrolled epilepsy in both pregnant and non-pregnant patients.

Perusquia: What are the physiological concentrations of 5β-reduced progesterone metabolites in the blood in relation to the concentrations of 5α-reduced compounds?

Bäckström: During the luteal phase of the menstrual cycle the concentration of 5α-pregnane-3,20-dione in serum is about one-third of the concentration of progesterone. We don't know the concentration of the 5β metabolite in blood (Bäckström et al 1986).

Baulieu: Do you cause fever when you inject 5β-pregnan-3α-ol-20-one?

Bäckström: We monitored temperature during the anaesthesia and for four hours afterwards, and saw no increase in temperature.

Baulieu: So you didn't confirm previous findings (Kappas et al 1958)?

Bäckström: When the 5β-pregnane steroids were injected previously they were always injected in some kind of oil, such as Cremophor-EL. A number of the effects of these injections, anaphylactic reactions in particular, are now considered to be caused by the vehicle.

Majewska: Have you noticed any differences in the patterns of steroids in the blood between the first trimester of pregnancy and the second or third trimesters, when the placenta takes over progesterone synthesis from the corpus luteum?

Bäckström: I think that seizure frequency increases in the later part of pregnancy. Seizure frequency during pregnancy is related to the frequency seen before pregnancy and also to compliance with medical treatment. There are many factors involved.

Gee: The anticonvulsant profile of 5α-pregnan-3α-ol-20-one in animal models suggests that it's effective against partial seizure, but not effective against seizures induced by maximum electroshock, so it would probably not be useful in the treatment of grand mal epilepsy.

Olsen: Benzodiazepines are effective against pentylenetetrazol-, bicuculline- and picrotoxin-induced seizures, which are generalized seizures.

Gee: Protection against pentylenetetrazol-induced seizures typically predicts effectiveness against petit mal epilepsy, whereas protection against maximum electroshock predicts effectiveness against grand mal. You can prevent maximal electroshock-induced seizure using 5α-pregnan-3α-ol-20-one, but only at concentrations high enough to cause anaesthesia.

Simmonds: The relative potency of those pregnane derivatives against epilepsy compared with their anaesthetic potency is an interesting question. What information is available on this?

Bäckström: We had some indication in our cat model of focal epilepsy that pregnanedione was not effective in inhibiting the epileptic activity from the focus, whereas 5β- and 5α-pregnan-3α-ol-20-one seem to have pronounced effects, similar to each other, and both were more potent than clonazepam or progesterone (Landgren et al 1987).

Karavolas: I wanted to mention, Dr Bäckström, some of our findings on the effect of oestrogen on the uptake of progesterone by rat cerebral cortex and cerebellum that may be relevant to your findings, especially those showing inverse relationships with oestrogen levels. In the same *in vivo* studies noted in our paper (p 30), but not discussed, we observed that after oestrogen treatment, selective accumulation of progesterone by these neural tissues was halved, compared to that in non-oestrogen-treated groups.

Kubli-Garfias: It may be important to distinguish between the physiological and pharmacological action of C-5-reduced progestins. In Dr Bäckström's model of anaesthesia, 5α-pregnan-3α-ol-20-one and 5β-pregnan-3α-ol-20-one have similar potencies, but in more physiological models, such as loss of the righting reflex (Selye 1942, Atkinson et al 1965) or brain electrical changes (Gyermek 1967, Kubli-Garfias et al 1976), the 5β-reduced progesterone metabolites are more potent than the 5α forms, where lack of effectiveness is observed, for example with allopregnanedione (5α-pregnane-3,20-dione). Alphaxalone is a potent anaesthetic and it might be interesting to compare it with natural progestins from the physicochemical point of view.

Regarding the clinical picture, it is likely that women suffering seizures during pregnancy have altered progesterone metabolism, because normal pregnancy is associated with sleepiness and feelings of well-being. Thus from the experimental data it seems to me that steroid hormones and their reduced metabolites are modulating cellular excitability to some extent by increasing the seizure thresholds. Therefore, the onset of seizures during pregnancy, as happens in eclampsia for instance, might be related to low levels or altered metabolism of the sex steroids.

Bäckström: We have given women who suffered from partial epilepsy intramuscular injections of medroxyprogesterone in doses that produce amenorrhoea. Similar studies have been done by Richard Mattson in New Haven. Both of us have seen a definite reduction in the number of seizures experienced by these women and some of them have, for the first time in their lives, been completely free of seizures (T. Bäckström, unpublished results; Mattson & Cramer 1985).

I should point out that medroxyprogesterone has an anaesthetic potency much lower than that of progesterone, so its anaesthetic action in the brain is weak. It is possible that its anti-epileptic effect is exerted through interruption of ovarian oestradiol and progesterone production.

Dr Kubli-Garfias said that 5β-reduced metabolites of progesterone are more potent substances in humans than the 5α-reduced compounds. I would dispute that. In humans the 5β pathway is found mainly in the liver and is used for the reduction of steroids there, but the unglucuronized metabolites are not appreciably released into the circulation. The glucuronized steroids are not thought to pass the blood–brain barrier. In the rest of the body, including the brain, it is mainly the 5α-reductase pathway that is used. I would therefore doubt whether 5β-pregnan-3α-ol-20-one is of physiological importance in humans. The concentration of 5α-pregnane-3,20-dione that we have measured during the menstrual cycle is quite high, about a third of the concentration of progesterone.

Kubli-Garfias: The presence of 5β-reduced compounds was established long ago (Dorfman & Ungar 1965, Briggs & Brotherton 1970). Moreover, several years ago, the presence of 5β-pregnanediol in urine was used as a test for pregnancy because it is very abundant in that physiological state. This compound is derived from pregnanolone (5β-pregnan-3β-ol-20-one), which comes from pregnanedione (5β-pregnane-3,20-dione). In any case, I am not denying the existence of 5α-reduced compounds.

Bäckström: 5β-Pregnanediol, being a diol, has a different chemical structure from the potent pregnanolones; also, it's conjugated with glucuronic acid. Progesterone is metabolized in the liver by the 5β-reductase pathway to 5β-pregnanediol and this is conjugated with glucuronic acid. Only after conjugation is it released into the circulation and then excreted in the urine.

Simmonds: We have been talking mainly about steroids produced by the ovary or placenta. Is there a change in neurosteroids during pregnancy?

Baulieu: There has been only one study on this that has been published. Dr Jan-Ake Gustafsson has found that the concentration of the cytochrome *P*-450 enzyme is increased during pregnancy in rat. These results were obtained in biochemical experiments using whole brain homogenates (Warner et al 1989).

Karavolas: We have also studied the neuroendocrine metabolism of progesterone in the rat during pregnancy (Marrone & Karavolas 1981). We observed changes during different days of pregnancy in the 3α-, 5α- and 20α-reduction of progesterone by the pituitary and hypothalamus.

Majewska: Is it possible that epilepsy or PMS could be due to inborn errors in steroid-metabolizing enzymes such as 5α-reductase or 3α-hydroxysteroid oxidoreductase? If there were a deficiency in these enzymes, even if there were high levels of progesterone during pregnancy the anxiolytic/anticonvulsant reduced metabolites could not be formed. This could result in increased neuronal excitability (and seizures or anxiety). As far as I know, no one has yet accurately measured the concentration of tetrahydroprogesterone in blood, so we cannot talk about deficiencies until we can measure levels of this compound.

Bäckström: Inborn errors in steroid-metabolizing enzymes do exist. There is a condition called testicular feminization syndrome, which is sometimes due to lack of the 5α-reductase enzyme. Males with this condition acquire a female phenotype because they can't convert testosterone to 5α-dihydrotestosterone. It is likely that similar and less extreme errors could exist in steroid-metabolizing enzymes in females, so an inborn error of metabolism could well exist.

Martini: I wonder whether we are oversimplifying. I think, for instance, that we should also consider the role of adrenal cortex hormones in epilepsy; it is known that both gluco- and mineralocorticoids influence brain function. The secretion of hydrocortisone during the day shows a 24-hour pattern; is there any indication that in epilepsy there might be a 24-hour cycle, in addition to the 28-day cycle that you showed?

Bäckström: In petit mal epilepsy the seizures usually occur in the morning.

Martini: This is when there are higher levels of hydrocortisone.

Bäckström: In endogenous depression the mood changes during the day. Symptoms of depression are seen mainly in the morning.

Simmonds: I understand that in some cases of childhood epilepsy it is the practice to treat with large doses of prednisolone or prednisone.

Bäckström: ACTH is now used. Treatment with prednisolone has stopped because it was found that ACTH is more effective in decreasing the seizures.

Bernardo Dubrovsky has been studying adrenocorticoids and has found that 5α-THDOC alters the activity in the rat brain. Production of 5α-reduced steroids can be induced by treatment with ACTH (T. Bäckström, unpublished results).

Dubrovsky: Dr K. J. Penry reported a higher incidence of seizures concomitant with elevated dehydroepiandrosterone (DHEA) levels in patients with secreting adrenal adenomas (unpublished). Experimentally, Heuser (1967) showed that intravenous or intraperitoneal injections of DHEA in the 100 mg/kg range induced seizure activity in cebus monkeys, and Dr Majewska referred earlier (p 100) to the excitatory effects of DHEA sulphate. Dr Penry's work and that of Heuser would suggest that DHEA can cross the blood–brain barrier; this is supported too by Dr Majewska's work (personal communication).

Majewska: DHEA sulphate acts as an antagonist at the GABA receptor.

Baulieu: Dehydroepiandrosterone sulphate essentially doesn't pass the blood–brain barrier, so I do not know how to interpret the data. Also, if there is an adrenal tumour, the concentration of other steroids, such as cortisol, may be increased, so these observations should be interpreted with caution.

Su: Dr Bäckström has shown that the progesterone level in the rat cerebral cortex during the luteal phase is 300-fold higher than it is during the other phases. We have found a high level of σ receptor ligand binding in human cerebral cortex. Cowan et al (1979) have compared the abilities of three types of opioid receptor ligands (μ, κ and σ selective) to affect the threshold for induced seizures in rats. They found the σ receptor ligand d-SKF-10047 raised the seizure threshold dramatically. Because of these two findings, I would like to speculate that the epileptogenic effect of progesterone in humans might involve an action at the σ receptor. I wonder if haloperidol, which binds to the σ receptor, might be effective in the treatment of PMS.

Bäckström: I don't think treatment of PMS with haloperidol has ever been tried.

Simmonds: GABA antagonists act as convulsants, but subconvulsant doses have an anxiogenic profile in animal models (Pellow & File 1984). Could both PMS and catamenial epilepsy be related to the interactions of progesterone metabolites with the GABA system? They might be withdrawal reactions from the GABA-potentiating effects of these steroids.

Bäckström: That is a very interesting hypothesis which we are currently investigating.

Majewska: I had thought that some of the symptoms of PMS, particularly those associated with the fall of progesterone levels just before menstruation, might be due to the withdrawal of endogenous anxiolytic progesterone metabolites. However, this cannot be the cause of PMS, because Dr Bäckström has observed the symptoms at the time of peak progesterone levels.

Bäckström: The symptoms of PMS are already severe before progesterone levels begin to decrease and they continue to increase in severity during the last few days of the menstrual cycle. The symptoms actually start to increase in severity at the time of ovulation, when the corpus luteum starts to develop, and they rise more or less in parallel with the initial progesterone rise (Bäckström et al 1983).

Ramirez: We should remember that progesterone can have biphasic actions. Sawyer & Everett (1959) showed that progesterone facilitates ovulation in the rabbit during the first six hours after administration and then has an inhibitory effect 24 hours later. We have shown similar biphasic effects of progesterone on the dopaminergic striatal system of rats. In the first six hours after the initial injection of progesterone the amphetamine-evoked release of dopamine is potentiated, but by 24 hours amphetamine-evoked dopamine release is inhibited. In the premenstrual syndrome, progesterone initially (during the first six or so hours after administration) seems to enhance some of the symptoms, but then it has the opposite effect. Perhaps progesterone itself has a stimulatory effect initially but its metabolites have an opposite, inhibitory effect. Is that possible?

Bäckström: Yes. Professor Martini's comment about substances that are produced by the corpus luteum is also relevant to this point. We have measured progesterone concentrations in women with PMS because we have an assay for progesterone, but we know that numerous steroids are produced by the corpus luteum and many of them are 5α-reduced. We do not know exactly what type or concentration of steroids are produced or whether the steroids that are produced can affect the $GABA_A$ receptor, or if they have other effects in the brain. Also, we don't know whether any of these steroids are altered in patients with PMS. A lot of research needs to be done.

Most of the steroids that we have assayed in women with PMS show plasma concentrations more or less in parallel with each other during the luteal phase. So, when we see a relationship between progesterone levels and the development of a symptom, that symptom could be due to the effect of another steroid or protein that is produced by the corpus luteum in parallel with progesterone.

Majewska: Dr Glowinski's and Dr Joubert-Bression's data indicate that oestradiol interacts with dopamine receptors in the brain and pituitary. Since the dopaminergic system is important in the control of mood, varying oestrogen levels may be important in the aetiology of PMS.

Bäckström: We measured the concentration of oestradiol and progesterone in blood samples taken during the luteal phase of two consecutive menstrual cycles from 18 patients with PMS. The mean severity of these patient's symptoms differed in the two cycles and the changes in severity of the symptoms between the cycles correlated with the oestradiol concentration during the luteal phase more closely than with the progesterone concentration (Hammarbäck et al 1989).

Majewska: Perhaps the ratio of oestradiol to progesterone is the important factor.

Bäckström: Yes, or perhaps progesterone has some kind of permissive action on a dose-dependent effect of oestradiol, similar to its effects on uterine prostaglandin production, where the stimulatory influence of oestradiol on prostaglandin production is dose dependent only in the presence of progesterone (Downie et al 1974, Abel 1979). So there are other biological systems in which the interaction of oestrogen and progesterone is important. We are only at the beginning of a new understanding of the relationship between steroids and the CNS, but I hope we shall soon know how PMS arises.

Smith: A wide array of symptoms, both somatic and psychological, are reported from women experiencing cyclical discomfort during the premenstrual period. The global aspect of this symptomatology suggests that multiple hormone effects on a variety of substrates may be responsible. More specifically, the anxiety that is sometimes associated with the premenstrual syndrome has been correlated with low and rapidly falling levels of progesterone relative to other ovarian steroids (Dennerstein et al 1985); administration of progesterone, which has been shown to be anxiolytic in humans and in animal models of anxiety (Herrman & Beach 1978, Rodriguez-Sierra et al 1984), can alleviate these symptoms. These anxiolytic actions of this steroid are indeed consistent with the GABA-enhancing action of its 5α-reduced metabolites.

References

Abel MA 1979 Production of prostaglandins by the human uterus: are they involved in menstruation? Res Clin Forums 1:33–37

Andersch B, Wendestam C, Hahn L, Öhman R 1986 Premenstrual complaints. I. Prevalence of premenstrual symptoms in a Swedish urban population. J Psychosom Obstet Gynaecol 5:39–49

Atkinson RM, Davis B, Pratt MA, Sharpe MH, Tomich EG 1965 Action of some steroids on the central nervous system of the mouse. II. Pharmacol J Med Chem 8:426–432

Bäckström T, Sanders D, Leask R, Davidson D, Warner P, Bancroft J 1983 Mood, sexuality, hormones and the menstrual cycle. II. Hormone levels and their relationship to the premenstrual syndrome. Psychosom Med 45:503–507

Bäckström T, Andersson A, Baird DT, Selstam G 1986 5α-pregnane-3,20-dione in peripheral and ovarian vein blood of women of different stages of the menstrual cycle. Acta Endocrinol 111:116–121

Briggs MH, Brotherton J 1970 Steroid biochemistry and pharmacology. Academic Press, London & New York

Cowan A, Geller EB, Adler MW 1979 Classification of opioids on the basis of change in seizure threshold in rats. Science (Wash DC) 206:465–467

Dennerstein L, Spencer-Gardner C, Gotts G, Brown JB, Smith MD, Burrows GD 1985 Progesterone and the premenstrual syndrome: a double blind crossover trial. Br Med J 290:1617–1621

Dorfman RI, Ungar F 1965 Metabolism of steroid hormones. Academic Press, London & New York

Downie J, Poyser N L, Wunderlich M 1974 Levels of prostaglandins in human endometrium during the normal menstrual cycle. J Physiol (Lond) 236:465–469

Gyermek L 1967 Pregnanolone: a highly potent naturally occurring hypnotic-anesthetic agent. Proc Soc Exp Biol Med (NY) 125:1058–1062

Hammarbäck S, Bäckström T, Holst J, von Schoultz B, Lyrenäs S 1985 Cyclical mood changes as in the premenstrual tension syndrome during sequential estrogen-progestagen postmenopausal replacement therapy. Acta Obstet Gynecol Scand 64:393–397

Hammarbäck S, Damber J-E, Bäckström T 1989 Relationship between symptom severity and hormone changes in patients with premenstrual syndrome. J Clin Endocrinol Metab 68:125–130

Herrman WM, Beach RC 1978 Experimental and clinical data indicating the psychotropic properties of progestogens. Postgrad Med J 54:82–87

Heuser G 1967 Induction of anesthesia, seizures and sleep by steroid hormones. Anesthesiology 28:173–182

Janz D, Dam M, Richens A, Bossi L, Helge H, Schmidt D 1982 Epilepsy, pregnancy and the child. Raven Press, New York

Kappas A, Hellman L, Fukushima D, Gallagher TF 1958 The thermogenic effect and metabolic fate of etiocholanolone in man. J Clin Endocrinol 18:1043–1050

Kubli-Garfias C, Cervantes M, Beyer C 1976 Changes in multiunit activity and EEG induced by the administration of natural progestins to flaxedil immobilized cats. Brain Res 114:71–81

Landgren S, Aasly J, Bäckström T, Dubrovsky B, Danielsson E 1987 The effect of progesterone and its metabolites on the interictal epileptiform discharge in the cat's cortex. Acta Physiol Scand 131:33–42

Marrone BL, Karavolas HJ 1981 Progesterone metabolism by the hypothalamus, pituitary and uterus of the rat during pregnancy. Endocrinology 109:41–45

Mattson R, Cramer J 1985 Epilepsy, sex hormones and antiepileptic drugs. Epilepsia 26 Suppl 1:S40-S51

Pellow S, File SE 1984 Multiple sites of action for anxiogenic drugs: behavioural, electrophysiological and biochemical correlations. Psychopharmacology 83:304–315

Rodriguez-Sierra JF, Howard JL, Pollard GT, Hendrickes SE 1984 Effect of ovarian hormones on conflict behavior. Psychoneuroendocrinology 9:293–300

Sawyer CH, Everett JW 1959 Stimulatory and inhibitory effects of progesterone on the release of pituitary ovulating hormone in the rabbit. Endocrinology 65:644

Selye H 1942 Correlation between the chemical structure and pharmacological actions of the steroids. Endocrinology 30:437–453

Smith SS 1989 Estrogen administration increases neuronal responses to excitatory amino acids as a long-term effect. Brain Res 503:354–357

Warner M, Tollet P, Strämstedt M, Calström K, Gustafsson JA 1989 Endocrine regulation of cytochrome P-450 in the rat brain and pituitary gland. J Endocrinol 122:341–349

Early and late effects of steroid hormones on the central nervous system

B. Dubrovsky, D. Filipini, K. Gijsbers* and M. K. Birmingham

Laboratories of Neurophysiology and Steroid Biochemistry, McGill University, 1033 Pine Avenue West, Montreal, Quebec, Canada H3A 1A1 and *Psychology Department, Stirling University, Stirling, FK9 4LA, UK

Abstract. Steroids have fast and probably partly GABA-mediated central anaesthetic effects for which a strict structure–function correlation is required. They also affect short- and long-term activity in the CNS in other ways. One of these is long-term potentiation (the persistent facilitation of synaptic transmission), which occurs particularly in the hippocampus after repetitive stimulation of a fibre pathway. Two clearly distinguished components of the evoked response can be studied in the hippocampus: the excitatory postsynaptic potential (EPSP) which denotes the graded depolarization of the somadendritic region of the neuron and the population spike (PS), a manifestation of the all-or-none discharge of the cell action potential. Corticosterone had a significant depressant effect on the EPSP component of the evoked response immediately and 15 min after injection. Thereafter EPSP amplitudes were within normal values. Corticosterone significantly decreased the PS immediately after the train, the component remaining low 30 min after the train. 5α-Dihydrocorticosterone (a ring A-reduced metabolite of corticosterone) significantly reduced the PS component of the response at all times after injection. 18-Hydroxydeoxycorticosterone and deoxycorticosterone significantly decreased both EPSP and PS components of the evoked response from the time of infusion. Contrary to expectation, tetrahydrodeoxycorticosterone was ineffective in decreasing, and if anything, enhanced the development of long-term potentiation. 18-Hydroxydeoxycorticosterone 21-acetate behaved like vehicle, except for the first 30 min after injection, when the EPSP was decreased. Different steroids can selectively affect different parts of a neuron and appear to show a different structure–function correlation for long-term potentiation from that required for anaesthesia.

1990 Steroids and neuronal activity. Wiley, Chichester (Ciba Foundation Symposium 153) p 240–260

Steroid anaesthesia was first reported in experimental animals by Selye in 1941 and introduced into clinical use in 1955. From the beginning it was recognized that certain structural constraints were necessary for the steroid molecule to exert its anaesthetic effects. These conformational requirements indicate that steroid membrane lipophilicity cannot be the only mechanism mediating this effect. Current studies suggest that the anaesthetic effects of some steroids may depend on their capacity to behave in some measure as barbiturate-like ligands of the GABA receptor–chloride ion channel complex (Harrison et al 1987), or to modulate the GABA receptor complex at a site distinct from barbiturates (Turner et al 1989).

These developments, and the fact that a minimal change in the structure of a steroid anaesthetic molecule (e.g. the introduction of a double bond in the D ring of the steroid nucleus; Richards & Hesketh 1975) renders it ineffective, challenge the Meyer-Overton lipid solubility rule: 'The narcotizing substances enter into loose physicochemical combination with the vitally important lipoids of the cell . . .'. It is believed that an effective interaction between anaesthetics and the cells is mediated through the formation of non-covalent hydrophobic bonds (Miller & Roth 1986).

However, besides the recently established effects *in vitro* of adrenal steroids on the GABA receptor–chloride ion channel complex (Harrison et al 1987, Turner et al 1989, Turner & Simmonds 1989), steroids exert a multiplicity of effects on the nervous system involving modulation of neurotransmitter systems as well as regulation of protein synthesis. Many of these effects, but not all, are probably mediated via genomic induction (McEwen et al 1986).

That these effects have important behavioural consequences is revealed by behavioural and clinical work. Thus a frequent manifestation of Cushing's disease is affective disorder, mostly in the form of depression (Jeffcoate et al 1979). In turn, a significantly large population of patients (44% with major depression and 50% with melancholia) show signs of adrenal hyperactivity, with non-suppression in the dexamethasone-suppression test (Arana & Mossman 1988). However, in neither case is the magnitude of the psychological disturbance related linearly to cortisol levels in blood; mild depressions can be accompanied by high cortisol levels, and vice versa (Arana & Mossman 1988). This should not be surprising, because cortisol is one of many steroid compounds secreted by the adrenal cortex, and in a state of adrenal hyperactivity there is hyper-secretion of several of these compounds. As Holzbauer et al (1985) wrote: 'The endocrinologist sees the adrenal cortex primarily as a source of hormones capable of modifying carbohydrate metabolism, of controlling inflammatory processes and of conserving body sodium. The extent to which this gland contributes hormones not confined to so-called gluco- and mineralocorticoid activities is much less readily considered and deserves attention. These include steroids commonly associated with the ovary such as progesterone or pregnenolone, as well as other steroids devoid of gonadal or corticoid activity, which may nevertheless have a biological role, possibly related to their anaesthetic action.'

The hypercortisolaemia of depressed patients was thought to be secondary to a deficit in catecholamine levels (Maas & Garver 1975), because catecholamines were thought to inhibit the parvicellular zone of the paraventricular nucleus (PVN) which secretes ACTH-releasing factor. Hence a lowering of catecholamine levels would be accompanied by a disinhibition of the PVN, excess ACTH and excess cortisol. But this view of hypercortisolaemia in depression as secondary to catecholamine deficit can no longer be maintained, because the available data support the view that catecholamines have an excitatory impact on the PVN (Negro-Vilar et al 1987).

Both Cushing's disease and depressive disease present characteristic memory impairments. In depression, patients tend to remember the negative aspects of their lives (Dunbar & Lishman 1984). In certain kinds of depression these disturbances can become a central focus of the disease. We therefore asked whether steroid hormones could be involved in the establishment and biasing of memories. The reasons for asking this question were that the hippocampus, a crucial structure in memory mechanisms, is also a main target for adrenal steroid hormones (McEwen et al 1986), and that these selective memory disturbances in Cushing's disease and in depressive patients are relieved by treatment of the adrenal hyperactivity of these patients.

We are trying to answer this question at both the experimental and clinical levels. This report relates mainly to the experimental work, in which we chose to study the effects of steroid hormones and their ring A-reduced metabolites on long-term potentiation. We selected this phenomenon for investigation because it is a well-established and quantifiable index of neuronal plasticity related to memory.

In the early 1970s, Bliss & Lomo (1973) described the enhancement of synaptic transmission in a monosynaptic path in the hippocampus after a tetanic priming stimulation. They termed this enhancement, which can last from hours to weeks, long-term potentiation (LTP). The length of the process, and the fact that it can be even more easily elicited by using as priming stimuli a sequence of naturally occurring bursts, led to the speculation that these electrophysiological changes could underlie memory and learning functions in the nervous system (Bliss & Lynch 1988).

These speculations were supported by various experiments that implied a causal relationship between LTP and learning. In one study it was possible to link changes in LTP with the age-related decline in the learning of spatial relations in a task known to involve the hippocampus. The amount of synaptic enhancement was statistically correlated with this behavioural ability. Moreover, LTP was maintained in young animals for at least 14 days, whereas in senescent rats it declined after the first high frequency priming sessions (Bliss & Lynch 1988).

Other workers have attempted to relate factors that enhance learning, such as post-trial stimulation of the mesencephalic reticular formation, to LTP.

It was found that the magnitude of LTP in the dentate gyrus of rats with chronically implanted electrodes was increased by stimulation of the reticular formation and that the time when reticular stimulation was most effective (10 seconds after tetanic stimulation) was also the time when learning was most effectively enhanced after trials (Bliss & Lynch 1988).

Recently the effects of exposure to a complex environment on potentials evoked by perforant path stimulation in the hippocampus were examined. Experiments in intact rats with implanted electrodes, as well as experiments in which these potentials were subsequently examined *in vitro*, showed similar results: increases in the amplitude of the two components of the evoked potential, the excitatory postsynaptic potential (EPSP) which denotes graded depolarization of the somadendritic region of the neuron, and the population spike (PS), a manifestation of the all-or-none discharge of the cell action potential (Bliss & Lynch 1988).

An important experiment showing a causal relation between LTP and learning in rats was reported by Morris et al (1986). They found that the antagonist of N-methyl-D-aspartate (NMDA), AP5 (2-amino-5-phosphonopentanoic acid), which blocks LTP without affecting synaptic transmission, severely impaired the acquisition of spatial learning in a water maze, a task mediated by the hippocampus. Performance of a visual discrimination task in the same animal, a task not believed to be mediated by the hippocampus, was not affected (Morris et al 1986). For all these reasons we feel it appropriate to study the effects of steroids on LTP.

Methods

To avoid saturation of putative corticosteroid receptors and binding sites we used adult male Sprague-Dawley rats that were adrenalectomized. Adrenalectomies were performed in our laboratories two days before the LTP experiments.

Animals were anaesthetized with chloral hydrate. The femoral artery and vein of one side were cannulated for blood pressure monitoring and drug infusion respectively. The temperature was monitored with a rectal thermometer and kept at 37 °C with a DC heating pad. A non-concentric bipolar electrode was positioned in the region of the perforant path parallel to the direction of the nerve fibres. The perforant path constitutes the main body of hippocampal afferents. A tungsten microelectrode (3–5 MΩ) was positioned in the zone of the dentate gyrus for recording. Stimulation was effected via an S8 stimulator with bipolar pulses to prevent electrode polarization. The priming tetanic stimulation used consisted of five trains of impulses of a total duration of one second, of train rate 0.03 Hz; the frequency in each train was 400 Hz, with a pulse duration of 50 μs in each half wave. Applied current intensities ranged from 100 to 600 μA. We avoided the effects of the circadian rhythm on LTP

(Dana & Martinez 1984) by doing all experiments at the same time of day, in the early afternoon. The data were analysed by paired two-tailed *t*-test analysis.

Perforant path evoked responses

Stimulation of the perforant path evoked a characteristic response in granular cells of the dentate gyrus (Fig. 1). A short latency potential (about 1.1 ms)

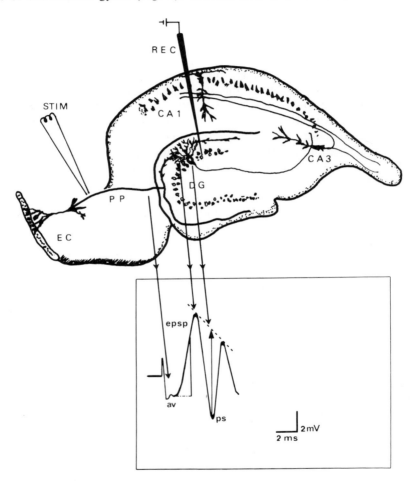

FIG. 1. Schematic diagram of mammalian hippocampus showing the stimulating electrode (STIM) in the perforant path (PP) and the recording electrode (REC) in the granular cells of the dentate gyrus (DG). EC, enthorhinal cortex. Inset, evoked potential generated in DG by stimulation of PP is illustrated, showing the afferent volley (av), excitatory postsynaptic potential (epsp) and population spike (ps) with their respective field generators.

reflecting the presynaptic volley could be observed, although not in all cases. A second component with a latency of 1.6–2.5 ms was reliably observed. It is generated by the flow of synaptic current around the granule cells and is thus known as the population excitatory postsynaptic potential (EPSP). With sufficiently strong stimulation, a spike-shaped wave form superimposed on the EPSP appears. It is the envelope of the action potentials generated in the granule cells and is termed the population spike (PS).

The latency and amplitude of the PS were more variable than those of the population EPSP. Moreover, the population EPSP and the PS can change independently of each other; for example, they are differently affected by selective depletion of monoamines or by the action of hormones (Bliss & Lynch 1988, Dubrovsky et al 1987, Morimoto & Goddard 1985).

One important problem in evaluating the effects of steroids on the CNS has been to find a suitable vehicle, because many of the agents used, such as ethanol, themselves have central effects. The C-21 esters have been used to increase water solubility (e.g., hydroxydione in the anaesthetics Viadril and alphalodone in Althesin). Solvents used to increase steroid solubility have included Cremophor-EL and propylene glycol, but they are not inert. In contrast, Nutralipid not only behaves as an inert solvent but further enhances the entry of steroids into the brain. We compared the entry into the brain of labelled [3H] progesterone when administered intravenously in Nutralipid and in ethanol/saline (1:9). At tracer concentrations, 0.066% was recovered and at maximal (9 mg/ml) concentrations 0.18% was recovered from ethanol/saline. In contrast, 0.82 and 0.91% was recovered from Nutralipid at tracer and maximal concentrations respectively (Murphy et al 1986). We therefore used 10% Nutralipid as vehicle in our studies.

Results and discussion

The effects of corticosterone and 5α-dihydrocorticosterone were examined first. Our previous work revealed that corticosterone increased the discharge rate of tonically firing neurons in the pontine brainstem reticular formation, whereas its 5α-reduced metabolite, 5α-dihydrocorticosterone, decreased it (Dubrovsky et al 1985). It was also shown then that the two molecules—parent compound and metabolite—can counteract each other's effects.

In relation to the evoked potential components of LTP, corticosterone significantly decreased the amplitude of the EPSPs for the first 15 min after the train of stimuli but matched control values (with Nutralipid) thereafter (Fig. 2). After corticosterone injection, the PS showed a decrease immediately after the train, remaining low up to 30 min after (Fig. 3). Thus the response to corticosterone shows effects exerted at different times and at different neuronal loci.

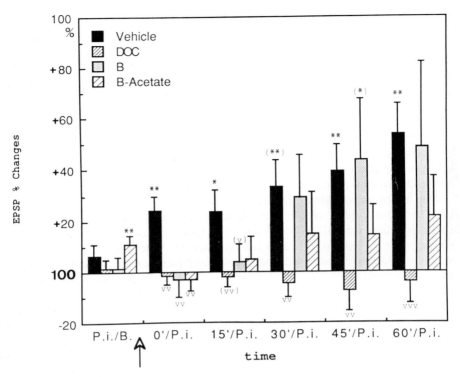

FIG. 2. Bar diagram showing the relative changes in time of the amplitude of the excitatory postsynaptic potentials (EPSPs) during the development of long-term potentiation after i.v. injection of corticosterone (B), corticosterone acetate (B-Acetate) and deoxycorticosterone (DOC) in adrenalectomized rats. Arrow denotes priming tetanic stimulation. Injection precedes stimulation by 2 min. Statistical significance: *, intrinsic; ^{v}, *versus* vehicle. $^{(*)}P<0.1$; $^{(**)}P<0.02$; $*P<0.05$; $**P<0.01$; $^{(v)}P<0.1$; $^{(vv)}P<0.02$; $^vP<0.05$; $^{vv}P<0.01$; $^{vvv}P<0.001$.

Hall (1982) had reported dissociated effects on neuronal excitability induced by methylprednisolone. This steroid lowered the threshold in the initial segment and increased it in the somadendritic region. The timing of the effects (up to 15 min in the EPSPs and up to 60 min after injection in the PSs) showed an overlap with the time course of the two components of LTP (early and late), as recently described by Davies et al (1989). According to these authors, both presynaptic and postsynaptic mechanisms contribute to the maintenance of the LTP, but in a temporally distinct manner. Postsynaptic sensitivity, which changes the late component of LTP, cannot be detected for at least 15 min after induction and takes about two hours to reach maximum development. This implicates presynaptic mechanisms in the early stages of LTP. It can be recalled here that steroids can act at presynaptic sites (Turner & Simmonds 1989) and

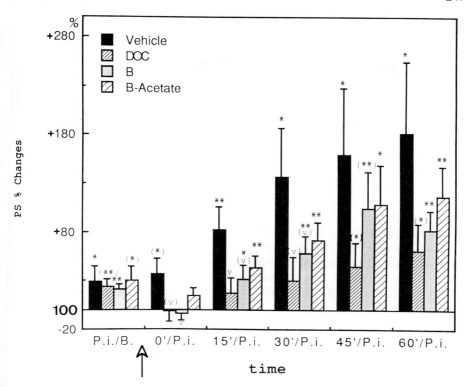

FIG. 3.   Bar diagram showing the relative changes in time of the amplitude of the population spike (PS) during the development of LTP after i.v. injection of corticosterone, corticosterone acetate and deoxycorticosterone. Arrow, priming tetanic stimulation.

that 5α-reductase, the rate-limiting enzyme for steroid metabolism, is found in larger amounts in white than in grey matter (Celotti et al 1987). It is conceivable, then, that adrenal steroids can affect both early and late components of LTP, via pre- and postsynaptic mechanisms.

5α-Dihydrocorticosterone impaired the development of the PS component of the LTP from time zero after priming stimulation throughout the experiment (Dubrovsky et al 1987).

Corticosterone acetate, in turn, decreased EPSP excitability, 15 min after the train of stimuli (Fig. 2). The effect of this steroid on PS was equivocal in relation to vehicle (Fig. 3).

These results seem to imply that structural characteristics of the corticosteroid play an important role in modulating a plastic phenomenon in the hippocampus such as LTP. This premise was substantiated by further work on the effects of 18-hydroxydeoxycorticosterone (18OHDOC) and its 21-acetate form on LTP in the rat hippocampus. 18OHDOC is the most abundant mineralocorticoid hormone in the rat. Addition of a hydroxyl group at C-18 modifies the biological properties of some pregnane derivatives, such as the inhibitory effect of deoxycorticosterone (DOC) on pituitary–adrenal function, as well as obliterating the glycolytic effects of DOC, progesterone and corticosterone in the adrenal gland.

Our previous work showed that 18OHDOC decreases CNS excitability for a short period, up to 30 min after injection, starting at 10–15 min (Dubrovsky et al 1986). In the case of LTP, a long-term phenomenon, 18OHDOC affected both components of the evoked time potential responses in the dentate gyrus.

Immediately after injection and throughout the recording period of 60 min the excitatory postsynaptic potential decreased significantly from control levels, reaching its lowest levels at 60 min. The population spike was also significantly depressed after the train stimulus, throughout the experiment (K. Gijsbers & B. Dubrovsky 1989, unpublished work) (Fig. 4).

In contrast to these effects of 18OHDOC, its 21-acetate form significantly decreased the EPSP component of the EP for only the first 30 min after the train of stimuli (Fig. 4). PS was not affected by 18OHDOC acetate in relation to vehicle (Fig. 4). This is in keeping with the notion that steroids do not act just by combining with 'lipoids' in the cell wall. The 21-acetate derivative of 18OHDOC will have an enhanced lipophilicity imparted by masking of the 21-hydroxyl group. This notwithstanding, its effects on LTP were minimal.

DOC and its ring A tetrahydroderivative, 5α-pregnane-3α,21-diol-20-one (allotetrahydrodeoxycorticosterone) were also examined. We already know the depressant effects of both these steroids on CNS activity, and that, at the single-neuron level, the onset latency of the effect of the ring A-reduced metabolite of DOC was significantly shorter than that for DOC itself (Dubrovksy et al 1982). Our results revealed that DOC significantly impaired the development of LTP and that this impairment, observed in both components of the evoked potential (EPSP and PS), increased with time in the EPSP, and was not significant after 30 min in the PS (D. Filipini & B. Dubrovsky 1989, unpublished work). (Figs. 2 & 3).

Contrary to expectation, alloTHDOC not only did not decrease the evoked potentials of LTP, but even marginally increased the amplitude of both its EPSP and PS components (D. Filipini & B. Dubrovsky 1989, unpublished work). As GABA can block the induction of LTP (Scharfman & Sarvey 1985), and as, jointly with 5α-pregnan-3α-ol-20-one (3α-OH-DHP), alloTHDOC is one of the two steroid metabolites that most potently enhance GABA responses (Harrison et al 1987), this appears to be a surprising result. However, a closer look at GABAergic effects in the hippocampus can explain this apparent paradox. Some of the excitatory (i.e. disinhibitory) effects of GABA on hippocampal neurons can be due to the inhibition of GABAergic interneurons by GABAergic terminals (Milner & Bacon 1989). AlloTHDOC could enhance the synaptic contacts on

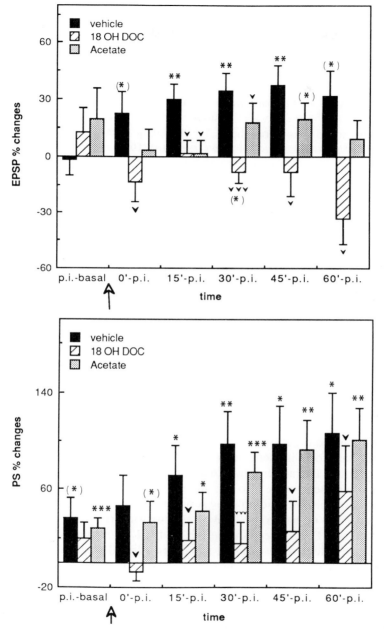

FIG. 4.   Bar diagrams showing the relative change in amplitude of the EPSP and PS during the development of long-term potentiation under the influence of 18-hydroxydeoxycorticosterone (18OHDOC) and 18OHDOC acetate (Acetate).

GABAergic interneurons, and in this way increase the amplitude of hippocampal responses during LTP.

Besides direct activation of the chloride ion channel, GABA also induces phospholipase C activation (Corradetti et al 1987), while phospholipase C is known to mediate the activation of protein kinase C. Inhibition of the latter enzyme inhibits the development of LTP (Akers et al 1986), but it is not yet known if this phospholipase activation by GABA is also enhanced by steroids.

Steroids could also modulate LTP by being part of the mechanisms of activation of protein kinase C. Liu & Greengard (1976) have identified a cytosolic protein whose extent of phosphorylation is regulated by both cyclic AMP and steroid hormones. This protein, called SCARP ('steroid and cyclic AMP regulated phosphoprotein'), has been suggested to be the regulatory subunit of protein kinase C: if so, regulation of the phosphorylation of this protein could affect the activity of protein kinase C, and hence LTP.

The effect of the steroid hormones in decreasing the phosphorylation of SCARP was specific for their respective target tissues (e.g. 17β-oestradiol for uterus; cortisol, liver; testosterone, ventral prostate and seminal vesicle). Further, a protein synthesis inhibitor, cycloheximide, abolished the effect of the steroid hormones, but not of cyclic AMP, on the endogenous phosphorylation of SCARP.

The modulation of the GABA receptor by steroids shows both stereospecificity and dose-dependence. Both 5α- and 5β-pregnanes display this response. Essential features of the steroid structure appear to be a 3α-hydroxyl group and a ketone group at position C-20; 3β-OH derivatives are inert in this respect (Harrison et al 1987).

Structural requirements for effects of steroid molecules on LTP were revealed in our studies on 18OHDOC and its 21-acetate form. Whereas significant depression of both EPSP and PS components was observed with 18OHDOC, the 21-acetate form induced depression of the EPSP only for the first 30 min after injection. Thereafter, amplitude values were the same as for controls and the PS components were also not significantly different from controls.

In addition, 5α-reduction of ring A of the corticosterone molecule produced a very different effect on the LTP components in experimental animals. Ring A reduction of DOC reverses the effect on the LTP response from depressant to excitatory. However, while ring A-reduced adrenal pregnanes have powerful effects on CNS excitability, some of them appear to be devoid of feedback effects. At a dose of 1 mg/100 g injected subcutaneously, both corticosterone and DOC reduced stress levels (obtained after half an hour of immobilization) of serum corticosterone from 21.4 ± 2.3 µg per 100 ml to 6.4 ± 0.7 and 6.4 ± 2.0 µg, respectively, while 5α-dihydro-DOC (18.9 ± 1.9) and 5α-dihydrocorticosterone (18.5 ± 1.8) had no effect (Kraulis et al 1975, Dubrovsky et al 1985).

As the effects of a hormone or neurotransmitter become specified only by the response induced at the receptor site, the message is therefore not necessarily determined by the messenger itself, so a particular steroid molecule acting on different neuronal loci could have different effects. This is in keeping with what has become an evolutionary norm in endocrinology, that steroids, like other hormones, were originally biological regulatory molecules and their present-day hormonal role came about by target organ specialization and not by the evolution of the molecules themselves (Sandor & Mehdi 1979).

Steroid hormones differentially affect the two components of the LTP response (EPSP and PS). As these components represent the activity of different neuronal sites, the EPSP representing somadendritic depolarization and the PS representing the action potential of the initial segment, the selective effects of hormones on the EPSP and PS could represent selective effects of steroids on distinct neural loci.

Reminiscent of these phenomena are the data of Feldman (1981) on the modification of responses to sensory and hippocampal stimuli in the hypothalamus of rats in the presence of cortisol. It was shown that whereas tonic activity was not altered by iontophoretically applied cortisol in succinate form, neuronally evoked responses were affected by the hormone. That is, mechanisms related to tonic discharge in the rat mediobasal hypothalamus were unaffected by the application of cortisol, but mechanisms related to neuronal responsiveness were significantly modified. Of particular significance were a group of hypothalamic cells which are normally silent and respond to afferent stimulation with inhibition of glutamate stimulation. In the presence of cortisol, the inhibitory responses of these neurons were reduced or became excitatory.

Our studies of the short- and long-term effects of adrenal steroids on neuronal excitability touch upon this problem too. Whereas we evaluated short-term excitability changes by measuring firing rates and constructing interval histograms of tonically discharging neurons in the pontine brainstem (Dubrovsky et al 1982, 1985), we studied long-term effects by evaluating changes in a hippocampal response triggered in the nervous system by a priming stimulus, as described here. Distinct neuronal processes are involved in generating tonic activity and evoked responses during LTP, a phenomenon intimately linked to memory (Bliss & Lynch 1988), and these processes are differentially affected by steroid compounds and their ring A-reduced metabolites, as we have shown.

The reduction of the double bond between carbon atoms 4 and 5 of steroid molecules is the first step in a sequence of reactions leading to the production of water-soluble conjugates which are excreted. It also results in the formation of compounds of key biological importance. There is considerable evidence that Δ^4 reduction is the rate-limiting step in steroid metabolism: when the reductases have performed their actions, other enzymes, in particular the 3α- and 3β-hydroxysteroid dehydrogenases, reduce the ring A-saturated steroids to 3α- and 3β-hydroxysteroids that are the substrates for glucuronyltransferases and sulphokinases. Thus, any altered rates of steroid reduction can lead to changes in the amount of native hormone available for the expression of its activity and that of its metabolites. For example, administration of ACTH to humans decreases the formation of 5α-reduced metabolites from injected cortisol by decreasing reductase activity. Other situations exist where the extent to which adrenal steroids are metabolized to tetrahydro metabolites is decreased, with a corresponding increase in the production of metabolites such as 6-hydroxycortisol, which is more polar and can be excreted in a free or unconjugated state. One of these situations is Cushing's syndrome.

As already mentioned, there is a positive correlation between hyperactivity of the adrenal cortex and memory disturbances in patients suffering from Cushing's disease and depressive diseases. We have seen dramatic improvements in depressive patients showing hypercortisolaemia who were treated with ketoconazole, an inhibitor of steroid synthesis (B. Dubrovsky, D. Spiguel & P. Gabay, unpublished observations). Memory bias in Cushing's patients is also relieved when the endocrine disorder is treated.

Could it be that a particular hormonal spectrum, with particular adrenal steroids acting through the hippocampus, enhances in a specific way the laying down of positively or negatively charged memories? We would argue that our memory of processes that have negative connotations may be enhanced by a specific hormonal spectrum, to which certain adrenal compounds may contribute. This is in keeping with the accepted notion that hormones play a role in establishing particularly vivid memories that develop when a stressful event occurs.

If a specific hormonal spectrum accompanies a particularly stressful event that has negative connotations, the maintenance or reactivation of that internal milieu will be an important factor in creating or recreating the mood of that state. The effect of context on memory is well recognized, and one very powerful source of this context effect in memory is mood. We propose that one of the effects of disinhibition of the hypothalamo-hypophysial-adrenal axis observed in patients with Cushing's disease and in depressive patients could be a setting of the mood that affects memory mechanisms, so characteristically biased in these patients. This could be effected via the action of adrenal steroids on the hippocampus, one of the main structures mediating their behavioural effects. The steroid biasing of memory mechanisms, by setting a background against which to evaluate present events, could set the conditions for cognitive models of depression. In these models, negative thinking is seen not as a symptom, as classically regarded in psychiatry, but as causally related to depression.

Different steroids may affect the processing of positive or negative memories in different ways. If their effects counteract each other, we may be able to design new pharmacological strategies for the therapy of CNS disorders where steroid imbalance can play a role, as in Cushing's disease and depressive diseases.

As described (p 250), we have shown that certain ring A-reduced metabolites, such as 5α-dihydrocorticosterone and 5α-dihydroDOC, although endowed with powerful effects on CNS excitability, lack feedback effects on ACTH secretion. There are instances, such as in Addison's disease, where one aspect of nervous activity is enhanced (e.g. sensitivity) while other aspects (e.g. neural discrimination) are decreased. For example, the detection threshold for salt in Addison's patients falls by several orders of magnitude. But, in spite of the lowered threshold for sensory stimuli, the Addisonian patient exhibits an impairment of judgement and of the ability to discriminate sensory inputs.

Dose-dependent effects, either sedation or seizures, have been described with various steroids, including 11-deoxycortisol, dehydroepiandrosterone (Heuser 1967), and alphaxalone (File & Simmonds 1988). In the short term (5–20 min), alloTHDOC decreased the neural excitability of tonically firing mesencephalic reticular formation cells, while enhancing the hippocampal responsiveness of LTP—a circuit phenomenon—at a later time (15–60 min). In contrast, Morimoto & Goddard (1985) showed that thyrotropin-releasing hormone (TRH) increases dentate gyrus responses to perforant path stimulation immediately after injection, but depresses LTP expression at a later stage—that is, it depresses the same responses. Thus hormonal effects on excitability are dose, time, state and site dependent. It may be possible to extend to neuroendocrinology a widely held notion in neurophysiology, that nervous systems process signals (chemical and/or physical) in parallel.

Thus, in contrast to the classically held notion that the brain processes signals only in a sequential mode, where, at each step in a neural path, all signals collectively are further analysed and specified, an alternative way may be parallel brain processing, where different brain regions process different aspects of sensory system signals. This concept depends on the fact that the emergence of phylogenetically new neural structures, derived from earlier ones during evolution, appears to be related to the development of new functions as well as the refinement of existing ones, as carried out by the ancestral structures. Almost without exception the invasion of a new ecological niche requires behavioural changes, and these behavioural changes are followed by structural ones. Moreover, as already postulated by William James, it is now clear that two aspects of the visual world, form and space, have a different evolutionary history, anatomy, and physiology in nervous systems. Thus a group of fibres project from the retina directly to the superior colliculus, a mesencephalic structure; the path continues to a diencephalic target, the pulvinar nucleus, and from here mainly to parastriate and striate cortex (Fig. 5). Lesions in this pathway severely impair visual spatial orientation without significantly affecting visual form discrimination. In contrast, lesions of the path from the retina to the lateral geniculate nucleus, which projects to the striate cortex (Fig. 5), preferentially impair visual form discrimination, while visual spatial orientation behaviour remains essentially unchanged. It is therefore possible to speak of two

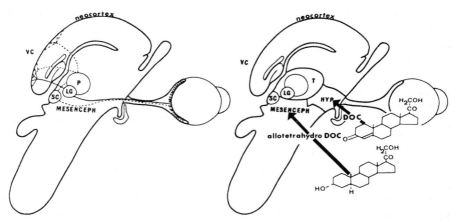

FIG. 5. Schematic diagram showing (*left*) the parallel processing of visual signals. The evolutionary ancestral path from retina to superior colliculus (SC) to the pulvinar nucleus (P) and to cortex relates to visual spatial orientation. The derived path from retina to lateral geniculate (LG) to cortex relates to form discrimination. Parallel processing of a hormonal chemical signal, deoxycorticosterone (DOC) is also shown (*right*). In the hypothalamic-hypophysial region, DOC acts on feedback neuroendocrine mechanisms. In mesencephalic regions, a ring A-reduced DOC derivative such as allotetrahydro-deoxycorticosterone acts on brain excitability as an anxiolytic and anaesthetic agent.

visual systems, for spatial and for form discrimination. And their evolutionary history is also distinct: the spatial orientation path is ancestral to the derived form discrimination path. This description clearly implies complementarity of the two aspects; its bases have been reliably established, at both experimental and clinical levels (Dubrovsky & Garcia-Rill 1971).

We believe the same principle can be applied to the processing of hormonal signals by nervous systems. In the words of Peter Medawar (1953): 'Endocrine evolution was not an evolution of the hormones but an evolution of the uses to which they are put'—that is, how a hormone is metabolized and interacts at different loci. We should take into account the evolutionary history of each hormonal receptor at different sites if we wish to understand the mode of operation of the receptors in each region.

Finally, these dissociated properties of hormones and their metabolites can provide the basis for rational treatments of neuropsychiatric disorders, such as the affective diseases produced by adrenal hyperactivity. We have shown that while deoxycorticosterone and corticosterone affect both brain excitability and feedback regulatory mechanisms, their ring A-reduced metabolites affect only CNS excitability. The biological processing of the chemical signal—the hormone—will determine its final action. As we have also shown, the effects of excitatory and depressant steroids can in many instances counteract each other in the CNS. Coupled with the dissociation between the effects of the hormones and their metabolites, these fundamental notions can serve as a basis for physiological therapeutics in neuroendocrine and psychiatric disorders produced by endocrine imbalance.

Acknowledgements

I would like to thank Dr I. Kraulis for her uninterrupted and cooperative work and Miss K. Smith for her excellent typing assistance. I would also like to thank the G. Stairs Foundation for its financial support.

References

Akers RF, Lovinger DM, Colley PA, Linden DJ, Routtenberg A 1986 Translocation of protein kinase C activity may mediate hippocampal long-term potentiation. Science (Wash DC) 231:587–589

Arana BW, Mossman D 1988 The dexamethasone suppression test and depression. Approaches to the use of a laboratory test in psychiatry. Endocr Metab Clin North Am 17:21–39

Bliss TVP, Lomo T 1973 Long lasting potentiation of synaptic transmission in the dentate area of the anaesthetized rabbit following stimulation of the perforant path. J Physiol (Lond) 232:331–356

Bliss TVP, Lynch MA 1988 Long term potentiation of synaptic transmission in the hippocampus: properties and mechanisms. In: Landfield PW, Deadwyler SA (eds) Synaptic potentiation in the brain. A critical analysis. Alan R Liss, New York, p 1–38

Celotti F, Melcangi RC, Negri-Cesi P, Ballabio M, Martini L 1987 Differential distribution of the 5α-reductase in the central nervous system of the rat and the mouse: are the white matter structures of the brain target tissue for testosterone action? J Steroid Biochem 26:125–129

Corradetti R, Ruggiero M, Chiarugi VP, Pepeu G 1987 GABA-receptor stimulation enhances norepinephrine-induced polyphosphoinositide metabolism in rat hippocampal slices. Brain Res 411:196–199

Dana RC, Martinez Jr JL 1984 Effect of adrenalectomy on the circadian rhythm of LTP. Brain Res 308:392–395

Davies SN, Lester RAJ, Reymann KG, Collingridge GL 1989 Temporally distinct pre- and postsynaptic mechanisms maintain long-term potentiation. Nature (Lond) 338:500–503

Dubrovsky B, Garcia-Rill E 1971 Convergence of tectal and visual input in cat motorsensory cortex. Exp Neurol 33:475–484

Dubrovsky B, Williams D, Kraulis I 1982 Effects of deoxycorticosterone and its ring A-reduced derivatives on the nervous system. Exp Neurol 78:728–739

Dubrovsky B, Williams D, Kraulis I 1985 Effects of corticosterone and 5α-dihydro-corticosterone on brain excitability in rat. J Neurosci Res 14:118–127

Dubrovsky B, Illes J, Birmingham MK 1986 Effects of 18-hydroxydeoxycorticosterone on central nervous system excitability. Experientia 42:1027–1028

Dubrovsky B, Liquornik M, Noble P, Gijsbers K 1987 Effect of 5α-dihydrocorticosterone on evoked potentials and long-term potentiation. Brain Res Bull 19:635–638

Dunbar GC, Lishman WA 1984 Depression, recognition-memory and hedonic tone. A signal detection analysis. Br J Psychiatry 144:376–382

Feldman S 1981 Electrophysiological effects of adrenocortical hormones on the brain. In: Fuxe K et al (eds) Steroid hormone regulation of the brain. Pergamon Press, Elmsford, NY, p 175–190

File SE, Simmonds MS 1988 Myoclonic seizures in the mouse induced by alphaxalone and related steroid anaesthetics. J Pharm Pharmacol 40:57–59

Harrison NL, Majewska MD, Harrington JW, Barker JL 1987 Structure-activity relationships for steroid interaction with the γ-aminobutyric acid$_A$ receptor complex. J Pharmacol Exp Ther 241:346–353

Heuser G 1967 Induction of anesthesia, seizures and sleep by steroid hormones. Anesthesiology 28:173–182

Holzbauer M, Birmingham MK, De Nicola AF, Oliver JT 1985 In vivo secretion of 3α-hydroxy-5α-pregnan-20-one, a potent anaesthetic steroid, by the adrenal gland of the rat. J Steroid Biochem 22:97–102

Hall ED 1982 Glucocorticoid effects of central nervous excitability and synaptic transmission. Int Rev Neurobiol 23:165–195

Jeffcoate WJ, Silverstone JT, Edwards CRW, Besser GM 1979 Psychiatric manifestations of Cushing's syndrome. Response to lowering of plasma cortisol. Q J Med 48:465–472

Kraulis I, Foldes G, Dubrovsky B, Traikov H, Birmingham M 1975 Distribution, metabolism and biological activity of deoxycorticosterone in the central nervous system. Brain Res 88:1–14

Liu AYC, Greengard P 1976 Regulation by steroid hormones of phosphorylation of specific proteins common to several target organs. Proc Natl Acad Sci USA 73:568–572

Maas JW, Garver DL 1975 Linkage of basic neuropharmacology and clinical psychopharmacology. In: Arieti S (ed) American handbook of psychiatry. Basic Books, New York, vol 6: 427–459

McEwen BS, De Kloet ER, Rostene W 1986 Adrenal steroid receptors and actions in the nervous system. Physiol Rev 66:1121–1188

Medawar PB 1953 Some immunological and endocrinological problems raised by the evolution of viviparity in vertebrates. In: Evolution (Symp Soc Exp Biol, vol 7) Cambridge University Press, Cambridge, p 320–338

Miller KW, Roth SH 1986 Inside the 'black box'. In: Roth SH, Miller KW (eds) Molecular and cellular mechanisms of anesthetics. Plenum Press, New York & London, p 261–266

Milner TA, Bacon CE 1989 GABAergic neurons in the rat hippocampal formation: ultrastructure and synaptic relationships with catecholaminergic terminals. J Neurosci 9:3410–3427

Morimoto K, Goddard GV 1985 Effects of thyrotropin-releasing hormone on evoked responses and long-term potentiation in dentate gyrus of rat. Exp Neurol 90:401–410

Morris RGM, Anderson E, Lynch GS, Baudry M 1986 Selective impairment of learning and blockade of long term potentiation by an N-methyl-D-aspartate receptor antagonist AP5. Nature (Lond) 319:774–776

Murphy BEP, Barta A, Dubrovsky B, Singer S, Kraulis I 1986 Anesthetic effects of some progesterone metabolites in the male rat using Nutralipid as vehicle. The Endocrine Society, 68th Annual Meeting, Anaheim, CA. Abstracts, p 204

Negro-Vilar A, Johnston G, Spinedi E, Valenza M, Lopez F 1987 Physiological role of peptides and amine on the regulation of ACTH secretion. Ann NY Acad Sci 512:218–236

Richards CD, Hesketh TR 1975 Implications for theories of anaesthesia of antagonism between anaesthetics and non-anaesthetic steroids. Nature (Lond) 256:179–182

Sandor T, Mehdi Z 1979 Steroids and evolution. In: Barrington EJW (ed) Hormones and evolution, vol 6. Academic Press, New York, p 1–71

Scharfman H, Sarvey JM 1985 Postsynaptic firing during repetitive stimulation is required for long term potentiation in hippocampus. Brain Res 331:267–274

Turner JP, Simmonds MA 1989 Modulation of the $GABA_A$ receptor complex by steroids in slices of rat cuneate nucleus. Br J Pharmacol 96:409–417
Turner DM, Ransom RW, Yang JSJ, Olsen RW 1989 Steroid anesthetics and naturally occurring analogs modulate the γ-aminobutyric acid receptor complex at a site distinct from barbiturates. J Pharmacol Exp Ther 248:960–967

DISCUSSION

McEwen: Several studies show that the most sensitive period during which LTP can be elicited is the waking period, in rats and in squirrel monkeys—in other words, after the period of elevation of glucocorticoid concentration that precedes waking (Barnes et al 1977, Dana & Martinez 1984). In one study, bilateral adrenalectomy in the rat resulted in a 12-hour shift in the peak of LTP elicitability (Dana & Martinez 1984). I wonder how that would fit into your scheme? Perhaps the phasic elevation of glucocorticoid concentrations is one of the factors that trigger the maximum sensitivity to elicitation of LTP.

Dubrovsky: In a study using tissue slices from the dentate gyrus obtained from normal rats at various times in the light–dark cycle, Harris & Teyler (1983) showed that the relative increase in population spike (PS) amplitude after tetanic stimulation was greatest during the dark phase; furthermore, a rhythmicity of LTP was not seen during development until there was a circadian rhythm of plasma corticosterone. In contrast, the experiments in adrenalectomized animals by Dana & Martinez (1984) that you mention showed the reverse effect, namely that adrenalectomized rats demonstrated more LTP during the light period than intact controls.

These results suggest that adrenal hormones play a role in regulating the circadian rhythm of LTP. To avoid these effects of circadian rhythm on LTP, we did all experiments at the same time of the day, in the early afternoon.

McEwen: That effect of stress on LTP has been shown to be an opiate effect; it can be blocked with naloxone. I don't think the stress effect on LTP is totally dependent on glucocorticoids (see Shors et al 1990).

Glowinski: To answer your question, Dr McEwen, data obtained in the hippocampus have indicated that when the noradrenergic innervation is destroyed by 6-hydroxydopamine, the LTP is considerably reduced. In fact, LTP in the hippocampus is regulated both by cholinergic and by noradrenergic neurons, originating respectively from the septum and the locus ceruleus. There is considerable diurnal variation in the activity of noradrenergic neurons, and these neurons are sensitive to glucocorticoids. This could provide one explanation for the observation that LTP is affected by glucocorticoids.

Baulieu: Are the levels of 18-hydroxydeoxycorticosterone in the human higher in blood during stress? I would be interested to know the concentrations.

Majewska: 18-OHDOC seems to be an 'equivalent' to DOC, which is the precursor of the GABA-agonistic steroid, tetrahydrodeoxycorticosterone, in dogs and rats.

Baulieu: But rats do not possess 17α-hydroxylase, and the patterns of steroids which are found are completely different in rat and human. Rats do not have cortisol, but they put out a lot of DOC. To my knowledge, human DOC levels are insignificant, and 18OHDOC is also insignificant in terms of concentration in the blood in humans.

Dubrovsky: You can increase the levels of 18OHDOC in stress in man.

Baulieu: You mean higher than cortisol levels?

Dubrovsky: 18OHDOC is under the control of both ACTH and the renin-angiotensin system. The hormone has mineralocorticoid properties and can be produced by human adrenals (De Nicola & Birmingham 1968, Melby et al 1971). Moreover, in humans, plasma levels of 18OHDOC are exquisitely sensitive to ACTH and exhibit increases of an order of magnitude, greatly in excess of the relative rise evoked by ACTH in the levels of plasma cortisol (Williams et al 1976, Chandler et al 1976, Mason et al 1979).

In the rat, corticosterone rather than cortisol is the major glucocorticoid; the absolute amount of 18OHDOC secreted under maximal stress can equal that of corticosterone in normal rats (Birmingham et al 1973) and exceed it in rats having a mammotropic tumour, nine weeks after implantation (De Nicola et al 1973). Finally, Bartova (1979) showed that the rat brain retains considerable amounts of 18OHDOC (30% of the plasma concentration) and that this amount fluctuates with the physiological state and shows some gross regional differentiation, with high levels in the septum (8.2 ± 1.92 ng/g of tissue) and lower levels in the hypothalamus (2.3 ± 0.73 ng/g of tissue). As I described, our work revealed that 18OHDOC can significantly modulate LTP.

Feldman: The hippocampus has the lowest epileptic threshold in the brain and hydrocortisone has been shown to lower the convulsive threshold for electroshock in rats. We therefore injected hydrocortisone into the lateral ventricle in cats and saw electrical epileptic phenomena as well as convulsive seizures produced initially in the hippocampus (Feldman 1966). We later infused hydrocortisone into various subcortical regions in cats and confirmed the highest susceptibility of the hippocampus in the generation of epileptic phenomena (Feldman 1971).

We have also used rats, with electrodes chronically implanted into the pontine reticular formation, the dorsal hippocampus, the lateral septum and the anterior hypothalamus. We stimulated these regions to elicit convulsive phenomena before and after hydrocortisone injection (5 mg) and obtained prominent epileptic activity in the brain about half an hour after hormone injection, particularly after stimulation of the hippocampus. Thus, with dorsal hippocampal stimulation, in 14 out of 29 experiments, there were pronounced seizures, with low stimulating voltages. This effect was not observed with higher voltages from the other brain regions (Conforti & Feldman 1975). So the hippocampus is a very interesting organ, in terms of learning, of neuroendocrine control, and also epilepsy. At least for hydrocortisone, the primary site of action, in relation to epilepsy, is probably the hippocampus.

Looking back to my experience as a young doctor, we used a lot of hydrocortisone in non-neurological patients and we saw convulsions in some of them. Nowadays, other glucocorticoids are used to treat such patients, including prednisone and dexamethasone, but we don't see more than an occasional patient with convulsions. I don't know if there are studies of epileptic thresholds with either of these drugs, but clearly hydrocortisone is a convulsive substance, and it should be remembered that if used in high dosages in patients with neurological disorders, and probably in other medical conditions, it may have a convulsive effect, and the primary focus is most probably the hippocampus.

McEwen: In relation to this point, and also to the issue of the natural effects of the adrenal steroids, Dr Maureen Gannon in our laboratory has been studying the calcium/calmodulin-regulated form of adenylate cyclase *in vitro*, at different times in the natural diurnal cycle. She finds an elevation of calcium/calmodulin cyclase activity in the hippocampus but not in the cerebral cortex, during the waking phase of the diurnal cycle of the rat. So there appears to be a diurnal variation in the activity of this enzyme, which is abolished by adrenalectomy. We don't know whether only adrenal steroids are responsible because it is difficult to do a replacement study if you are trying to replace a cycle. The adrenal medulla could be involved as well, for all we know.

References

Barnes C, McNaughton B, Goddard G, Douglas R, Adamec R 1977 Circadian rhythm of synaptic excitability in rat and monkey central nervous system. Science (Wash DC) 197:91–92

Bartova A 1979 Endogenous levels of 18-OH-DOC and related steroids in the brain. In: Jones MT et al (eds) Interaction within the brain-pituitary-adrenocortical system. Academic Press, London, p 213–220

Birmingham MK, De Nicola AF, Oliver JT et al 1973 Production of steroids *in vivo* by regenerated adrenal glands of hypertensive and normotensive rats. Endocrinology 93:297–310

Chandler DW, Tuck M, Mates DM 1976 The measurement of 18-hydroxy-11-deoxycorticosterone in human plasma by radioimmunoassay. Steroids 27:235–246

Conforti N, Feldman S 1975 Effect of cortisol on the excitability of limbic structures of the brain in freely moving rats. J Neurol Sci 26:29–38

Dana RC, Martinez JL Jr 1984 Effect of adrenalectomy on the circadian rhythm of LTP. Brain Res 308:392–395

De Nicola AF, Birmingham MK 1968 Biosynthesis of 18-hydroxycorticosterone from deoxycorticosterone-4^{14}C by the human adrenal gland. J Clin Endocrinol Metab 28:1380–1381

De Nicola AF, Dahl V, Kaplan S 1973 Transformation of [^{14}C]pregnenolone and production of corticosteroids by adrenal glands from rats bearing a transplantable mammotropic pituitary tumor. J Steroid Biochem 4:205–215

Feldman S 1966 Convulsive phenomena produced by intraventricular administration of hydrocortisone in cats. Epilepsia 7:271–282

Feldman S 1971 Electrical activity of the brain following cerebral microinfusion of cortisol. Epilepsia 12:249–262

Harris KM, Teyler T 1983 Age differences in a circadian influence on LTP. Brain Res 261:69–73

Mason PA, Fraser R, Semple PF, Morton JJ 1979 The interaction of ACTH and angiotensin II in the control of corticosteroid plasma concentration in man. J Steroid Biochem 10:235–239

Melby JC, Dale SL, Nilson TE 1971 18-Hydroxydeoxycorticosterone in human plasma. Circ Res 28 (Suppl II):143

Shors T, Levine S, Thompson RF 1990 Effect of adrenalectomy and demedullation on the stress-induced impairment of long-term potentiation. Neuroendocrinology 51:70–75

Williams GH, Braley LM, Underwood RH 1976 The regulation of plasma 18-hydroxy-11-deoxycorticosterone in man. J Clin Invest 58:221–229

Final general discussion

Use of adrenal corticosteroids in sports

Johnston: I would like to alert people to the apparently increasing use of cortisol in sport. There has been much publicity about the use of anabolic steroids in various sports. We have tested the main one that was in use for a long time, namely stanozolol. In our tests on guinea pig ileum tissue it behaves just like a glucocorticoid, enhancing GABA responses at low (pM) concentrations and blocking them at high (µM) concentrations (J. Richardson & G. A. R. Johnston, unpublished). We find that athletes who take stanozolol, particularly weight-lifters, experience acute euphoric effects which help their performance.

Colleagues in Sydney have been approached by the International Olympic Committee, warning them of the possible use of cortisol by athletes to increase performance. We are now trying to produce tests that would stand up in court by which to detect athletes using cortisol. It's a difficult analytical problem, but some solution is needed, in view of the possible recent surge in exogenous cortisol use. Presumably endogenous cortisol is allowable!

Baulieu: Some time ago I was administering cortisol to leukaemic patients and measuring the tetrahydro reduced metabolites (Baulieu et al 1956). When the amount of cortisol was increased, the ratio of 11β-hydroxy reduced metabolites to 11-keto reduced metabolites increased. Also there are more 11β-hydroxysteroids than 11-keto metabolites in Cushing's disease with high cortisol secretion. Probably, the oxidation of 11β-hydroxysteroids is a limiting step, and we may be able to use it to detect steroid users.

Johnston: Yes. We intend to look at as many cortisol metabolites as we can by gas chromatography and mass spectrometry and then try to pick out the important ones; but that is a good suggestion.

Baulieu: Do the athletes take the steroid by mouth, or by injection?

Johnston: By mouth.

Baulieu: So you would have more chance to find expected changes, since the liver is the most important metabolizing organ.

McEwen: What about measuring other substances than steroids, such as ACTH or endorphins, or even imaging the adrenals? The adrenal glands should become smaller if the individual athlete is taking enough steroids to suppress his or her endogenous steroid production by negative feedback.

Johnston: Measuring adrenal size might be difficult in the sporting context, but we could consider sampling for ACTH.

Baulieu: In humans, it would be easier, and as significant, to measure blood endorphins.

Johnston: That is a good idea.

261

Steroids and anaesthesia

Lambert: The question arises of whether the steroid effects on the GABA$_A$ receptor that we have shown are relevant to anaesthesia. There is a reasonably strong case that GABA modulation is the mechanism by which certain steroids, such as alphaxalone, produce anaesthesia. We haven't found anything else that the reduced metabolites of progesterone do, and it makes sense that potentiation of a major inhibitory transmitter will cause central depression and anaesthesia.

We have looked at about 20 steroids and find a good correlation between their GABA potentiating actions and their ability to produce a measure of anaesthesia in mice. The anaesthetic effect can occur rapidly, within a few seconds after intravenous injection, so we are looking for some rapid molecular mechanism. We feel that, for the steroids, the GABA$_A$ receptor must play an important role. It's more complicated for barbiturates and other intravenously administered general anaesthetics, which clearly have actions on other systems, such as calcium channels and excitatory amino acid receptors.

Johnston: Steroid effects on excitatory amino acids must certainly be taken into account. For years we thought that barbiturates work only on GABA receptors, yet it's now reasonably clear that they have an important action on glutamate release (Skerritt & Johnston 1984), so I would caution against over-emphasis on the effects of steroids on any one particular neurotransmitter system.

Kubli-Garfias: My comments are also related to anaesthesia. Progesterone gives rise to two kinds of derivatives, 5α and 5β. Kawahara et al (1975) showed the production of 5β-progestins in the dog's brain and Raisinghani et al (1968) showed this in the rat, so it is important to remember that these compounds are produced in many tissues. In the cat we studied the effects in several brain structures of 5β-pregnane-3,20-dione (pregnanedione), 3β-hydroxy-5β-pregnan-20-one (pregnanolone) and 3α-hydroxy-5β-pregnan-20-one (epipregnanolone) and progesterone (Kubli-Garfias et al 1976). We found changes in the brain electrical activity with slow waves and a fall in the multi-unit activity. In the rat those changes were also observed, along with deep hypnotic effects (Kubli-Garfias et al 1985). Interestingly, progesterone was the least effective compound. The latencies were 25–30 s for epipregnanolone and 60 s for pregnanedione, so the effect was almost immediate, whereas allopregnanolone (3β-hydroxy-5α-pregnan-20-one) had a latency of about 3 min. Thus it is possible that the latter steroid might be converted to 5β-reduced products.

Bäckström: I am surprised to hear that a 3β-hydroxypregnane compound has any effects on brain excitability at all.

Kubli-Garfias: Regarding the importance of C-3, C-5 and C-17 substituents of 4-en and C-5-reduced compounds, it was interesting to study their chemical structure and biological activity by comparing progestins with androgens which lack the chain at C-17. In depressing neuronal activity, androgens with the 3α-hydroxy-5α configuration are slightly more active than their 5β-epimers, but all of them are lower in potency that 5β-progestins (Kubli-Garfias et al 1982), suggesting than substitutions at C-17 are important for the non-genomic effects.

We used another model in order to show more clearly the effects of 5α and 5β progestins and androgens, namely contractions of the rat uterus *in vitro* (Kubli-Garfias et al 1979, 1980). Again 5β-progestins were the most active in producing myometrial relaxation among the androgens and progestins tested; pregnanolone was by far the most effective. Moreover, in this model another steroid family, namely corticosterone and deoxycorticosterone with the Δ^4 configuration, has a poor relaxant effect, even showing an excitatory effect with deoxycorticosterone at doses of 10^{-9} M (Perusquia et al 1986).

We have explored the possible mechanisms of action of 5β-progestins in rat brain slices. These compounds were shown to inhibit noradrenaline release (Kubli-Garfias et al 1983). In our rat uterus model, contractions elicited by depolarization with high potassium are depressed by 5β-progestins and this is reversed by calcium ionophores, which suggests a calcium-blocking action by C-5-reduced steroids (Perusquia et al 1990).

Su: Eckhart Weber used the guinea pig ileum as a σ receptor model (Campbell et al 1989). He believes that σ is related to the 5-HT$_3$ system. We approached this from another direction, and he seems to be right. However, we have a problem with the solubility of progesterone. What solvent do you use?

Kubli-Garfias: We use propylene glycol as solvent.

Martini: Incidentally, the brain of birds contains a 5β-reductase in addition to the 5α-reductase. Birds might therefore be a good model in which to dissect out some of the effects of the 5α-reduced as against the 5β-reduced derivatives of progesterone and of testosterone.

Baulieu: I would just like to add a caution about the 5α/5β discussion. It is difficult to generalize, because if we have different systems, I don't think we shall get any clue from the study of the steroids themselves. We have to do biology and not chemistry, at this stage.

Role of steroids in the brain

Karavolas: In this meeting I have been especially pleased to see the many lines of evidence indicating the several different effects that the various reduced metabolites of progesterone have on a number of progesterone-sensitive processes. The evidence would seem to support the general concept that I spoke about earlier, namely that a metabolite might be inactive on one biological effect but active on another and that the diverse neuroendocrine effects of progesterone might be due in part to these various reduced metabolites, whether produced *in situ*, or produced elsewhere and then taken up from the circulation. This array of metabolites could then provide the physiological adaptation to meet the ever-changing needs of the host animal.

These concepts are not new. In a sense, they have been reiterated frequently during the entire sixty-year history of steroid biology. A number of steroid biologists (chemists, biochemists, neuroscientists, etc.) have helped to develop and bring together these concepts. We should not forget to give credit to these earlier contributions and ideas. It seems that we need to revisit these ideas every 10 years or so to integrate new information. This conference is most timely now, with this exciting confluence of neurobiology with steroid biology. This is an excellent time to be sorting out these neural effects of steroids and their relationships.

Besides these earlier contributions, which we noted in our paper only in a general way with citations to reviews, I also want to recognize the contributions to steroid metabolism made by fellow researchers—those here (Bruce McEwen, Luciano Martini and Etienne Baulieu) and those absent, especially Margarethe Holzbauer.

Baulieu: We can consider that there are actually two sources of steroids in the brain. One pool consists of steroids derived from various glands (ovary, adrenal), and I would include the steroid metabolites that you describe. Then there are steroids that are made in the brain (neurosteroids). Some, such as pregnenolone, can be produced both by brain cells and peripherally, by the adrenals for instance, and so the same steroid may come from two different sources. There is a big difference between steroids which reach the brain from distant sources and are in relatively low concentrations in the blood, and then also presumably in the brain extracellular fluid, and steroids that are made locally in the CNS and can provide a high local concentration to the adjacent cells (parahormones).

The significance of steroids from the two groups may therefore be completely different, because we have seen how high the concentrations of steroids are that are needed for certain effects. I would stress that there may be two brain pools of specific steroids. For example, progesterone itself and even its metabolites are entering the brain at low concentration, and they may have a different significance from progesterone and its metabolites made in the brain, which could be in much higher concentration. Conceptually this is important for devising new experiments. In addition, pregnenolone and dehydroepiandrosterone sulphates cannot easily cross the blood–brain barrier, so one should be very careful when interpreting data.

Karavolas: This question of a concentration gradient is very important. It may be that certain steroids are produced in a particular chemical form in order to provide easy entry to certain tissues or cell membranes, as with most steroids. Once having arrived, the steroids can be metabolized to another chemical form that keeps the transformed steroid(s) at these target sites and/or prevents exit from the target cell. Thus, these various processing steps may be the means by which these steroids gain entry and are retained. For example, processes such as metabolite formation, hydroxylation and esterification of the parent steroid may help in sequestering steroids within these target sites against a much lower concentration gradient of the parent steroid.

Consider an analogy to the uptake of glucose. In many cell types, glucose freely enters and leaves by diffusion, but once glucose (within the cell) is phosphorylated or converted to other forms such as sorbitol, this effectively 'locks' the glucose in the cell. Similarly, very small amounts of circulatory steroids could be delivered to these end organs. In addition, these amounts are also enriched by classical sequestration mechanisms (binding proteins, receptors) and then 'locked' into certain intracellular compartments. Many of the effects that we see in target sites usually do come about from apparently low circulating concentrations.

Baulieu: However, when a male animal is castrated, the level of testosterone in the blood goes down immediately, and concentrations of testosterone sulphate and testosterone fatty esters also fall. In the brain, the concentration of testosterone rapidly decreases to an undetectable level (contrary to the pregnenolone and dehydroepiandrosterone concentrations; Corpéchot et al 1981, 1983, Baulieu et al 1987). Therefore, although I agree in principle with your point, the actual data do not suggest that the concept is correct! I can differentiate what is made in the CNS from what is entering the brain from the periphery.

Genomic or non-genomic?

Baulieu: I have the impression from the symposium that at present it is difficult to speak of non-genomic actions as a single, homogeneous group of effects. Diversity is probably the best word to use for what we have heard. For example, we have heard about $GABA_A$ receptors. I wish I could add here more on the muscarinic receptor (preliminary data of Martine El Etr) and possibly other neurotransmitter receptors which are functionally influenced by steroids, but we lack information in these areas. We heard from Dr Hall about the extraordinary corticosteroid analogues and derivatives which do not bind to intracellular receptors, and membrane perturbation has been evoked, which is also a completely different non-genomic mechanism from the neurotransmitter receptor systems. Who knows if there are other membrane receptors which are neither neurotransmitter receptors nor membrane perturbation systems?

Finally, and to come back to the discussion initiated by Bruce McEwen at the beginning of the symposium, it seems that you can start from steroid activity on the genome, and obtain membrane effects via changes in the synthesis of channels, receptors, G proteins, and so on. Thus, we always have to define what end-point we are analysing; if we are a little late, we see a membrane effect, but in fact it was initially a genomic mechanism.

Conversely, the response can start at the membrane and go to the genome. This is the mechanism which is used by all growth factors, and I believe is also used by some steroids, possibly via adenylate cyclase or protein kinase C. So what we really have when we speak of non-genomic versus genomic effects, as was implicit in Bruce McEwen's paper, is that there are probably always the two aspects—surface and genes. Which comes first? This is what concerns people who are interested in mechanisms. It is very important in terms of drug design, because probably the most specific point at which one may modify a phenomenon at the cellular level is where the informational molecule reaches the receptor; that is the *first* interaction of biological importance, whether at the membrane or the genomic level. So we have to be very critical in terms of the definition of the phenomenon we are analysing and ask whether it is a primary or a secondary effect.

References

Baulieu EE, De Vigan M, Jayle MF 1956 Les 11-oxysteroids: étude de l'equilibre entre 11-β-hydroxy et 11-cétosteroides. Elimination urinaire du cortisol, de la cortisone, du tétrahydrocortisol et de la tétrahydrocortisone après administration de cortisol et d'ACTH à l'homme. C R Soc Biol 150:971–973

Baulieu EE, Robel P, Vatier O, Haug M, Le Goascogne C, Bourreau E 1987 Neurosteroids: pregnenolone and dehydroepiandrosterone in the brain. In: Fuxe K, Agnati LF (eds) Receptor–receptor interactions. Macmillan, Basingstoke, vol 48: 89–104

Campbell BG, Scherz MW, Keana JFW, Weber E 1989 Sigma receptors regulate contractions of the guinea-pig ileum longitudinal muscle/myenteric plexus preparation elicited by both electrical stimulation and exogenous serotonin. J Neurosci 9:3380–3391

Corpéchot C, Robel P, Axelson M, Sjovall J, Baulieu EE 1981 Characterization and measurement of dehydroepiandrosterone sulfate in the rat brain. Proc Natl Acad Sci USA 78:4704–4707

Corpéchot C, Synguelakis M, Talha S et al 1983 Pregnenolone and its sulfate ester in the rat brain. Brain Res 270:119–125

Kawahara FS, Berman ML, Green DC 1975 Conversion of progesterone 1,2-3H to 5β-pregnane-3,20-dione by brain tissues. Steroids 25:459–463

Kubli-Garfias C, Cervantes M, Beyer C 1976 Changes in multiunit activity and EEG induced by the administration of natural progestins in flaxedil immobilized cats. Brain Res 114:72–81

Kubli-Garfias C, Medrano-Conde L, Beyer C, Bondani A 1979 *In vitro* inhibition of rat uterine contractility induced by 5α and 5β progestins. Steroids 34:609–619

Kubli-Garfias C, Lopez-Fiesco A, Pacheco-Cano MT, Ponce-Monter H, Bondani A 1980 *In vitro* effects of androgens upon the spontaneous rat uterine contractility. Steroids 35:633–641

Kubli-Garfias C, Canchola E, Arauz-Contreras J, Feria-Velazco A 1982 Depressant effect of androgens on the cat brain electrical activity and its antagonism by ruthenium red. Neuroscience 7:2777–2782

Kubli-Garfias C, Azpeitia E, Villaneuva-Tello T, Ponce-Monter H 1983 Inhibition of noradrenaline release by 5β-progestins in cerebral cortex slices. Proc West Pharmacol Soc 26:135–138

Kubli-Garfias C, Rocha-Arrieta L, Melgarejo-Salgado A, Hoyo-Vadillo C, Perusquia M, Valadéz-Rodriguez J 1985 Electroencephalographic and behavioral changes produced by 5β-progestins and its antagonism by 4-aminopyridine. Arch Invest Med 16 (Suppl 3):133–141

Perusquia M, Hoyo-Vadillo C, Kubli-Garfias C 1986 Biphasic effect of corticosteroids on the contractions of isolated rat uterus. Arch Invest Med 17:203–209

Perusquia M, Garcia-Yañez E, Ibañez R, Kubli-Garfias C 1990 Non-genomic mechanism of action of Δ4 and 5-reduced androgens and progestins on the contractility of the isolated rat myometrium. Life Sci, in press

Raisinghani KH, Dorfman RI, Forchielli E, Gyermek L, Genther G 1968 Uptake of intravenously administered progesterone, pregnanedione and pregnanolone by rat brain. Acta Endocrinol 57:395–404

Skerritt JH, Johnston GAR 1984 Modulation of excitant amino acid release by convulsant and anticonvulsant drugs. In: Fariello RG et al (eds) Neurotransmitters, seizures and epilepsy II. Raven Press, New York, p 215–224

Summing-up

M. A. Simmonds

Department of Pharmacology, School of Pharmacy, University of London, 29/39 Brunswick Square, London WC1N 1AX, UK

I shall relate my summing-up to the questions I posed in the Introduction, but I shall need to go beyond that, because a number of matters that I did not foresee featured in our discussions.

The first question concerned the extent to which structure–activity relationships have been determined for various non-genomic effects of steroids. It has become clear that the area where we have the best information is that of steroid interactions with the $GABA_A$ system. The indications are that a universally applicable profile is unlikely. This is because there are variations in the composition of the $GABA_A$ channel, with different subunit combinations in different brain areas. So we must be prepared for several different structure–activity profiles for steroid modulation of this receptor system. There are also gender differences in the sensitivity of the $GABA_A$ receptor to drugs that interact with it. Therefore, we have to take into account the influence of the endogenous steroid patterns in the animal on which we do the study or from which the experimental tissue is taken. Besides gender, there is the operator-induced variable of stress in handling the animal at the time of the experiment. The whole problem of the endogenous steroids and how they will influence the apparent structure–activity profiles of acutely applied steroids in the experimental situation is a considerable one.

With regard to other receptor systems, the σ site has been discussed, and also the question of steroid interaction with oxygen free radicals. In both those cases the structure–activity profile, even on the limited data available, will be quite different from that for the $GABA_A$ receptor. Matters are less clear for the pituitary and modulation by steroids of the release of LHRH and the amphetamine-induced release of dopamine. We do not have enough structure–activity information yet to comment on whether steroid–GABA interactions are involved in these effects.

On the second question, concerning the extent to which perturbations of the lipid structure of cell membranes by steroids may underlie some of their effects, we have been shown how a fairly distinct structure–activity relationship to steroids can exist simply for the perturbation of lipids. We therefore do not have to assume that the steroids are interacting directly with a protein binding site. However, it may well be that perturbation of the lipids does, in turn, affect the function of specific proteins within the lipid bilayer, and that in the end it is the change in properties of these membrane proteins that is important for some of the non-genomic effects of steroids. If this is so, it may be only one leaflet of the membrane bilayer that is crucially involved. For example, alphaxalone was shown not to affect the $GABA_A$ system if it is put inside the cell. The implication of this finding is that if alphaxalone is primarily perturbing the membrane lipids with secondary consequences for the $GABA_A$ protein, it is only having this effect at the level of the outer leaflet.

Account must also be taken of the interactions of steroids with prostaglandins, to the extent that they may influence interactions between proteins and lipids in the bilayer.

Rather little has been said about the third question, of whether existing classes of drugs mimic or antagonize particular non-genomic effects of steroids. An example of what I had in mind was the possibility that steroids and barbiturates might have a common site of action. The data presented indicate that barbiturates and steroids are strongly synergistic in the potentiation of GABA, suggesting that they have separates sites of action, even though the ensuing mechanisms are very similar. I do not see any evidence from this symposium for specific classes of drug acting through the sites of steroid action that we have been discussing, apart from the steroids themselves.

The fourth question concerned the physiological relevance of steroid modulation of specific transmitter systems. Data have been presented on the effects of adrenalectomy or ovariectomy in animals and the subsequent replacement, or partial replacement, of steroids, and on the effects of gender, particularly on the $GABA_A$ system. My impression is that endogenous steroids do, indeed, modulate the overall activity of the $GABA_A$ system, but to different extents in different neuronal populations according to the circumstances.

For the human, we have heard about events related to the menstrual cycle and to pregnancy, particularly the clinical signs and symptoms of epilepsy and how these correlate with changes in levels of progesterone, and presumably of its metabolites, plus changes in oestrogen levels. If these phenomena are to be partially explained by interactions with the GABA system, here again would be evidence that steroidal interaction with the GABA system is physiologically relevant.

The other important aspect of that fourth question is whether the concentrations of the steroids that we use in our experimental systems are relevant to physiology. This is often difficult to resolve because of redistribution of the steroids from the aqueous medium into lipids. Also, there is a paucity of information on endogenous levels of the metabolites of progesterone and the corticosteroids that are of particular interest. With regard to pregnenolone sulphate, we were assured that the amounts present in brain do not make unreasonable the concentrations found to be active *in vitro*.

The fifth and last question concerned the possibility of distinguishing the genomic and non-genomic neuronal actions of steroids, and Etienne Baulieu has summarized the position very clearly in the final discussion. This has developed into a major theme of the symposium. We have looked at the question of the separation of genomic from non-genomic effects on the basis of timing. My impression is that there exists a large grey area where both effects may overlap, the latency of the genomic effect ranging from a few minutes to an hour or two, depending on the conditions. Conversely, a non-genomic effect of an administered steroid may be delayed in its onset because of the formation of an active metabolite of that steroid. These are confounding factors in the interpretation of latencies. We also discussed the question of whether an initial non-genomic effect might switch on a more persistent secondary response that could be confused with a genomic effect.

Most interesting was the variety of mechanisms suggested for a genomic effect following on from a non-genomic one, and the implication that a genomic effect does not necessarily involve the steroid reaching the nucleus. For example, there is the possibility that genomic effects could result from an action of a steroid at the cell membrane being transmitted via intracellular messenger systems, including the phosphoinositide system, calcium and protein kinase C, to regulate the expression of specific proteins.

Other points have arisen in the meeting that I find particularly interesting. One of these is the morphological changes that can be induced by steroids; in particular, the development of spines on dendrites under the influence of progesterone and oestrogens, and the remarkable speeding up of the spread of oxytocin sites into the dendrites of neurons in the ventromedial nucleus of the hypothalamus by adding progesterone after oestrogen priming.

Another interesting aspect is the ability of glial cells to synthesize progesterone and to metabolize it to reduced compounds which we now know have their own activities in the brain. The functional role of glial cells in this respect still has to be explored. We need to know what is controlling progesterone synthesis within the glial cell and more particularly its release; does it just diffuse out of the cell or is it under some more active control? That will be a very interesting area to follow up.

Finally, the work on the effect of steroids on the synthesis of G proteins is another extremely interesting area which I am sure is due for much further development.

I hope that the text of this symposium will convey something of the exciting resurgence of interest in the effects of steroids on central nervous system function. In particular, some of the important effects that do not involve the genome now seem to be explicable by modulation of the inhibitory $GABA_A$ receptor system. Still to be explored are the possibilities of analogous steroid interactions with other transmitter systems. However, studies on the perturbation of the lipid structure of artificial bilayers may provide the first indications of a common fundamental mechanism of action whereby steroids can influence the function of specific membrane proteins. Such effects, together with the genomic control of intracellular processes, seem likely to allow both circulating and locally synthesized steroids a major regulatory influence in the central nervous system.

Index of contributors

Subject index